REVIEW OF VASCULAR SURGERY

REVIEW OF VASCULAR SURGERY

WILLIAM C. KRUPSKI, M.D.

Professor and Chief, Vascular Surgery Section
University of Colorado Health Sciences Center
Denver, Colorado

W. B. SAUNDERS COMPANY
A Division of Harcourt Brace & Company
PHILADELPHIA/LONDON/TORONTO/MONTREAL/SYDNEY/TOKYO

W. B. SAUNDERS COMPANY

A Division of Harcourt, Brace & Company

The Curtis Center
Independence Square West
Philadelphia, PA 19106

Library of Congress Cataloging-in-Publication Data

Review of vascular surgery / [edited by] William C. Krupski.
p. cm.
ISBN 0-7216-4843-6
1. Blood-vessels—Surgery. 2. Blood-vessels—Diseases. I. Krupski, William C.
[DNLM: 1. Vascular Diseases—surgery. 2. Vascular Surgery. WG
500 R454 1995]
RD598.5.R48 1995
617.4'13—dc20
DNLM/DLC

94-10941

REVIEW OF VASCULAR SURGERY ISBN 0-7216-4843-6

Printed in the United States of America.

Last digit is the print number: 9 8 7 6 5 4 3 2 1

Contributors

M. SAMY ABDOU, M.D.
Los Angeles, California

ERIC R. ASHBY, M.D.
Los Angeles, California

J. DENNIS BAKER, M.D.
Sepulveda, California

WILLIAM H. BAKER, M.D.
Maywood, Illinois

DENNIS F. BANDYK, M.D.
Tampa, Florida

DENIS D. BENSARD, M.D.
Bexley, Ohio

JOHN J. BERGAN, M.D.
La Jolla, California

VICTOR M. BERNHARD, M.D.
Tucson, Arizona

FRED BONGARD, M.D.
Torrance, California

DAVID C. BREWSTER, M.D.
Boston, Massachusetts

T. J. BUNT, M.D.
Phoenix, Arizona

JOHN A. BUTLER, M.D.
Orange, California

GARY R. CAPUTO, M.D.
San Francisco, California

STEPHEN W. K. CHENG, MB, BS, FRCS
San Francisco, California

KENNETH J. CHERRY, JR., M.D.
Rochester, Minnesota

RICHARD W. CHITWOOD, M.D.
Portland, Oregon

G. PATRICK CLAGETT, M.D.
Dallas, Texas

ALEXANDER W. CLOWES, M.D.
Seattle, Washington

STANLEY N. COHEN, M.D.
Los Angeles, California

ANTHONY J. COMEROTA, M.D.
Philadelphia, Pennsylvania

TIMOTHY P. CONNALL, M.D.
Orange, California

DANIEL P. CONNELLY, M.D.
San Francisco, California

JOSEPH S. COSELLI, M.D.
Houston, Texas

ENRIQUE CRIADO, M.D.
Chapel Hill, North Carolina

JACK L. CRONENWETT, M.D.
Hanover, New Hampshire

BRUCE S. CUTLER, M.D.
Worcester, Massachusetts

RICHARD H. DEAN, M.D.
Winston-Salem, North Carolina

JOSEPH R. DURHAM, M.D.
Chicago, Illinois

JAMES M. EDWARDS, M.D.
Portland, Oregon

ERROL E. ERLANDSON, M.D.
Ann Arbor, Michigan

D. PRESTON FLANIGAN, M.D.
Orange, California

THOMAS J. FOGARTY, M.D.
Palo Alto, California

RICHARD J. FOWL, M.D.
Cincinnati, Ohio

JULIE A. FREISCHLAG, M.D.
Milwaukee, Wisconsin

JAMES C. A. FUCHS, M.D.
Baltimore, Maryland

RAJU H. GANDHI, M.D.
New York, New York

BRUCE L. GEWERTZ, M.D.
Chicago, Illinois

JOSEPH M. GIORDANO, M.D.
Washington, D.C.

PETER GLOVICZKI, M.D.
Rochester, Minnesota

MICHAEL F. X. GLYNN, M.D.
Toronto, Ontario, Canada

JERRY GOLDSTONE, M.D.
San Francisco, California

MICHAEL J. V. GORDON, M.D.
Denver, Colorado

FRANK A. GOTTSCHALK, M.D.
Dallas, Texas

LAZAR J. GREENFIELD, M.D.
Ann Arbor, Michigan

VLADIMIR HACHINSKI, M.D., D.SC.
London, Ontario, Canada

JOHN W. HALLETT, JR., M.D.
Rochester, Minnesota

PROFESSOR JOHN P. HARRIS
Sydney, Australia

NORMAN R. HERTZER, M.D.
Cleveland, Ohio

TOSHIO INAHARA, M.D.
Portland, Oregon

KAJ JOHANSEN, M.D., PH.D.
Seattle, Washington

GEORGE JOHNSON, JR., M.D.
Chapel Hill, North Carolina

STEPHEN P. JOHNSON, M.D.
Denver, Colorado

DARRELL N. JONES, PH.D.
Denver, Colorado

SHELDON E. JORDAN, M.D.
Santa Monica, California

JOHN W. JOYCE, M.D.
Rochester, Minnesota

JEFFREY L. KAUFMAN, M.D.
Springfield, Massachusetts

ANDRIS KAZMERS, M.D.
Detroit, Michigan

RICHARD F. KEMPCZINSKI, M.D.
Cincinnati, Ohio

LAWRENCE L. KETCH, M.D.
Denver, Colorado

WILLIAM C. KRUPSKI, M.D.
Denver, Colorado

DAVID A. KUMPE
Denver, Colorado

STEPHEN G. LALKA, M.D.
Indianapolis, Indiana

RAYMOND W. LEE, M.D.
Portland, Oregon

HERBERT I. MACHLEDER, M.D.
Los Angeles, California

NEIL A. MARTIN, M.D.
Los Angeles, California

PROFESSOR JIM MAY
Sydney, Australia

KENNETH E. MCINTYRE, M.D.
Tucson, Arizona

ROBERT H. MEIER, III, M.D.
Denver, Colorado

D. CRAIG MILLER, M.D.
Stanford, California

TIMOTHY A. MILLER, M.D.
Los Angeles, California

MAX B. MITCHELL, M.D.
Denver, Colorado

GREGORY L. MONETA, M.D.
Portland, Oregon

WESLEY S. MOORE, M.D.
Los Angeles, California

MARK R. NEHLER, M.D.
Portland, Oregon

KENNETH OURIEL, M.D.
Rochester, New York

WILLIAM PEARCE, M.D.
Chicago, Illinois

MALCOLM O. PERRY, M.D.
Lubbock, Texas

JOHN M. PORTER, M.D.
Portland, Oregon

WILLIAM QUIÑONES-BALDRICH, M.D.
Los Angeles, California

SESHADRI RAJU, M.D.
Jackson, Mississippi

DANIEL J. REDDY, M.D.
Detroit, Michigan

THOMAS S. RILES, M.D.
New York, New York

ERNEST J. RING, M.D.
San Francisco, California

STEVEN P. RIVERS, M.D.
Bronx, New York

THOM W. ROOKE, M.D.
Rochester, Minnesota

STEVEN C. ROSE, M.D.
Seattle, Washington

ROBERT J. ROSEN, M.D.
New York, New York

ROBERT B. RUTHERFORD, M.D.
Denver, Colorado

GEORGE E. SARRIS, M.D.
Stanford, California

PROFESSOR P. M. SATCHELL
Sydney, Australia

SHIGEHIKO SHIONOVA, M.D.
Nagoya, Japan

DONALD SILVER, M.D.
Columbia, Missouri

LOUIS L. SMITH, M.D.
Loma Linda, California

JAMES C. STANLEY, M.D.
Ann Arbor, Michigan

GREG VAN STIEGMANN, M.D.
Denver, Colorado

STEPHEN W. SUBBER, M.D.
Denver, Colorado

DAVID S. SUMNER, M.D.
Springfield, Illinois

ROY L. TAWES, M.D.
Burlingame, California

LLOYD M. TAYLOR, JR., M.D.
Portland, Oregon

PROFESSOR JOHN TERBLANCHE
Cape Town, Republic of South Africa

ERWIN R. THAL, M.D.
Dallas, Texas

BRIAN L. THIELE, M.D.
Hershey, Pennsylvania

ROBERT W. THOMPSON, M.D.
San Francisco, California

M. DAVID TILSON, M.D.
New York, New York

JONATHAN B. TOWNE, M.D.
Milwaukee, Wisconsin

WILLIAM W. TURNER, JR., M.D.
Dallas, Texas

FRANK J. VEITH, M.D.
Bronx, New York

HEINZ W. WAHNER, M.D.
Rochester, Minnesota

PHILIP J. WALKER, M.D.
Herston, Queensland, Australia

CHARLES W. VAN WAY, III, M.D.
Kansas City, Missouri

THOMAS A. WHITEHILL, M.D.
Denver, Colorado

WALTER M. WHITEHOUSE, JR., M.D.
Ann Arbor, Michigan

ANTHONY D, WHITTEMORE, M.D.
Boston, Massachusetts

SAMUEL ERIC WILSON, M.D.
Orange, California

CHARLES L. WITTE, M.D.
Tucson, Arizona

MARLYS H. WITTE, M.D.
Tucson, Arizona

JAMES S. T. YAO, M.D.
Chicago, Illinois

CHRISTOPHER K. ZASRINS, M.D.
Stanford, California

GERALD B. ZELENOCK, M.D.
Ann Arbor, Michigan

R. EUGENE ZIERLER, M.D.
Seattle, Washington

Foreword

I have long felt that *Vascular Surgery* has evolved, like the specialty itself, to the point where it deserves a companion review book. This project was belatedly agreed upon as the third edition of the text was in production, but by that time, the contributors to the book had no enthusiasm for the additional work it represented. It was decided that for this fourth edition the review book would be prepared parallel with the preparation of each chapter of the text. In the interim, however, I was elected to the American Board of Surgery and was made chairman of the Vascular Surgery Examination Committee. Even though the primary intent, and the different question format, of the companion review book do not violate the board's policies on this subject, I still thought that some people might perceive a conflict of interest in these two roles. Furthermore, the additional chore of preparing both books in parallel would have been prohibitive. My dilemma was nicely resolved by my associate Bill Krupski, who agreed to take on this task. His in-depth knowledge of the literature and his logical, precise way of thinking made him particularly well suited to serve as the editor of this review book. As I look over the final product, it is clear that the circumstances which led to this solution were fortuitous, both for me and for this book. It has turned out better than I had originally hoped it would, and I am certain the reader will find it the valuable educational resource I envisioned.

ROBERT B. RUTHERFORD, M.D.

Preface

This review has been designed to provide surgical residents, vascular fellows, and practicing surgeons with a comprehensive, expedient, and effective method for self-evaluation and critique within the field of general vascular surgery. The book has been specifically written to help readers verify their understanding of vascular diseases, identify areas of relative weakness, and introduce new concepts in vascular surgery. In addition to facilitation of personal appraisal, this companion to *Vascular Surgery*, edited by Robert B. Rutherford, M.D., is intended to encourage and stimulate discussion on important topics in peripheral vascular disease at teaching conferences.

The book is divided into nineteen chapters corresponding to the sections in *Vascular Surgery*, 4th edition. In general, the questions are in chronological order with respect to the chapters in consecutive sections of the textbook. The questions are true/false and multiple choice in format. In many instances, *more than one* correct answer is possible. Each question is accompanied by an answer, a paragraph explanation, and references to specific pages in the text, should the reader need additional information.

The contributors to this work are authorities in their fields, who furnished not only questions but also thorough explanations of correct answers. They have provided questions on subjects that they consider of major importance in their chapters.

Although conventional didactic lectures, interactive seminars with workshops, and local/regional/national conferences are important components of learning, home study is probably the most common technique by which students and physicians assimilate new information. Testing retention after exposure to topical material is one of the most effective methods of medical education. Optimally, the learner should write down the answers to each question and, after completing each chapter, check his or her answers against those supplied. In order to provide an opportunity for the learner to truly ascertain his or her knowledge, explanations of answers follow the various sets of questions. Perhaps the most important part of the educational process involves review of these discussions, whether or not the correct answer was marked.

Finally, I wish to thank the contributors and several individuals whose input and hard work has made publication of the review possible. Hazel Hacker of W. B. Saunders Company was instrumental in ensuring that this review was published in a timely manner, accompanying the revision of the text. I'd like to give special thanks to Donna Fay for administrative assistance and the preparation of manuscripts.

I hope you will find this text a useful tool in your professional education.

William C. Krupski, M.D.

Contents

1

General Considerations

1. Chronic extremity swelling:
   - **A.** Demonstrates "pitting" edema only when cardiac in origin.
   - **B.** Is completely relieved by extremity elevation *only* when it is of venous origin.
   - **C.** Is rarely equal bilaterally.
   - **D.** Involves the feet and toes when due to lymphedema.
   - **E.** Is associated with pigmentation and cicatricial changes around the ankle only with chronic venous insufficiency.

2. Chronic leg ulcers:
   - **A.** Are almost always due to either arterial or venous insufficiency.
   - **B.** Are usually located near the malleoli if venous in origin.
   - **C.** Are not associated with pain unless secondarily infected.
   - **D.** Can almost always be diagnosed *as to origin* by physical examination alone.
   - **E.** Have an unpredictable spontaneous healing potential.

3. Extremity pain of vascular origin:
   - **A.** Can usually be diagnosed by taking a careful history.
   - **B.** If nocturnal, is usually associated with leg cramps.
   - **C.** Is arterial in origin if precipitated by exercise.
   - **D.** Is significantly affected by leg elevation.
   - **E.** Is a harbinger of limb loss if a vascular reconstructive procedure is not successfully performed.

4. Claudication:
   - **A.** Is derived from the name of the Roman emperor Claudius, who suffered this disorder.
   - **B.** Carries a risk of major amputation with expectant medical management of only 5% in five years.
   - **C.** Distance may be doubled by frequently exercising to the point of pain.
   - **D.** Usually requires arteriography for management.
   - **E.** Justifies infrainguinal bypass because of its current low risk and high long-term patency.

5. The postthrombotic syndrome is a form of chronic venous insufficiency:
   - **A.** In which stasis sequelae (dermatitis, ulceration) result from slow or stagnant venous flow when the patient is in the upright position.
   - **B.** That results in stasis ulcers in 50% of patients after five years if untreated.
   - **C.** That is inevitable after deep venous thrombosis (DVT).
   - **D.** That can be controlled by elastic stockings and intermittent elevation in over 90% of compliant patients.
   - **E.** That can be controlled in over 90% of patients by venous reconstructive surgery.

6. "Limb salvage":
   - **A.** Is a term applied to operations carried out to relieve chronic critical ischemia.
   - **B.** Is achieved if a pain-free functional foot is preserved or restored.
   - **C.** Is applicable to any procedure that lowers the anticipated level of amputation.
   - **D.** Is achieved by infrainguinal bypass in only one third of cases after five years.
   - **E.** Is achieved at a rate significantly higher than the graft patency rate after infrainguinal bypass.

1

Answers

1. The answers are **C, D, E** (Rutherford, 4th ed., pp. 8–9).

Pitting edema is typically produced by cardiac failure but is also present when edema is produced by severe hypoproteinemia. Edema due to heart failure, as well as venous edema, can be relieved by extremity elevation and disappears overnight; however, in the former setting the mobilization of fluid may produce orthopnea, paroxysmal nocturnal dyspnea, and nocturia. Congestive heart failure frequently causes bilateral edema as compared to venous edema or lymphedema, but even it is usually asymmetrical, commonly being worse on the left. Lymphedema typically involves the toes, feet, ankles, and leg in ascending fashion. Cardiac edema and other orthostatic edemas (e.g., hypoproteinemia) also can involve the feet to a degree, but venous edema almost never does. Venous edema, and sometimes edema of heart failure, produces pigmentation from the breakdown of extravasated erythrocytes, but only venous edema progresses to subcutaneous fibrosis and cutaneous atrophy in response to the extravasated red blood cells and plasma proteins. In the late stage of lymphedema ("elephantiasis") areas of pigmentation may develop, but the skin becomes hypertrophic and the subcutaneous tissues remain full because various-sized "lakes" of lymph accumulate.

2. The answers are **B, D** (Rutherford, 4th ed., pp. 9–10).

The vast majority of chronic leg ulcers are of *arterial, venous*, or *neuropathic* origin. Venous ulcers are usually located near the malleoli or at least in the "gaiter" distribution. Arterial and neuropathic ulcers are usually located on the foot, although any bony prominence or pressure point is susceptible to the latter. Neurotrophic ulcers are often not painful, whereas infected and uninfected ischemic ulcers are usually associated with ischemic "rest" pain. However, the more painful the venous ulcer, the greater the likelihood of secondary infection. The underlying cause of chronic leg ulcers is usually apparent from location, appearance, and associated physical signs (e.g., absent pulses, signs of chronic venous insufficiency, or detectable neuropathy). Healing potential of leg ulcers can be predicted on the basis of noninvasive testing (e.g., segmental pressures, plethysmography, capillary oxygen tension) *and* the ability to control the underlying cause (e.g., venous hypertension for venous ulcers, focal pressure points in neuropathic ulcers, and, for ischemic ulcers, successful revascularization).

3. The answers are **A, D** (Rutherford, 4th ed., pp. 2–6).

Extremity pain of vascular origin is usually so characteristic that it can be readily suspected even before physical examination. The nature and location of the pain and the effect of exercise, rest, or elevation offer immediate clues. Calf cramping with exercise relieved by rest is typical of arterial claudication, but nocturnal cramps are common in elderly patients without vascular disease. Nocturnal ischemic pain is located in the forefoot and is relieved by dependency. *Venous* claudication is a rarer form of vascular leg pain produced by exercise and relieved by rest. It is caused by severe venous outflow obstruction and secondary ambulatory venous hypertension, which increases rapidly because exercise induces increased arterial inflow. This pressure-induced pain is *not* promptly relieved by stopping the exercise, as is arterial claudication. Venous hypertension is relieved by leg elevation; ischemic rest pain is precipitated or made worse by leg elevation, and claudication does not occur during leg elevation (no exercise, no leg pain). Most extremity pain of vascular origin can be treated nonoperatively without risk of limb loss; persistent ischemic rest pain with or without ulceration/gangrene is the only major exception. Claudication is greatly ameliorated by exercise programs and cessation of smoking, with 5% or less risk of limb loss in five years. Well over 90% of chronic venous insufficiency can be controlled by elastic stockings and frequent leg elevation in compliant patients.

4. The answers are **B, C** (Rutherford, 4th ed., pp. 2, 11–14).

Claudication is derived from the Latin stem *claudicatio,* "to limp." Around 5% of all claudicators risk limb loss in five years, but this outlook is improved by stopping smoking (e.g., 2% for those who stop, 12% for those who don't). Those with lower ankle brachial indexes (e.g., ABI <0.3) have a significantly worse prognosis, but they also have a higher risk with arterial reconstruction. All 27 clinical trials have shown a benefit of exercise therapy for claudication. In the nine controlled trials, peak walking times increased from 25 to 183% (average 100%) or double the distance. Noninvasive studies detect, localize, and gauge the severity of the responsible occlusive lesions with such high accuracy (>95%) that arteriography is reserved for *therapeutic* indications, i.e., intent to treat. One can screen for discrete localized lesions amenable to endovascular interventions by color duplex scanning. Even though it can be performed under epidural anesthesia with minor blood loss and hemodynamic changes, infrainguinal bypass carries as high a mortality risk as aortic surgery (2–3%) but a lower patency—around 75% five-year patency in the best scenario of the claudicator with good runoff using a vain graft.

5. The answer is **D** (Rutherford, 4th ed., pp. 9–10, 12).

The postthrombotic syndrome results from involved venous segments that either remain obstructed or recanalized but contain malfunctioning valves. The resulting venous reflux and/or obstruction causes ambulatory *venous hypertension*, which, more than slow flow, is the final common denominator in determining stasis sequelae. This venous hypertension forces serum and erythrocytes out into the extravascular tissue spaces, resulting in brawny edema, subcutaneous inflammation and fibrosis, cutaneous atrophy, and pigmentation, which together characterize "stasis dermatitis" and are the forerunners of venous ulceration. Although Bauer's classic study in 1942 estimated the five-year incidence of stasis dermatitis and ulceration at 45% and 20% respectively, more recent studies indicate the incidence of these complications is significantly less. The postthrombotic syndrome with its stasis sequelae is not inevitable. In fact, 20% of patients with documented DVT are normal on follow-up noninvasive testing. Furthermore, over 90% of *compliant* patients can be quite adequately treated by wearing good elastic support stockings and frequently elevating their legs (e.g., ankles above heart level for 10 minutes every 2 hours). On the other hand, the results of venous reconstructive surgery, though admittedly performed on more severe cases, has not reached the same level of benefit (only about 70% clinical improvements, which correlates poorly with noninvasive studies). Therefore, venous reconstruction should be considered in those very few patients who are truly unable to control the stasis sequelae despite compliance with a good postphlebitic regimen.

6. The answers are **A, B, E** (Rutherford, 4th ed., pp. 12–14).

"Chronic critical ischemia" refers to persistent ischemic rest pain, nonhealing ischemic ulcers, and/or digital gangrene resulting from severe diffuse pedal ischemia. "Limb salvage" operations are directed at these forms of ischemia and imply that major amputation would be inevitable without successful revascularization. Actually, up to 40% of such cases may achieve initial limb salvage by nonoperative management (use of dependency, topical care, antibiotics, rheologic agents, improved cardiac function, etc.). The term "limb salvage" is somewhat of a misnomer. Only preservation or restoration of a painless functional foot truly qualifies for this definition. Simply lowering the amputation level does not suffice. Infrainguinal bypass, using autogenous vein graft, salvages over 80% of such limbs for five years, although this success rate may be 30% or less if prosthetic grafts are used and are carried below the knee to tibial arteries. Limb salvage rates generally exceed graft patency rates by 10–20% because, even if the bypass graft fails after healing has taken place, pain, ulceration, and gangrene do not necessarily return. In such cases, the revascularization procedure has temporarily provided the higher flows needed for healing.

2

Hemodynamics and Diagnosis of Arterial Disease

1. Which of the following statements are correct concerning steady flow in a frictionless fluid system?
   A. Pressure rises as velocity increases.
   B. Pressure falls as velocity increases.
   C. Fluid always moves from a point of high pressure to a point where the pressure is lower.
   D. Hydrostatic pressure and gravitational potential energy are equivalent, but have opposite signs.

2. Which of the following statements concerning Poiseuille's law are accurate?
   A. The pressure gradient between two points is directly related to fluid viscosity.
   B. For a given flow rate, the pressure gradient is inversely proportional to the fourth power of the radius.
   C. The law is generally applicable to flow situations encountered in the human body.
   D. The length of a stenosis has as much effect on pressure gradient as its radius.

3. Which of the following statements are true?
   A. Critical stenosis is defined as a 50% reduction in arterial diameter and is independent of flow rate.
   B. Resting blood flow in tissues distal to a stenosis is maintained at near normal levels largely as a result of collateral development.
   C. Tissues become ischemic when autoregulation is no longer capable of compensating for a decreased perfusion pressure.
   D. The drop in ankle pressure observed during and just after exercise in patients with arterial obstruction is due to a decrease in blood flow through the stenotic segment and the parallel collateral bed.
   E. Reflected waves from the periphery are largely responsible for the reversal of flow seen in early diastole in normal arteries during resting conditions.

4. Which of the following statements are true?
   A. Due to the Bernoulli effect, normal blood vessels tend to constrict when the velocity of flow increases.
   B. Sympathectomy has a greater effect on peripheral blood flow in limbs with arterial stenosis than it does in normal limbs.
   C. Bypass grafting is particularly efficacious as a method for treating arterial obstruction because it reduces segmental resistance to near normal levels.
   D. Stress on the arterial wall is directly related to intraluminal pressure and the arterial radius, and is inversely proportional to wall thickness.

5. With regard to pulse plethysmography, which of the following is *not* true? The contour of the peripheral arterial pressure pulse is influenced by:
   A. Left ventricular contraction.
   B. Intraluminal pressure.
   C. Interstitial pressure.
   D. Arterial wall elasticity.
   E. Proximal arterial obstruction.

6. In instruments employing duplex ultrasonography, which of the following is correct?
   A. The transmitting frequency used is usually between 15 MHz and 20 MHz.
   B. The ultrasound source emits a constant sound wave into the tissues.
   C. It is not possible to localize the site of sampling for the Doppler component of the instrument.
   D. The ultrasound source emits sound waves intermittently.
   E. Gray Scale is a method used to measure the blood flow velocity.

7. Which of the following features associated with Gray Scale spectra is used to determine the degree of stenosis in carotid arterial disease?
   A. Acceleration time to peak systole.
   B. Peak spectral broadening in systole.
   C. Peak systolic frequency.
   D. Peak spectral broadening in diastole.
   E. Peak diastolic frequency.

8. Potential sources of error in the measurement of arterial systolic pressure using a pneumatic cuff and Doppler flow detector include:
   A. Use of a Doppler instrument with a low transmitting frequency (i.e., 5 MHz).
   B. Medial calcification, which prevents compression of the arteries by the cuff.
   C. Use of a pulsed rather than a continuous-wave-type Doppler device.
   D. Changing the site of Doppler flow detection distal to the cuff.
   E. Use of a cuff that is narrow relative to the diameter of the limb at the site of measurement.

9. Which of the following statements about duplex scanning with color-flow imaging are true?
   - **A.** Color-flow imaging is not subject to artifacts from aliasing.
   - **B.** The color-flow image displays peak systolic frequencies just as reliably as spectral wave forms.
   - **C.** The color-flow image provides a display of velocity information for the entire B-mode image.
   - **D.** Direction of flow with respect to the ultrasound transducer is readily determined from the color-flow image.
   - **E.** The velocities represented in the color-flow image are independent of the ultrasound beam-to-vessel angle.

10. The treadmill exercise test for intermittent claudication would be useful in which of the following clinical situations?
    - **A.** A patient with ischemic rest pain and an ankle/brachial index of 0.2 on the affected side.
    - **B.** A patient with occasional hip and calf pain on walking and an ankle/brachial index of 0.75 on the affected side.
    - **C.** A patient with bilateral nocturnal muscle cramps and ankle/brachial indexes of 0.98.
    - **D.** A patient who reports shortness of breath and chest pain on walking one block.
    - **E.** A patient with calf pain after walking three blocks and an ankle/brachial index of 0.6 on the affected side.

11. In which of the following clinical situations would measurement of toe pressure be more valuable than measurement of ankle pressure?
    - **A.** A diabetic patient with medial calcification of the tibial arteries.
    - **B.** A patient with intermittent claudication based on a positive exercise treadmill test.
    - **C.** A patient with a foot ulcer and an ankle/brachial index of 0.6 on the affected side.
    - **D.** A patient who requires a toe amputation.
    - **E.** A patient being followed after a femoral-tibial in situ saphenous vein bypass graft.

12. Which of the following statements about arterial duplex scanning is correct?
    - **A.** Widening of the frequency band (spectral broadening) represents turbulent flow, and an increased peak systolic frequency represents a high-velocity jet within a stenosis.
    - **B.** Because flow disturbance is associated with arterial lesions that occur along long segments of the arterial system, only a few representative spectral samples are required during an examination.
    - **C.** Color-flow imaging cannot be used as an alternative to spectral wave form analysis for identifying stenotic arterial lesions.
    - **D.** When combined with B-mode imaging, the pulsed Doppler and continuous-wave Doppler provide similar wave forms.
    - **E.** When color-flow imaging is used, spectral wave forms are no longer required for accurate disease classification.

13. Which of the following statements regarding the diagnostic criteria for arterial duplex scanning is correct?
    - **A.** Renal artery lesions are characterized by comparing the end diastolic velocity in the renal artery to the peak systolic velocity in the aorta.
    - **B.** End-diastolic frequencies are useful in characterizing high-grade stenoses of the internal carotid artery.
    - **C.** Spectral broadening is an important component of the noninvasive diagnosis of a 60–70% iliac artery stenosis.
    - **D.** A renal–aortic peak systolic velocity ratio of 2.8 indicates a 60–70% renal artery stenosis.
    - **E.** A proper arterial duplex examination of the lower extremities is best performed following two minutes of walking on a treadmill at 1.5 mi/hr.

14. Magnetic resonance angiography (MRA) is a rapidly developing technique used to evaluate the arterial system. Which of the following statements is *incorrect* regarding MRA?
    - **A.** The same technique of image acquisition (time-of-flight) for the evaluation of luminal lesions (stenosis) can be used for the study of perigraft fluid, as in a patient with suspected graft infection.
    - **B.** The brightness of the vessel is directly dependent on the rate at which blood enters the area of acquisition; therefore, contrast is velocity dependent.
    - **C.** MRA can visualize most vessels, but images can be obscured by overlying bone, bowel gas, or dense vascular calcifications.
    - **D.** A T1-weighted spin-echo image is most similar to computed tomography (CT) in its information content.
    - **E.** A high-grade carotid stenosis demonstrated by conventional angiography is shown as a segmental occlusion on MRA.

15. Computed tomography (CT) is helpful for the evaluation of abdominal aortic aneurysms and can identify each of the following *except:*
    - **A.** An inflammatory aneurysm.
    - **B.** A contained rupture of an abdominal aortic aneurysm.
    - **C.** Visceral artery aneurysms.
    - **D.** Stenosis of the origin of the superior mesenteric artery.
    - **E.** Mycotic aneurysms.

16. Identification of *severe* arterial stenoses by duplex scanning depends primarily on which of the following features?
    - **A.** Visualization of atherosclerotic plaque on the B-mode image.
    - **B.** Finding a localized high-velocity jet with broadening of the spectral wave form.
    - **C.** Localized broadening of the spectral wave form without a change in velocity.
    - **D.** Accentuation of the diastolic reverse-flow phase distal to the stenotic site.
    - **E.** Damping of the spectral wave form proximal to the stenotic site.

17. Which of the following characteristics are useful for differentiating between the internal and external carotid arteries during duplex scanning of the carotid bifurcation?
    - **A.** The external carotid is typically located anteromedially.
    - **B.** The walls of the internal carotid artery produce brighter echoes than the external.
    - **C.** The external carotid spectral wave form contains a reverse-flow component.
    - **D.** The internal carotid spectral wave form shows forward flow throughout the cardiac cycle.
    - **E.** The external carotid artery has no branches within the neck.

18. CT findings of an aortic dissection include:
    - **A.** Displacement of intimal calcium.
    - **B.** Double contrast-filled lumen separated by an intimal flap.
    - **C.** Left lower lobe atelectasis.
    - **D.** Enhancing hyperemic rim with chronic dissection.
    - **E.** All of the above.

19. Because of its high specificity, the CT scan is the diagnostic modality of choice in aortic dissections. **True** or **false?**

20. For extraluminal arterial pathology of the popliteal fossa which techniques are most useful:
    - **A.** MRI.
    - **B.** CT.
    - **C.** Arteriography.
    - **D.** Ultrasound.

21. Time-of-flight magnetic resonance angiography:
    - **A.** Pulses radio waves into an imaging slice so it becomes dark.
    - **B.** Is the technique of choice to depict small vessels with slow in-plane blood flow.
    - **C.** Relies on "inflow phenomena" to provide contrast between the blood vessels and soft tissue.
    - **D.** A and C only.
    - **E.** None of the above.

22. Phase-contrast magnetic resonance angiography:
    - **A.** Eliminates background without substantially saturating blood.
    - **B.** Employs two acquisitions with bipolar gradient pulses of opposite polarity, which when subtracted cause stationary tissue signal to disappear, while moving tissue has signal intensity dependent on its velocity.
    - **C.** Is employed for depicting the slow flow in dural venous sinuses and small collateral vessels.
    - **D.** All of the above.
    - **E.** A and C only.

23. Cardiac magnetic resonance imaging may be considered the primary diagnostic modality for the evaluation of:
    - **A.** Constrictive pericarditis.
    - **B.** Paracardiac and intracardiac masses.
    - **C.** Thoracic aortic disease.
    - **D.** Certain forms of congenital heart disease.
    - **E.** All of the above.

24. Phase-contrast velocity-encoded cine magnetic resonance angiography:
    - **A.** May be useful in assessing the hemodynamic significance of a peripheral vascular stenosis whose severity might be overestimated by using time-of-flight magnetic resonance angiography alone.
    - **B.** Demonstrates a triphasic wave form when a hemodynamically significant arterial obstruction (>50% reduction in diameter) occurs.
    - **C.** Has measured velocities in normal volunteers in the popliteal, anterior tibial, and peritoneal arteries that are not significantly different from those measured using color-coded sonography.
    - **D.** All of the above.
    - **E.** A and C only.

25. All of the following adverse effects are greater with conventional ionic high osmolar contrast agents than with nonionic low osmolar contrast agents *except:*
    - **A.** Vasodilation.
    - **B.** Adverse effects on erythrocytes.
    - **C.** Thromboembolic events.
    - **D.** Adverse effects upon capillary endothelium.
    - **E.** Arrythmias.

26. The following have been considered risk factors for contrast-induced nephropathy *except:*
    - **A.** Chronic renal insufficiency.

B. Diabetes.
C. Renal artery stenosis.
D. Dehydration.
E. Advanced age.

27. Which of the following are true concerning idiosyncratic reactions to contrast agents?
A. Dose dependent.
B. There is a reduced incidence of minor reactions with low osmolar contrast media.
C. An example is pruritus.
D. An example is contrast nephropathy.
E. A "test dose" of contrast is a safe, reliable test to predict the idiosyncratic response.

28. Which of the following statement(s) is/are *false* concerning axillary hematomas and brachial plexus palsy?
A. This complication is occurring much less frequently.
B. Presenting complaint is usually severe pain/sensory loss in the hand.
C. Distal pulses are usually diminished.
D. A visible hematoma is almost always present.
E. Treatment is usually compression of the puncture site.

29. Contrast angiography:
A. Has been replaced by noninvasive imaging techniques such as ultrasound and magnetic resonance arteriography.
B. Can be competently performed by one who is familiar with basic concepts and standard protocols.
C. Has been refined to the point where associated risks are nonexistent.
D. Remains a mainstay of vascular diagnosis and therapy.

30. Compared to conventional film-screen techniques, DSA is:
A. Preferable in all respects.
B. Safer and faster.
C. Cheaper and faster.
D. More sensitive.

31. Guidewires and catheters:
A. Are usually preferable to direct needle angiography.
B. Are better if custom formed by the angiographer.
C. Are available in a wide variety of materials and standard configurations.
D. Are inappropriate for certain specialized intravascular studies.

32. When vessels are superimposed over bone, visibility can be improved by the following *except:*
A. Repositioning.
B. Increasing the contrast volume.
C. Using high-kilovoltage technique.
D. Using DSA.

2

Answers

1. The answers are **B, D** (Rutherford, 4th ed., pp. 18–20).

Bernoulli's principle states that the total fluid energy is the same from one point to another further downstream in a closed system, provided there are no frictional losses and the flow is steady (nonpulsatile):

$$P_1 + \rho g h_1 + \tfrac{1}{2}\rho v_1^2 = P_2 + \rho g h_2 + \tfrac{1}{2}\rho v_2^2$$

Because the sum of the pressure (P), the gravitational potential energy (ρgh), and the kinetic energy ($\tfrac{1}{2}\rho v^2$) at point 1 (upstream) on the left-hand side of the equation must equal the sum of the same parameters at point 2 (downstream) on the right-hand side of the equation, an increase in velocity (e.g., the tube narrows) must be accompanied by a decrease in pressure, provided the gravitational potential energy remains constant. If the upstream point is higher relative to the earth's surface than the downstream point, fluid may move from a point of low pressure to a point where the hydrostatic pressure is higher. This is possible because hydrostatic pressure and gravitational potential energy are both given by ρgh, but have opposite signs. In other words, the increase in hydrostatic pressure at the lower point is canceled by a decrease in gravitational potential energy.

2. The answers are **A, B** (Rutherford, 4th ed., p. 20).

Poiseuille's law states that the pressure drop ($P_1 - P_2$) between two points in a straight tube with a circular cross section is directly proportional to the flow rate (Q), the length (L) of the tube, and the viscosity of the fluid (η), and is inversely proportional to the fourth power of the radius (r):

$$P_1 - P_2 = Q\frac{8L\eta}{\pi r^4}$$

provided the flow is steady (nonpulsatile) and laminar and the tube is long enough for a parabolic flow profile to develop—conditions seldom, if ever, observed in blood vessels. Thus, Poiseuille's law invariably underestimates the pressure drop for a given flow rate. The length of a stenotic segment has far less effect on the pressure drop than does its radius.

3. The answers are **C, E** (Rutherford, 4th ed., pp. 24–30).

A stenosis is said to be "critical" when it causes a perceptible drop in blood pressure and/or flow. Although this usually occurs at a diameter reduction of about 50% (75% reduction in cross-sectional area), the degree of stenosis necessary varies with the flow rate, occurring at a less severe degree of stenosis when the flow rate is high and at a greater degree of stenosis when the flow rate is low. In other words, a stenosis may become "critical" only during exercise.

In claudicants, peripheral blood flow is maintained at near-normal levels largely as a result of compensatory dilatation of the peripheral arterioles. Although collateral development also acts to reduce the inflow resistance, alone it is seldom sufficient to maintain normal perfusion. "Autoregulation" refers to the ability of the peripheral arterioles to dilate in response to a reduction in peripheral perfusion pressure. Thus, tissues become ischemic only when the arterioles are completely dilated and pressures drop below the level at which autoregulatory compensation is possible.

Due to exercise-induced dilatation of the intramuscular arterioles, blood flow through the stenotic segment and parallel collateral bed, which comprise the "segmental resistance" (R_{seg}), is actually increased during exercise even in claudicating limbs. Therefore, the drop in ankle pressure is caused by increased energy losses incurred as a result of increased flow through the relatively high and "fixed" segmental resistance:

$$P_2 = P_1 - QR_{seg}$$

In this formula, P_2 represents the ankle pressure, P_1 the inflow pressure, and Q the flow through the segmental resistance.

Flow waves in normal limbs are reflected all along the arterial tree but can be construed as being reflected from the high-resistance peripheral bed. Thus, under resting conditions, the reflected wave is responsible for the reversed flow component seen in the normal arterial flow wave form. During exercise, when the peripheral arterioles are dilated, the reversed-flow component disappears. It is also absent at rest in normal arteries, such as the carotid and renal arteries, which feed low-resistance peripheral vascular beds.

4. The answers are **C, D** (Rutherford, 4th ed., pp. 34–38).

Although, according to the Bernoulli principle, an increase in the velocity of flow is accompanied by a decrease in intraluminal pressure, the effect is small (only about a 1.0 mm Hg reduction in pressure for a velocity increase of 50 cm/sec). Therefore, the arterial diameter, which depends on the elasticity of the arterial wall and the intraluminal pressure, would change very little. (However, under certain circumstances, a velocity increase in low-pressure veins may cause the venous wall to collapse.) Because increased shear stress on the vascular wall releases endothelium-derived relaxing factor (EDRF), vessels tend to dilate in response to increased flow velocity.

Sympathectomy increases blood flow by decreasing the tone in arteriolar sphincters. Because the arterioles are already partially dilated in limbs with inflow obstruction, sympathectomy has less effect on flow in limbs with arterial disease than it does on flow in normal limbs.

Bypass grafting places a low-resistance conduit parallel to the high segmental resistance imposed by the stenotic or occluded artery and its parallel collaterals. Thus, a well-designed graft may return the segmental resistance to normal and, provided there is no distal obstruction, may restore normal circulation.

The hoop stress (τ) on a cylinder is given by:

$$\tau = P\frac{r_i}{\delta}$$

where r_i is the internal radius and δ is the wall thickness. This explains why aneurysms are more likely to rupture when they are large and when the patient is hypertensive.

5. The answer is **C** (Rutherford, 4th ed., pp. 45–48).

Pulse plethysmography is the technique used in pulse volume recordings to evaluate the status of the arterial circulation. It provides a means of sensing the arterial pressure pulse that is originally derived from left ventricular contraction and is also influenced by the intraluminal pressure and elasticity of the arterial wall. The presence of peripheral arterial obstruction results in dampening of this peripheral pressure pulse wave form and is the basis for its use in the diagnosis of arterial disease. Interstitial pressure is not influential in the contour of the peripheral arterial pressure pulse. Therefore, conditions associated with increases in interstitial pressure do not affect the sensitivity of this instrumentation.

6. The answer is **D** (Rutherford, 4th ed., pp. 48–52).

Whereas early duplex instruments used continuous-wave ultrasound for sampling the blood flow stream, modern instruments routinely use an ultrasound source that emits sound waves intermittently—termed pulsed Doppler ultrasound. The frequency at which these pulses are transmitted through the tissues is referred to as the pulse repetition frequency (PRF). The transmitting frequencies used for most instruments vary from 2.5 to 10 MHz because of the necessity to penetrate tissues of varying depths. In general terms, the deeper the tissue, the lower the transmitting frequency. Transmitting frequencies of 15 or 20 MHz can be used for instruments that are applied directly to vessels. The use of pulsed ultrasound enables the operator to define a particular depth at which the Doppler may be focused for sampling the flow stream. The fast Fourier-derived spectra obtained from the back-scattered Doppler information is depicted in Gray Scale format. This refers to the technique of displaying signals of varying amplitudes and does not refer to the technique for measuring the blood flow velocity.

7. The answer is **C** (Rutherford, 4th ed., pp. 56–58, 122).

The primary information contained in the Gray Scale spectra that is used to determine the degree of stenosis is the peak systolic frequency. Measurement of this parameter with conversion to velocity on the basis of the Doppler equation overcomes and provides a method of standardization for differences in transmitting frequency and angle of insonation. Acceleration time to peak systole is not used for the diagnosis of carotid disease, and the degree of spectral broadening, whether this occurs in systole or diastole, is not measured by most current instruments. *Peak* diastolic frequency is never used to estimate the degree of stenosis in the carotid arteries, although *end* diastolic frequency or conversion to end diastolic velocity is often used for the diagnosis of critical stenosis of the internal carotid artery.

8. The answers are **B, E** (Rutherford, 4th ed., pp. 65–76).

The Doppler transmitting frequency should not influence the results of pressure measurements, although lower frequencies are preferred for deeply located arteries, since tissue penetration by ultrasound is inversely proportional to the transmitting frequency. Either a pulsed or continuous-wave-type Doppler device can be used for pressure measurements; however, the continuous-wave type is usually more practical. Because blood flow past the cuff can be detected in any distal artery, the exact site of Doppler flow detection is not critical. For convenience, the posterior tibial or dorsalis pedis artery signals can be used for all lower-extremity pressure measurements. Medial calcification, which can render the underlying vessels incompressible, is the most common source of error with indirect peripheral pressure measurements, particularly in diabetic patients. This leads to artificially high pressure values. Use of a relatively narrow cuff can result in pressure values that are falsely high. This is especially likely to occur for thigh pressure measurements, with higher pressures in patients with large thighs and lower, more accurate pressures in patients with small thighs.

9. The answers are **C, D** (Rutherford, 4th ed., p. 85).

Since color-flow imaging is an alternative method for displaying pulsed Doppler information, it is subject to the *same* limitations as spectral wave form analysis. These include artifacts due to aliasing when the pulsed Doppler PRF is too low for accurate detection of the Doppler shift frequencies. Because the color assignments in the color-flow image are based on a mean or average frequency estimate, the peak frequencies seen with spectral wave forms are generally higher than the frequencies indicated by the color-flow image. Doppler frequency shift measurements by both color-flow imaging and spectral wave form analysis depend on the beam-to-vessel angle. The main advantage of the color-flow image is that it provides a real-time display of velocity information for the entire B-mode image. The direction of flow with respect to the ultrasound transducer can be determined from the color-flow image by using different colors to indicate flow in opposite directions.

10. The answers are **B, E** (Rutherford, 4th ed., pp. 93–97).

The treadmill exercise test is valuable for confirming the clinical impression of intermittent claudication and determining its severity under controlled conditions. Patients who have obvious critical ischemia with rest pain or tissue loss and very low ankle pressures should not require treadmill exercise testing. On the other extreme, treadmill exercise testing is not generally helpful in patients with normal ankle/brachial indexes and without exercise-induced symptoms. The treadmill exercise test should be used with extreme caution in patients who report symptoms of chest pain or shortness of breath during walking. Patients with true intermittent claudication will show a marked drop in ankle pressure with exercise to the point of muscle pain. If a patient is able to walk for five minutes on the treadmill without symptoms and with no drop in ankle pressure, then claudication is not present.

11. The answers are **A, C, D** (Rutherford, 4th ed., pp. 70–72, 97–99, 109–111).

Medical calcification does not appear to affect the digital arteries, so toe pressures are a reliable indicator of the physiologic severity of arterial occlusive disease when the ankle pressure measurements are artificially high. Toe pressures have also been more useful than ankle pressures for predicting healing of foot lesions and toe amputations. Measurement of toe pressures would not be likely to provide any important additional information in a patient with claudication only. The optimal method for follow-up of bypass grafts in the leg is duplex scanning.

12. The answer is **A** (Rutherford, 4th ed., pp. 85, 120–121).

Arterial duplex scanning uses spectral broadening (turbulent flow) to identify smaller degrees of stenosis and increased peak systolic frequencies, which represents a high-velocity flow through a narrowed segment of artery, to detect arterial disease. Since the flow disturbances associated with arterial lesions are best detected in the area of the stenosis, thorough evaluation with frequent spectral samples is required during the examination. Color-flow imaging is a new addition that can be used as an alternative to spectral wave form analysis for stenotic arterial lesions. The principal advantage of the color-flow display is that it presents flow information on the entire image, even though the amount of information on each site is reduced. Color-flow imaging can be helpful in identifying vessels, especially when they are small, deeply located, or anatomically complex. However, since the color assignments in the flow image represent mean (or mode) rather than peak velocities, it is difficult to determine disease severity based on the color-flow image alone. Therefore, even when color-flow imaging is used, spectral wave forms are required for accurate disease classification.

13. The answer is **B** (Rutherford, 4th ed., pp. 122–129).

Duplex scanning assesses the physiologic significance of vascular lesions and classifies the severity of disease according to relatively broad categories. The details of disease classification by duplex scanning differs for the various arterial segments studied. However, the underlying principles relating the severity of arterial disease to localized blood flow disturbances remain the same. Renal artery lesions are identified by comparing the ratio of the peak systolic velocity in the renal artery to the peak systolic velocity in the aorta (renal–aortic ratio). A renal–aortic ratio of ≥3.5 or a renal artery peak systolic velocity of ≥180 cm/sec indicates a ≥60% stenosis. End diastolic frequencies are required to characterize high-grade stenoses of the internal carotid artery. Generally, an end diastolic frequency of ≥4.5K Hz (velocity of 120 cm/sec) indicates a high-grade stenosis (≥80%) of the internal carotid artery. While spectral broadening is important in identifying lesser degrees of iliac artery stenosis, iliac stenosis of 60% or more is identified by a peak systolic velocity ≥100% relative to the adjacent proximal segment. These duplex examinations are performed in a patient at rest.

14. The answer is **A** (Rutherford, 4th ed., pp. 132–134, 142–144).

It is important to understand that magnetic resonance angiography (MRA) is quite different from conventional contrast arteriography. The similarity between an MRA and a conventional angiogram depends upon favorable blood flow conditions and well-chosen acquisition parameters. As an example, in the carotid system the MRA and conventional angiogram are often similar in carotid arteries with moderate disease. However, vessels with severe stenosis on the angiogram may be shown as a segmental *occlusion* on MRA (because of the lack of acquisition signals in the area of high-grade stenosis). Several techniques are well established for magnetic resonance imaging specific for the information required. The spin-echo technique does not produce an angiogram per se. However, it is frequently used to evaluate blood vessel size and the perivascular tissues. For example, it visualizes the true size of an aneurysm even when the aneurysm is thrombosed. A T1-weighted spin-echo image is most similar to computed tomography (CT) in its information content. A T2-weighted magnetic resonance image (MRI) is most frequently used to study perigraft fluid and patients with suspected graft infection. Time-of-flight is the most commonly applied method for angiography in most parts of the body. Protons, which are pulsed rapidly and repeatedly, lose their magnetization and therefore lose their signal on MRI. This process of suppressing the signal of tissues is called saturation. Tissues that have not been pulsed for several seconds recover their magnetization and again appear differently on MRI. This process is called relaxation. With repeated signal processing, images are stacked and projected to provide an angiogram-like image. The brightness of the vessels is directly dependent on the rate at which blood enters the area of acquisition. Therefore, the vascular contrast is velocity dependent.

15. The answer is **D** (Rutherford, 4th ed., pp. 131–132, 134–140).

The abdominal aorta from the diaphragm to the iliac bifurcation is well visualized with computed tomography (CT). The characteristic CT finding of an abdominal aortic aneurysm (AAA) is dilation of the calcified arterial wall. Disruption of the calcium with obliteration of adjacent soft tissue may represent rupture, and identifying a chronic but contained rupture has been helpful in planning surgical repair. CT scans are helpful in identifying the thickened, soft tissue surrounding inflammatory aneurysms and the presence of visceral aneurysms. Mycotic aneurysms have also been demonstrated and appear as eccentric thick aortic walls with intramural air. Standard CT is not useful to identify arterial stenoses, although the advent of "spiral" CT scan may change this.

16. The answer is **B** (Rutherford, 4th ed., pp. 120–122).

While B-mode imaging may be helpful in identifying the location of atherosclerotic plaque, it has not been useful for classifying the severity of stenotic lesions. The finding of a localized high-velocity jet and spectral broadening by Doppler spectral wave form analysis is the most accurate method for noninvasive identification of a severe arterial stenosis. Localized broadening of the spectral wave form without a change in velocity suggests a moderate (less than 50% reduction in diameter) stenosis. The diastolic reverse-flow phase is typically reduced or absent distal to a severe stenosis. Changes in the spectral wave form proximal to a stenosis are generally not helpful, since they are affected by the presence of branches and collateral flow.

17. The answers are **A, C, D** (Rutherford, 4th ed., p. 122).

The internal and external carotid arteries can be distinguished by their typical anatomic locations and the characteristic features of their flow patterns. Just distal to the level of the carotid bifurcation, the external carotid is located anteromedially, and the internal carotid is located posterolaterally. There is no appreciable difference in the echogenicity of the arterial walls of the various carotid branches. The triphasic external carotid wave form contains a reverse-flow component that is typical of peripheral arteries supplying a high-resistance vascular bed. The internal carotid flow pattern is characteristic of an artery supplying a low-resistance vascular bed with forward flow throughout the cardiac cycle. The external carotid artery has branches within the neck, which may be visualized during duplex scanning; the internal carotid artery has no cervical branches.

18. The answer is **E** (Rutherford, 4th ed., pp. 134–135).

Aortic dissection may be diagnosed on CT scan with a contrast-enhanced study. A dissection is seen as double contrast-filled lumens separated by the intimal flap. In a noncontrast study calcified fragments of the intima may be displaced due to the dissection. With chronic dissections, a hyperemic rim is seen. Potential pitfalls occur when the innominate vein fills with contrast and appears as a dissection at the aortic valve. Also calcium within a pre-existing thrombus may appear as a displaced calcified intima. In addition, with volume averaging, a larger segment of the aorta may be superimposed on a smaller portion, producing what appears to be a displaced calcium fragment.

19. The answer is **false** (Rutherford 4th ed., pp. 130–136).

A variety of different imaging modalities have been used to define aortic dissections. The complete scan provides a sensitivity similar to MRI and transesophageal echo (TEE). However, the specificity is lower when compared to the other modalities. The CT scan does not provide useful information regarding the aortic valve or the status of the coronary arteries. The MRI gives the ability to reconstruct the aorta in multiple planes. In the thoracic aorta this is particularly useful to define the longitudinal length. The drawback to the MRI, although it is more sensitive and more specific than the CT, is the long imaging times required in a potentially unstable patient. TEE offers a rapid technique that appears to be as sensitive and as specific as the MRI. The principal advantages are safety and ability to perform at the bedside. The major disadvantage is that extension at the dissection into the abdominal aorta cannot be determined.

20. The answers are **A, B, D** (Rutherford, 4th ed., pp. 136–137).

While arteriography is useful in defining arterial stenoses and runoff, adjacent soft tissue structures are not well defined. CT scan and MRI are useful in diagnosing arterial entrapment, popliteal artery cysts, and aneurysms. A popliteal cyst is seen as a cystic structure adjacent to the arterial lumen. Although ultrasound is able to define aneurysms, it identifies popliteal cysts with difficulty. In the young patient with claudication and suspected popliteal fossa pathology, CT scan is the diagnostic method of choice. Popliteal entrapment is characterized by a muscle band passing between the artery and vein in all the types except type V entrapment.

21. The answer is **D** (Rutherford, 4th ed., p. 143).

Time-of-flight magnetic resonance angiography (MRA) saturates the signal from soft tissues by pulsing radio waves into an imaging slice to suppress its signal. Blood outside this slice is bright, and as it flows through the slice the signal remains bright for several pulses before it too becomes suppressed. This process is called in-flow phenomena or flow-related enhancement. The spins in small vessels with slow in-plane flow are subjected to repetitive radio waves that saturate their signal. Therefore, using a phase-contrast technique is preferred.

22. The answer is **D** (Rutherford, 4th ed., p. 143).

Phase-contrast magnetic resonance angiography (MRA) achieves excellent background suppression by applying bipolar gradients pulses of opposite polarity on two sequential gradient echo acquisitions, and then subtracts the two acquisitions. Stationary tissue undergoes no net phase accumulation and subtracts out, whereas the moving spins accumulate a nonzero phase shift when subtracted—yielding bright signal intensity. Since phase-contrast MRA can be sensitized to different velocities, it is especially useful for depicting slow flow in dural venous sinuses and small collateral vessels.

23. The answer is **E** (Rutherford, 4th ed., pp. 144–149).

Cardiac magnetic resonance imaging (MRI) provides direct visualization of the pericardium, enabling the diagnosis of constrictive pericarditis to be made on the basis of pericardial thickness (>4 mm). Intracardiac thrombi, primary and metastatic tumors to the heart, as well as mediastinal tumors invading cardiovascular structures, have been effectively demonstrated by cardiac MRI. Cardiac MRI has a sensitivity and specificity in excess of 90% in the evaluation of suspected thoracic aortic disease. In the presence of aortic dissection, cardiac MRI clearly demonstrates the intimal flap and extent of dissection within the aorta. Cardiac MRI remains a secondary diagnostic technique to echocardiography in many congenital heart lesions. However, it can be considered the technique of choice in the pre- and postoperative evaluation of aortic arch and pulmonary arterial abnormalities.

24. The answer is **E** (Rutherford, 4th ed., pp. 143, 147–149, 150–151).

Phase-contrast velocity-encoded cine magnetic resonance angiography (MRA) has been utilized to assess the hemodynamic significance of a peripheral vascular stenosis whose severity might be overestimated by using MRA alone, which is subject to signal loss from turbulence and visual overestimation of the severity of a stenosis. When a hemodynamically significant arterial obstruction (>50% reduction in diameter) occurs, the triphasic wave form dampens in the artery, resulting in amplitude reduction and broadening of the systolic segment with absence of diastolic segments (monophasic wave form). In the presence of a more severe obstruction the pulsatility of the velocity wave form is completely absent. Therefore, answer B is incorrect. There was no significant difference between phase-contrast velocity-encoded cine MRA and color-coded sonographic velocity measurements in the popliteal, anterior tibial, and peritoneal arteries of normal volunteers.

25. The answer is **C** (Rutherford, 4th ed., pp. 165–168).

High osmolar conventional ionic contrast agents have a greater adverse effect on hemodynamics, erythrocytes, and capillary endothelium. Hemodynamic effects include vasodilatation, hemodilution, hypervolemia, and changes in pulmonary artery pressure, cardiac output, and systemic resistance. Adverse effects on erythrocytes include increased rigidity and decreased mobility resulting in tissue hypoxia. Adverse effects on capillary endothelium include increased capillary permeability, vasodilatation, and osmotic hypervolemia. Binding of calcium by ionic agents is felt to be the etiology of arrhythmias and myocardial depression. Less neurologic- and nephrotoxicity also has been reported with nonionic low osmolar agents. The nonionic low osmolar agents do have an increased propensity for clot formation and thus a higher risk of thromboembolic events.

26. The answer is **C** (Rutherford, 4th ed., pp. 168–170).

All of the above are risk factors for contrast-induced renal insufficiency except renal artery stenosis. Additional risk factors include the dose and administration of contrast and recent surgery/vascular interventional procedures. Multiple myeloma is no longer considered to be a risk factor as long as the patient is not dehydrated or has an elevated creatinine. The above risk factors may be additive. Contrast nephropathy is defined as a rise in creatinine of 1.0 mg/dl within 48 hours of contrast administration. Renal failure usually reverts back to baseline within 1–2 weeks, but oliguria/anuria lasting days and chronic renal failure requiring dialysis have been reported. Nonionic low osmolar agents should be used in high-risk groups because of their reported lower renal toxicity.

27. The answers are **B, C** (Rutherford, 4th ed., pp. 169–170).

Idiosyncratic reactions to contrast agents are anaphylactic-like reactions that are *not* dose dependent. Small amounts of contrast media may produce a severe reaction in susceptible patients; therefore, administering "test doses" of contrast are not reliable or safe methods of predicting the idiosyncratic response. Clinical symptoms of idiosyncratic reactions are classified as mild, moderate, and severe. Minor reactions include nausea, vomiting, urticara, pruritis, and diaphoresis. Moderate reactions include severe vomiting, profound urticaria, facial edema, laryngeal edema, and bronchospasm. Severe reactions include shock, pulmonary edema, and cardiopulmonary arrest. An overall decrease in all adverse pulmonary reactions from 12.6% in patients receiving ionic high osmolar contrast to 3.1% in those receiving nonionic low osmolar contrast has been demonstrated.

28. The answers are **A, C, D, E** (Rutherford, 4th ed., p. 173)

Brachial plexis palsy after arterial punctures is a compressive neuropathy from a focal hematoma. Angiographers and referring physicians must have a high index of suspicion because of the possible devastating consequences of this complication. The complication is likely to occur more frequently because of increased use of the axillary approach, larger angioplasty catheters, and thrombolytic/anticoagulation therapy. The first symptoms are usually severe pain and mild sensory loss in the hand. This may progress to profound sensory and motor loss. Motor loss usually involves the median and ulnar nerves, resulting in loss of dorsiflexion of hand, apposition of thumb and index finger, and diminished hand grip. A visible hematoma is not present in the majority of cases and correlates poorly with clinical outcome. The distal pulses are usually intact. Manual compression does not play a role in therapy. The patient may be observed if sensory symptoms are very mild, but prompt surgical decompression is imperative if there is a progression of sensory findings or any motor symptoms.

29. The answer is **D** (Rutherford, 4th ed., pp. 178–180).

Although noninvasive imaging techniques are excellent for many screening and diagnostic applications, contrast arteriography remains *the* best modality for accurate evaluation of most vascular disease processes, as well as providing a means for transcatheter therapy. While many "standard" arteriographic studies are straightforward and follow typical protocols, many variables are involved, and the complexity and technical demands of some cases, often unanticipated, can be very high. Rigorous training is required prior to performing anything beyond basic angiography. Despite technical advances and an appropriately high level of training and skill, inherent risks are associated with angiography and must be weighed against the anticipated benefits of the procedure.

30. The answer is **C** (Rutherford, 4th ed., pp. 181–182).

DSA offers many advantages over conventional angiography, but there are trade-offs. While higher-contrast sensitivity permits the use of less contrast for a given injection (lowering the risk related to the use of contrast), the higher radiation exposure needed for each digital image, as well as the greater number of images usually obtained, substantially increases the radiation exposure (with its attendant risks) to the patient. The relative safety of the two methods is not easily determined. A single film run at one station is faster using DSA, given the set-up and processing requirements of plain-film imaging. A femoral run-off arteriogram using DSA, however, requires separate injection and filming at each station, which can take longer and use more total contrast than a plain-film runoff using a single injection and step-table filming sequence. The contrast sensitivity of DSA permits delineation of vessels or flow patterns that may be poorly demonstrated on plain-film examinations, although conventional filming is more sensitive in demonstrating subtle structural abnormalities (e.g., intimal flaps), and diagnosis by DSA can easily be compromised by motion. Costs are greatly reduced with DSA due to reduced set-up, processing requirements, and film usage. DSA is becoming the angiographic imaging modality of choice, largely because of speed and reduced expense.

31. The answers are **A**, **C** (Rutherford, 4th ed., pp. 182–184).

Guidewires and catheters are essential for all but the simplest angiographic evaluations. While both guidewires and catheters may be hand formed into custom shapes when needed for specific situations, standard configurations are available and appropriate for most circumstances. A number of materials and a large choice of configurations permit the use of standard guidewires and catheters for most applications.

32. The answer is **B** (Rutherford, 4th ed., p. 186).

Repositioning the patient and changing the projection so that bone and vessel are no longer superimposed, if possible, are the simplest solutions. High-kilovoltage (low-contrast) technique, if not utilized to begin with, may improve assessment of vessels by reducing the opacity of the overlying bone. With DSA, the "background" bone density is subtracted from subsequent images, optimally showing only opacified vessels. Assuming an adequate initial contrast volume, using more will not improve vessel visibility.

3

Arterial Pathology

1. Increased arterial blood flow results in which of the following?
   A. Endothelial damage.
   B. Increase in the number of medial elastic lamellae.
   C. Lumen enlargement.
   D. Smooth muscle cell proliferation.
   E. Subintimal lipid accumulation.

2. The most important factor in localization of atherosclerotic plaque in the human carotid bifurcation is:
   A. Endothelial denudation.
   B. High wall shear stress.
   C. High total cholesterol level.
   D. Low and oscillatory wall shear stress.
   E. High blood pressure.

3. Which of the following hemodynamic factors is *least* likely to promote atherosclerotic plaque localization?
   A. Low wall shear stress.
   B. High wall shear stress.
   C. Oscillation of shear stress.
   D. Increased particle residence time.
   E. Flow separation.

4. Which pathobiologic feature of atherosclerosis is most likely to result in clinical symptoms?
   A. Artery enlargement.
   B. Erosion of the fibrous cap.
   C. Smooth muscle cell proliferation.
   D. Cholesterol crystallization in the plaque.
   E. Calcification of the plaque.

5. The *least* important factor in the pathobiology of plaque formation is:
   A. Lipid uptake by subendothelial macrophages.
   B. Monocyte adhesion to the endothelial surface.
   C. Smooth muscle cell proliferation.
   D. Smooth muscle cell migration.
   E. Endothelial denudation.

6. Which factor is *least* likely to be important in pathogenesis of aneurysm formation?
   A. Increased collagenase activity.
   B. Genetic predisposition.
   C. Increase in medial elastin.
   D. Atherosclerotic plaque degeneration.
   E. Artery enlargement.

7. All forms of serum cholesterol are potentially atherogenic and should be lowered in patients with atherosclerotic vascular disease. **True** or **false**?

8. For patients with severe elevations of LDL, which of the following drugs might be helpful?
   A. Dipyridamole.
   B. Cholestyramine.
   C. Lovastatin.
   D. Sulfinpyrazone.
   E. Ticlopidine.

9. For the average patient with atherosclerotic peripheral vascular disease, which of the following risk factors is most commonly present?
   A. Hypercholesterolemia.
   B. Hypertension.
   C. Cigarette smoking.
   D. Diabetes.
   E. Obesity

10. Which of the following criteria are important for clinical diagnosis of Buerger's disease?
    A. A history of cigarette smoking.
    B. Onset before the age of 50 years.
    C. Aortoiliac arterial occlusions.
    D. Infrapopliteal arterial occlusions.
    E. Hypercholesteremia.
    F. Either upper-limb involvement or phlebitis migrans.

11. Indications for lumbar sympathectomy in patients with Buerger's disease include:
    A. Trophic lesions of the skin.
    B. Intermittent claudication.
    C. Vasospastic symptoms, such as coldness or cold sensitivity.
    D. Prophylaxis for progression.
    E. Wet gangrene.

12. Which statements are true about angiography for Takayasu's disease?
  - **A.** Angiography is the principal means of establishing a diagnosis of Takayasu's arteritis.
  - **B.** Serial angiograms showing progressive stenosis in an artery with previously diagnosed disease is an indication of active arteritis.
  - **C.** New vascular lesions on serial angiography suggest active arteritis.
  - **D.** The arteries most commonly affected are subclavian, descending aorta, renal, carotid, mesenteric, ascending aorta, and abdominal aorta.

13. Which of the following statements about subclavian arterial involvement with Takayasu's disease are true?
  - **A.** The subclavian artery is the most commonly involved vessel.
  - **B.** Subclavian steal syndrome is commonly associated with Takayasu's disease of the subclavian artery.
  - **C.** Takayasu's disease usually involves long segments of the subclavian as well as the axillary artery.
  - **D.** Because subclavian involvement is commonly bilateral, accurate determination of blood pressure measurements is difficult.

14. The following statements about bypasses of obstructive lesions in patients with Takayasu's disease are true:
  - **A.** Proximal and distal anastomoses must always be performed in arteries free of disease on arteriography.
  - **B.** It is preferable to perform bypasses with anastomoses placed in sites that statistically have a low incidence of involvement.
  - **C.** Arteries that are normal on arteriograms predictably do not have microscopic evidence of disease.
  - **D.** Endarterectomy with patch graft is an option for obstructive lesions.

15. The most likely cause of stroke in patients with Takayasu's disease is:
  - **A.** Occlusion of a major extracranial carotid artery.
  - **B.** Embolization from a stenotic extracranial carotid artery.
  - **C.** Cardiac arrythmias.
  - **D.** Intra-cerebral arterial disease.
  - **E.** Intracranial hemorrhage.

16. Differences in the expression of infrarenal abdominal aortic aneurysmal (AAA) and atherosclerotic occlusive (ASO) disease include all of the following *except*:
  - **A.** The mean age of patients presenting with AAA is greater.
  - **B.** The male/female ratio is greater with AAA.
  - **C.** Genetic susceptibility is more important for ASO than AAA disease.
  - **D.** The enzymatic activity of AAA tissue is increased.

17. The arterial wall matrix component most responsible for tensile strength is:
  - **A.** Microfibrils.
  - **B.** Proteoglycans.
  - **C.** Elastin.
  - **D.** Collagen.

18. Infiltration of chronic inflammatory cells within aortic aneurysm walls has been most notable in the:
  - **A.** Adventitia.
  - **B.** Media.
  - **C.** Intima.
  - **D.** There is generally no significant inflammatory infiltrate within the vessel walls of aneurysms.

19. All of the following concerning anastomotic aneurysms are true *except:*
  - **A.** They result from any etiology that causes a separation between the graft and host artery.
  - **B.** They lead to the abandonment of arterial homografts.
  - **C.** The aneurysmal wall is composed of an intima, media, and adventitia.
  - **D.** They can be associated with the use of autologous vein.

20. Renal artery fibrodysplasia is the second most common anatomic cause of renovascular hypertension. The spectrum of disease involves:
  - **A.** Medial fibroplasia, affecting nearly 85% of cases with series of stenoses and intervening mural aneurysms.
  - **B.** Medial hyperplasia, accounting for 15% of dysplastic renovascular disease, involving mostly females.
  - **C.** Perimedial dysplasia, accounting for 10% of cases, and presenting with multiple mural aneurysms and excessive elastic tissue at the junction of the media and adventitia.
  - **D.** Intimal fibroplasia, affecting 20% of black females with dysplastic renal arteries.

21. The most common type and location of carotid artery fibrodysplasia is:
  - **A.** Intimal fibroplasia affecting the origin of the common carotid artery at the aortic arch.
  - **B.** Medial hyperplasia involving the intracranial internal carotid artery.
  - **C.** Medial fibroplasia involving the internal carotid artery adjacent to the second and third cervical vertebrae.
  - **D.** Perimedial dysplasia of the distal common carotid artery.

22. Intracranial aneurysms coexistent with extracranial carotid fibrodysplasia:
    A. Occur in almost all cases and are characterized by medial fibroplasia of the aneurysm wall.
    B. Affect 12 to 25% of patients and not necessarily in the same cerebral hemisphere affected by the extracranial dysplastic disease.
    C. Occur in a different distribution than the typical "berry" aneurysm distribution in patients unaffected by extracranial carotid fibroplasia.
    D. Are seen only in association with severe hypertension.

23. Medial fibroplasia of the external iliac artery occurs:
    A. In 50% of patients with renal artery fibrodysplasia.
    B. Usually in male patients.
    C. As serial stenoses with intervening mural aneurysms typically in the proximal third of the vessel.
    D. Usually in women during their third and fourth decades of life.

24. Intimal hyperplasia in healing vein grafts and carotid arteries after endarterectomy is the result of:
    A. Abnormal accumulation of smooth muscle cells (smooth muscle hyperplasia).
    B. Abnormal accumulation of endothelial cells (endothelial hyperplasia).
    C. Systemic hypertension.
    D. Both A and B.
    E. None of the above.

25. Intimal hyperplasia is an important cause of vascular graft thrombosis after surgery during the period:
    A. 0–1 month.
    B. 1–24 months.
    C. Later than 24 months.
    D. Only under unusual circumstances.

26. Platelet factors and platelet-derived growth factor (PDGF) are powerful stimulants of migration and proliferation of vascular smooth muscle cells in culture. In animal models of arterial injury, factors from platelets stimulate:
    A. Smooth muscle proliferation.
    B. Smooth muscle migration.
    C. Endothelial cell proliferation.
    D. Both smooth muscle migration and proliferation.
    E. Neither smooth muscle migration nor proliferation.

27. The development of bilateral arm effort fatigue simultaneously in a 58-year-old female secretary is best explained by:
    A. Mitral valve disease, atrial fibrillation, and emboli to both brachial arteries.
    B. Bilateral thoracic outlet compression of the subclavian arteries.
    C. Temporal arteritis involving the axillosubclavian arteries.
    D. Takayasu arteritis with subclavian artery involvement.

28. The diagnosis of the case described above can be confirmed by:
    A. An erythrocyte sedimentation rate exceeding 60 mm/hour.
    B. The presence of a normochromic, normocytic anemia and reactive thrombocytosis.
    C. Temporal artery biopsy.
    D. Retrograde aortography delineating the arch and upper-extremity arterial system.

29. A popliteal aneurysm is found in a 25-year-old man. Which of the following diseases would *not* typically be associated with the lesion?
    A. Popliteal artery entrapment.
    B. Thromboangiitis obliterans.
    C. Behcet's disease.
    D. Relapsing polychondritis.

30. Occlusive lesions of the abdominal aorta and its branches, causing both claudication and hypertension in young adults, include all but which of the following:
    A. Radiation fibrosis.
    B. Neurofibromatosis.
    C. Tuberous sclerosis.
    D. Takayasu arteritis.

3

Answers

1. The answer is **C** (Rutherford, 4th ed., pp. 204–211).

Arterial blood flow is the primary determinant of arterial lumen diameter. During fetal circulation the vascular channels with high flow enlarge, whereas those with small amounts of blood flow atrophy and disappear. In adult life, arteries are also able to change lumen caliber depending on changes in blood flow. For example, arteries supplying an amputated limb will diminish in caliber, and arteries supplying an arteriovenous fistula will enlarge. The flow of blood produces a drag force (shear stress), which is sensed by endothelial cells. Increased shear stress results in endothelial production of EDRF (nitric oxide) with resultant artery dilatation. Wall shear stress is directly related to blood flow. There is no evidence that changes in blood flow result in endothelial damage, change in the number of medial elastic lamelle, smooth muscle cell proliferation, or subintimal lipid accumulation.

2. The answer is **D** (Rutherford, 4th ed., pp. 211–214).

The human carotid bifurcation is particularly prone to plaque formation on the outer wall of the first portion of the internal carotid artery (carotid sinus). This is an area of flow separation with low and oscillatory wall shear stress. Low and oscillatory wall shear stresses are also important in plaque localization in other areas of the arterial tree. High wall shear stress inhibits plaque formation. While evidence exists that endothelial *dysfunction* may be an important feature of plaque pathogenesis, there is no evidence that endothelial denudation or disruption is an important feature in plaque initiation. In late stages of plaque formation gaps in the endothelium may appear, but these are not of prime importance in plaque initiation or localization. High total cholesterol is a factor in plaque pathogenesis but not a significant factor in plaquc localization. Similarly, high blood pressure is a risk factor for atherosclerosis but not a significant factor for plaque localization.

3. The answer is **B** (Rutherford, 4th ed., pp. 211–213).

Several hemodynamic factors have been identified that favor plaque formation. These include low wall shear stress, flow separation and stasis, oscillation of shear stress direction, and an increase in particle residence time. Each of these hemodynamic features is found in the carotid bifurcation along the outer wall of the carotid sinus, which is uniquely prone to plaque formation. High wall shear stress has a protective effect in inhibiting plaque formation in experimental models. In humans, plaques typically do not form in high shear stress regions such as the inner wall of the carotid sinus. Experimental evidence has demonstrated an inverse correlation between plaque formation and the level of wall shear stress.

4. The answer is **B** (Rutherford, 4th ed., pp. 215–218).

Atherosclerotic plaques usually consist of intimal deposits of proliferated smooth muscle cells with increased intra- and extracellular lipid. The plaque frequently becomes fibrotic and calcified, and the necrotic core of the plaque is covered with a fibrous cap. The fibrous cap serves to separate the necrotic core, including cholesterol crystals, from the lumen. Erosion of the fibrous cap results in extrusion of plaque contents and embolization and may leave a raw surface prone to thrombosis. Thus fibrous cap erosion can result in embolization and/or thrombosis, which may produce clinical symptoms of atherosclerosis. Artery enlargement, a compensatory response of atherosclerotic arteries, tends to preserve normal lumen caliber. Calcification does not cause clinical symptoms.

5. The answer is **E** (Rutherford, 4th ed., pp. 204–207).

Intimal plaque formation involves monocyte adhesion to the endothelial surface, smooth muscle cell proliferation, and migration and lipid uptake by subendothelial macrophages. While the older literature suggests that endothelial denudation may occur spontaneously or in response to chemical or hemodynamic stimuli and that such denudation may predispose to platelet deposition and plaque formation, no evidence has been provided to support this mechanism in vivo. The endothelium is intact in areas where lesions form. Endothelial *dysfunction* with demonstrable biologic and biochemical abnormalities may exist in areas of lesion formation, but this is not associated with frank denudation.

6. The answer is **C** (Rutherford, 4th ed., pp. 217–218).

A number of factors have been identified as being important in aneurysm formation, including a genetic predisposition. The action of proteolytic enzymes on both collagen and elastin is to break down the medial elastic lamellar architecture. Thinning of the media and loss of elastin are the most prominent histologic features of aneurysms. There is no increase in elastin content. There is a close association between atherosclerosis and aneurysm formation, and atherosclerotic plaques result in artery enlargement and thinning of the media. Both of these features of atherosclerotic artery wall degeneration are felt to predispose to aneurysm formation. Artery enlargement in atherosclerosis may predispose to subsequent aneurysm formation if plaque regression and degeneration occur.

7. The answer is **false** (Rutherford, 4th ed., pp. 223, 226–231).

Total serum cholesterol is a primary risk factor for atherosclerosis. This cholesterol is transported in lipoproteins. When individual lipoprotein fractions are analyzed, the low-density portion, or LDL, is directly related to incidence of atherosclerosis. The high-density lipoprotein, or HDL, on the other hand, appears to mobilize cholesterol from tissue pools and is inversely related to the development of arterial disease. Any maneuver to *elevate* the serum cholesterol in the HDL fraction is, therefore, desirable for prevention of atherosclerotic vascular disease.

8. The answers are **B, C** (Rutherford, 4th ed., pp. 226–231).

Drugs that interfere with cholesterol absorption (cholestyramine, a bile acid-binding resin) or those that block cholesterol synthesis (Lovastatin, an HMG-CoA reductase inhibitor) are successful in lowering LDL levels. Dipyridamole, Sulfinpyrazone, and Ticlopidine are agents that influence platelet function.

9. The answer is **C** (Rutherford, 4th ed., pp. 223–224, 232).

Although it may not be an *independent* initiating factor in atherogenesis, cigarette smoking is the greatest risk factor for the development of peripheral arterial occlusive disease. The progression of atherosclerosis from claudication to a stage requiring amputation will occur in a predictable rate in patients who continue to smoke. It is almost nonexistent in claudicants who stop smoking.

10. The answers are **A, B, D, F** (Rutherford, 4th ed., pp. 237–238).

The premature onset of arterial occlusion, severe ischemia of the lower extremity, systemic manifestations (upper limb involvement or phlebitis migrans), and the absence of atherogenic risk factors other than smoking are characteristic of Buerger's disease. The disease is self-limiting if patients discontinue tobacco use.

11. The answers are **A, C** (Rutherford, 4th ed., p. 243).

Sympathectomy produces cutaneous vasodilatation, prevents vasoconstruction, and is of value in patients with Buerger's disease. Sympathectomy remains a therapeutic modality for treatment of Buerger's disease because arterial reconstruction is not often feasible. Because circulation in muscle is not significantly improved by sympathectomy, this technique is not indicated for intermittent claudication.

12. The answers are **A, C, D** (Rutherford, 4th ed., pp. 246–247).

Arteriography remains the best modality to diagnose Takayasu's disease. The clinical features of the disease vary and are usually nonspecific. There are no laboratory tests specific for Takayasu's arteritis. The diagnosis is made by an arteriogram showing diffuse narrowing of major arteries, including the subclavian, descending aorta, carotid, renal, and mesenteric arteries. Active arteritis is diagnosed by serial angiograms showing new lesions developing in different areas of the arterial system (in addition to elevated erythrocyte sedimentation rates). An increase in stenosis in an artery with previously documented disease is not diagnostic of an active vasculitis because this may be due to scarring as the disease becomes more chronic (so-called "burned-out" disease).

13. The answers are **A, C, D** (Rutherford, 4th ed., pp. 245–248).

The subclavian artery is the vessel most commonly involved with Takayasu's disease. It is unusual for the disease to affect only the orifice of the subclavian; generally it involves a long segment of both the subclavian and axillary arteries. Because the disease affects the segment of the subclavian artery proximal and distal to the vertebral artery, subclavian steal syndrome is rare. The long involvement of the subclavian and axillary arteries accounts for the significant upper arm ischemia that these patients experience. Since both subclavian arteries are frequently involved, hypertension is difficult to diagnose. This has a profound effect on both the morbidity and mortality of patients with Takayasu's disease. At the time of arteriography central arterial pressures should be obtained in the aorta to determine accurate blood pressure. If the patient is significantly hypertensive, some authors have recommended subclavian artery bypass to follow and treat hypertension effectively.

14. The answers are **A, B** (Rutherford, 4th ed., p. 248).

Proximal and distal anastomoses should always be performed in arterial segments that appear normal on arteriogram. However, it should be noted that microscopic involvement at these sites has been documented, which may cause anastomotic stenoses at a later date. To minimize potential anastomotic problems later, bypasses preferably should be done in arterial segments that statistically have a low incidence of involvement. Therefore, it would be inappropriate to bypass a subclavian arterial stenosis with the proximal anastomosis originating from the common carotid since the common carotid artery is a frequently involved vessel. It is more appropriate to originate these bypasses from the ascending aorta, which has a low incidence of involvement. Endarterectomy is not recommended because the involvement of all three layers of the artery makes this technically difficult.

15. The answer is **A** (Rutherford, 4th ed., pp. 248–249).

The intima of an involved carotid artery is usually smooth and does not frequently give rise to peripheral emboli. Because the innominate, both carotid, and both subclavian arteries can all be involved concurrently, it is postulated that the occlusion of one of these arteries may precipitate a stroke. In the 1991 report from the George Washington University Medical Center, *all* patients who presented with a stroke had occlusion of one or more major arteries. It is postulated then that occlusion of cerebral arteries is the cause of stroke.

16. The answer is **C** (Rutherford, 4th ed., pp. 253–259).

The traditionally accepted role of atherosclerosis in the etiology of aneurysms has been a topic of much controversy over the past two decades. Although atherosclerotic plaque is frequently found in the walls of aneurysms, it may represent a sequelae of boundary layer separation and subintimal hyperplasia caused by abnormal hemodynamics found in aneurysmally dilated arteries. The genetic predisposition of aneurysmal disease has been well documented by numerous authors subsequent to Clifton's first report in 1977 of three brothers who had suffered abdominal aortic aneurysmal (AAA) rupture in the seventh decade of life. In 1986, Johansen and Koepsell found a sixfold increase in the risk-odds ratio of an AAA in first- degree relatives of probands. In addition, a plethora of clinical and biochemical differences have been defined between "dilating" aneurysmal disease and "constricting" atherosclerotic disease, including a significantly greater male/female ratio and average age of patients with AAA and altered biochemical profile associated with increased proteolytic activity in AAA tissues.

17. The answer is **D** (Rutherford, 4th ed., pp. 255, 259–260).

The major constituents of arterial wall matrix include collagen, elastin, microfibrils, and proteoglycans. Collagen imparts tensile strength to the vessel, with elastin conferring the elasticity required for normal vessel recoil. The microfibrils are thought to act as a scaffolding upon which collagen and elastin molecules are deposited and undergo crosslinking. Although proteoglycans are felt to "stabilize" matrix, their exact mechanisms of action have yet to be elucidated. The depletion of elastin in AAA is generally well accepted. However, collagen content in AAA has been variably measured in increased, decreased, and unchanged amounts by different investigators. These findings may in part be explained by the ability of adult tissue to synthesize collagen without having a comparable mechanism for elastin replacement.

18. The answer is **A** (Rutherford, 4th ed., p. 260).

Histologic examination of AAA tissue by Beckman in 1986 revealed significant infiltration of inflammatory cells in the adventitia of over two thirds of the specimens. In addition to confirming these results, studies in both Koch's and Tilson's laboratories have identified, using immunohistochemical and fluorescence-activated cell-sorting techniques, significant numbers of macrophages and T-cells. These inflammatory cells are capable of producing the battery of proteolytic activities observed in the tissues of aneurysms.

19. The answer is **C** (Rutherford, 4th ed., pp. 261–262).

Notwithstanding the architectural disruption of the various constituents of "true" aneurysm wall, there is preservation of the three components of normal arterial wall, which include the intima, media, and adventitia. Conversely, the wall of false or pseudoaneurysms is generally formed only by organized periadventitial tissue. Traumatic and anastomotic aneurysms are both examples of pseudoaneurysm. Traumatic aneurysms, the most common form of pseudoaneurysm, develop secondary to arterial punctures, which may be iatrogenic or secondary to blunt or penetrating trauma. Anastomotic aneurysms result from separation of the graft from the native artery. Pathogenetic factors known to be associated with these aneurysms include the use of silk sutures, suture line infection, inadequate suture purchase, and progression of atherosclerotic degeneration.

20. The answer is **A** (Rutherfad, 4th ed., pp. 264–276).

Medial fibroplasia is the most frequent type of renal artery fibrodysplastic process, comprising 85% of the cases. More than 90% of patients are women; this lesion, like all other forms of dysplasia, is very uncommon among black patients. The morphologic appearance ranges from a solitary focal stenosis to a series of stenoses with intervening mural aneurysms. *Medial fibroplasia* most often affects the distal main renal artery with extension into first-order segmental branches in 25% of cases. *Medial fibroplasia* is bilateral in 55% of cases, and if unilateral, affects the right side far more often than the left side. *Medial hyperplasia* is a very uncommon entity, accounting for less than 1% of dysplastic renovascular disease. Some investigators have even questioned its existence as a separate type. *Perimedial dysplasia*, accounting for 10% of renal artery dysplastic disease, involves excessive accumulation of elastic tissue at the junction of the media and adventitia. These lesions present as either focal stenoses or multiple constrictions involving the midportion of the main renal artery *without* intervening mural aneurysms. *Intimal fibroplasia* accounts for 5% of dysplastic lesions and occurs with no sex predilection in younger patients.

21. The answer is **C** (Rutherfard, 4th ed., pp. 276–281).

Arterial fibrodysplasia of the extracranial and intracranial cerebral vasculature is a well-recognized disease entity. It most commonly occurs as medial fibroplasia of the extracranial internal carotid artery, involving the 2- to 6-cm segment of the carotid artery adjacent to the second and third cervical vertebrae. Multiple stenoses with intervening mural aneurysms are characteristic. Bilateral disease occurs in 65% of the cases. Similar disease of the proximal internal carotid artery at its origin has not been described. Typical medial fibroplastic lesions of the intracranial arteries have been described but are extremely rare, and involvement of the external carotid artery and its branches has been reported, but it is also quite rare. Intimal fibroplasia, a secondary process in most cases, presents as smooth focal or long tubular narrowings or isolated webs affecting the proximal internal carotid artery, whereas perimedial dysplasia and medial hyperplasia of the carotid artery have not been described.

22. The answer is **B** (Rutherford, 4th ed., pp. 279–281).

Coexistent intracranial aneurysms with extracranial carotid fibrodysplasia have been documented in 12 to 25% of patients. A tendency for these aneurysms to develop on the same side as the extracranial disease has been reported. However, they do not necessarily develop in the involved vessel affected by the fibroplasia. They may evolve as part of a generalized dysplastic arteriopathy, manifested by vessel wall weakening at arterial branchings. The distribution of these berry aneurysms among patients with medial fibroplasia is the same as that in patients without extracranial carotid fibrodysplasia. Hypertension may contribute to these aneurysms but has not been identified as a major etiologic factor in their genesis.

23. The answer is **C** (Rutherford, 4th ed., pp. 281–283).

Medial fibroplasia of the external iliac artery typically presents with serial stenoses with intervening mural aneurysms in the proximal third of the vessel. The microscopic appearance is one of a medial fibroproliferative response alternating with areas of medial thinning. These lesions are identical to those of the renal artery and affect 1 to 6% of patients with renal artery fibrodysplasia. Most patients are women in their fifth or sixth decades of life. Hormonal influences are likely important in the pathogenesis of this lesion in addition to insufficient vasa vasorum and consequent mural ischemia.

24. The answer is **A** (Rutherford 4th ed., pp. 285–291).

All forms of arterial injury induce a reparative response that includes endothelial regeneration and smooth muscle cell migration and proliferation. If the injury is extensive, endothelial repair will be limited to 1–2 cm from the injury boundary. On the other hand, smooth muscle cell proliferation and accumulation will occur all along the zone of injury. Hence, smooth muscle mass will increase in injured arteries, whereas the number of endothelial cells will ultimately be the same or diminished compared to the uninjured vessel, depending upon the extent of injury.

25. The answer is **B** (Rutherford, 4th ed., pp. 286–287).

Vascular grafts are susceptible to thrombosis at all times after surgery, but the underlying mechanism appears to vary, depending upon the time interval. Thrombosis early after surgery is usually related to a technical complication such as a twist in the graft, an improperly sewn anastomosis, intimal flap, uncut valve leaflet, and poor outflow. Late failures are most often related to progression of atherosclerosis either proximal or distal to the graft in the native artery or in the graft itself. Intimal hyperplasia appears relatively early and is a significant cause of stenosis and thrombosis during the period 1–24 months.

26. The answer is **B** (Rutherford, 4th ed., pp. 288–291).

During the last decade considerable progress has been made in developing an understanding of specific mechanisms of wound healing in injured arteries. Although PDGF was first described as a growth factor for cultured smooth muscle cells, it possesses a number of other properties. Recent investigation has demonstrated that platelets and platelet factors (especially PDGF) have more to do with the migration of smooth muscle cells from the media to the intima than with smooth muscle proliferation. On the other hand, basic fibroblast growth factor (bFGF) is likely to be the major stimulant of smooth muscle cell proliferation immediately after injury.

27. The answer is **C** (Rutherford, 4th ed., pp. 296–297).

Simultaneous embolism to both arms is rare and would present as an acute rather than insidious event. Subclavian artery compression at the thoracic outlet usually produces aneurysm, and arm effort fatigue follows acute embolism to major and/or digital arteries. Stenosis is a less common occurrence. It would be uncommon for either stenotic or aneurysmal disease caused by outlet compression to produce synchronous symptoms bilaterally. The development of symptomatic occlusive disease simultaneously in paired proximal arteries of the upper and/or lower extremities over a few months is characteristic of extracranial temporal arteritis. This can also occur in Takayasu arteritis but is more often asymmetric and occurs in much younger patients.

28. The answers are **C, D** (Rutherfad, 4th ed., pp. 297–299).

An elevated sedimentation rate is seen in almost all cases of active temporal arteritis but may be normal if anti-inflammatory agents are being used by the patient. The sedimentation rate is supportive of the diagnosis but nonspecific. Normochromic, normocytic anemia and reactive thrombocytosis are common to many forms of vasculitis and infection, and although common in temporal arteritis, it is not diagnostic. Typical bilateral tapering stenosis with poststenotic dilations of the axillosubclavian system are characteristic of temporal arteritis. The lesions are often less typical in the femoropopliteal system and may be confused with atherosclerosis. Takayasu arteritis may have identical radiologic appearance, although stenosis of the subclavian arteries at their origins is far more common. Involvement of the aorta, common carotids, and other arteries and the patient's age define Takayasu arteritis. A temporal artery biopsy with characteristic histology defines temporal arteritis. On rare occasion the temporal artery is involved in Takayasu arteritis, and the histology is identical to temporal arteritis; age and angiographic features diffientiate the two syndromes.

29. The answer is **D** (Rutherford, 4th ed., pp. 300–301).

Poststenotic dilation and frank aneurysm formation are present in about a quarter of patients with popliteal artery entrapment. This disorder may be diagnosed clinically or found incidentally by arteriography. Aneurysms of the popliteal artery occur occasionally in thromboangiitis obliterans and may present with acute occlusion. The diagnosis of Buerger's disease is suggested by antecedent distal disease of both limbs and/or the upper extremity, a history of tobacco use, and the patient's age. Aneurysm formation, arterial thrombosis, and deep or superficial phlebitis are random, ubiquitous events in up to 25% of patients with Behcet's disease. Aneurysmal or thrombotic disease of the femoropopliteal system is well described. Two or more of the cardinal symptoms, which consist of aphthous ulcers of the mouth or genitals, uveitis, or meningoencephalitis, identify the syndrome. Relapsing polychondritis is manifest chiefly by inflammation and destruction of cartilage in the nose, ears, or tracheobronchial system. Aneurysm formation occurs in 10% of patients but is confined to the thoracic aorta.

30. The answer is **C** (Rutherford, 4th ed., pp. 296–299, 304–305, 307).

High-dose radiation therapy given in childhood for retroperitoneal tumors can cause aortic and renal artery fibrosis of enough magnitude to produce both claudication and renovascular hypertension (Fig. 16–9, p. 306). There is an increasing appreciation of arterial involvement by neurofibromatosis, and the most commonly observed lesion is tubular coarctation of the abdominal aorta and stenosis of the renal artery orifices. Pararenal coarctation of the abdominal aorta, with or without proximal renal artery stenosis, is a common manifestation of Takayasu arteritis. Hypertension is seen in tuberous sclerosis and is caused by replacement of the renal parenchyma by hamartomas. However, while aneurysmal disease is occasionally associated with this syndrome, occlusive lesions causing claudication have not been described.

4

Fundamental Therapeutic and Technical Considerations

1. The endothelium synthesizes which of the following?
   A. PGI_2.
   B. Thrombomodulin.
   C. Von Willebrand factor.
   D. Factor V.
   E. All of the above.

2. Which of the following is a complication of warfarin therapy?
   A. Osteoporosis.
   B. Dermal gangrene.
   C. Allergic reaction.
   D. Pulmonary insufficiency.
   E. None of the above.

3. When the heparin-induced thrombocytopenia syndrome is suspected in a patient receiving heparin, which of the following should be the next clinical step?
   A. Discontinue the current heparin therapy and restart the heparin infusion at a lower dose.
   B. Discontinue all heparin exposure, including intravenous and subcutaneous doses, and heparin-coated catheters.
   C. Switch from beef to porcine heparin.
   D. Platelet transfusion.
   E. Inhibit platelet function with aspirin.

4. Which of the following factors is important in determining blood viscosity?
   A. Fibrinogen level.
   B. Hematocrit.
   C. Platelet aggregation.
   D. Leukocyte aggregation.
   E. All of the above.

5. Which of the following factors have been reported in patients with symptomatic peripheral arterial disease?
   A. Elevated fibrinogen.
   B. Elevated hematocrit.
   C. Elevated leukocyte count.
   D. Increased platelet activation.
   E. All of the above.

6. Which of the following statements is true regarding the effects of pentoxifylline in patients with intermittent claudication?
   A. Pentoxifylline treatment results in improvement in walking distance reported by a majority of patients with intermittent claudication.
   B. Pentoxifylline treatment results in increased ankle brachial pressure ratio in the affected extremities of patients with intermittent claudication.
   C. Pentoxifylline treatment results in increased lower extremity blood flow in patients with intermittent claudication.
   D. Pentoxifylline treatment produces statistically significant improvement in treadmill walking distance in treated patients compared to placebo-treated controls.
   E. Pentoxifylline treatment results in discontinuance of medication in about 15% of patients due to intolerable side effects.

7. Which of the following statements about lower-extremity ischemic rest pain and ischemic ulcers is true?
   A. The presence of chronic ischemic rest pain and ischemic ulcers means that limb loss is inevitable without revascularization.
   B. Chronic ischemic rest pain and ischemic ulcers nearly always result in limb loss without revascularization, but a small percentage of patients (1–5%) may improve spontaneously without specific treatment.
   C. Most patients with chronic ischemic rest pain and ischemic ulcers improve spontaneously with nonspecific measures. Need for amputation is rare.
   D. Approximately one third (25–40%) of patients with chronic ischemic rest pain and ischemic ulcers improve spontaneously without specific therapy. The remaining two thirds will ultimately require amputation unless revascularization is achieved.
   E. Drug treatment with multiple prostaglandin analogs has been shown to result in improved rates of resolution of chronic ischemic rest pain and healing of ischemic ulcers when compared to placebo treatments.

8. Inhibitors of fibrinolysis are:
   A. Proteins that exhibit antiactivator activity.
   B. Proteins that exhibit antiplasmin activity.
   C. Molecules that block the binding of plasmin to fibrin.
   D. Sometimes secreted by human fibroblasts.
   E. All of the above.

9. The following statement is true regarding urokinase:
   - **A.** Neutralizing antibodies are present that block the activation of plasminogen by urokinase.
   - **B.** Urokinase combines with plasminogen to form an activator complex.
   - **C.** Urokinase contains lysine binding sites, which explains its affinity for fibrin.
   - **D.** Urokinase is a direct plasminogen activator with a half-life of 14 minutes.
   - **E.** Urokinase is a naturally occurring plasminogen activator.

10. Treatment of a patient undergoing regional fibrinolytic therapy who has a significant hemorrhagic complication should consist of:
    - **A.** ε-aminocaproic acid.
    - **B.** Discontinuation of the drug.
    - **C.** Administration of fresh-frozen plasma or cryoprecipitate.
    - **D.** Tranexamic acid.
    - **E.** All of the above.

11. Pulmonary emboli during intra-arterial or intravenous fibrinolytic therapy:
    - **A.** Occur more often with lytic therapy than with heparin therapy.
    - **B.** Should lead to cessation of lytic therapy in all cases.
    - **C.** Occur in up to 30% of the cases, but has been found to be of little clinical consequence.
    - **D.** Are an indication for placement of a vena cava filter.
    - **E.** None of the above.

12. Tissue plasminogen activator (t-PA):
    - **A.** Is a direct plasminogen activator working through the process of exogenous fibrinolysis.
    - **B.** Has a half-life of 26 minutes.
    - **C.** May bind and be activated on platelet surfaces.
    - **D.** Has been shown to have decreased bleeding complications compared to urokinase and streptokinase.
    - **E.** Will achieve in vitro lysis of fibrin directly through release of d-disulfide covalent bond.

13. Percutaneous transluminal angioplasty is more successful when lesions are:
    - **A.** Short length instead of long.
    - **B.** Ostial instead of distal.
    - **C.** Eccentric instead of concentric.
    - **D.** Single instead of multiple.
    - **E.** Stenoses rather than occlusions.

14. The potential benefits of atherectomy over percutaneous transluminal angioplasty (PTA) include:
    - **A.** Improved technical success of recanalization in cases of occlusion.
    - **B.** Smoother posttreatment lumen.
    - **C.** Minimal injury to the media.
    - **D.** Effective debulking.
    - **E.** Long-term results that have proved to be superior to angioplasty alone.

15. The only stent approved by the FDA for intravascular use is:
    - **A.** Wallstent.
    - **B.** Palmaz Expandable Stent.
    - **C.** Strecker Stent.
    - **D.** Gianturco Z Stent.
    - **E.** Nitinol Spring Coil Stent.

16. Stents have proved to be an important adjunct in management in all the following circumstances *except:*
    - **A.** Malignant SVC syndrome.
    - **B.** Angioplasty-induced dissections of iliac arteries.
    - **C.** Improved long-term patency in superficial femoral artery lesions.
    - **D.** Eccentric lesions of iliac arteries postangioplasty.
    - **E.** Chronic iliac artery occlusions.

17. End-to-end anastomosis:
    - **A.** Was the first anastomotic technique employed clinically.
    - **B.** Is the most common technique used in arterial bypass surgery.
    - **C.** Is the most common technique used in arterial reconstruction for aneurysmal disease.
    - **D.** Can produce anastomotic narrowing if performed with continuous suture.
    - **E.** Should not be used for repair of small-caliber vessels.

18. End-to-side anastomosis:
    - **A.** Is ideal for interposition grafts.
    - **B.** Should enter at 30–45°.
    - **C.** Should equal the diameter of the recipient vessel.
    - **D.** Should be started at the most inaccessible point in its circumference.
    - **E.** Is not used in thoracoabdominal aneurysm repair.

19. For suturing vessels and performing anastomoses:
    - **A.** Silk sutures should not be used.
    - **B.** Monofilament sutures tend to break, so braided sutures should be used in prosthetic anastomoses.
    - **C.** Only interrupted sutures must be used in children to allow anastomotic growth.
    - **D.** The depth and separation (travel) of continuous suture placement should generally be equal in dimension.
    - **E.** The needle should travel "outside in on the artery, inside out on the graft" when anastomosing prostheses to arteriosclerotic arteries.

20. Successful microsurgical anastomosis for free tissue transfer in the lower extremity:
    A. Requires interposition vein grafting.
    B. Should be accomplished at a distance from side branches.
    C. Is best performed at a site of flexible normal vessel outside an area of disease or injury.
    D. May be completed by a synthetic bypass graft.
    E. All of the above.

21. Reduced risk of arterial thrombosis and increased venous patency of a microsurgical anastomosis may be achieved by:
    A. Vasodilators.
    B. Dextran infusion.
    C. Aspirin.
    D. Heparinization.
    E. None of the above.

22. Nonhealing, neurotrophic ulcers and associated osteomyelitis in the feet of dysvascular, diabetic patients:
    A. Are nonsalvageable despite the ability to bypass inframalleolar occlusive disease.
    B. Inevitably progress to amputation if complicated by extensive tissue loss and gangrene.
    C. Demonstrate small vessel occlusive disease, which precludes preservation.
    D. Treated with prior distal revascularization and subsequent microvascular free tissue transfer may result in as high as a 90% salvage rate.
    E. Progresses to amputation in 20 to 40% of cases following inframalleolar bypass.
    F. Can sustain ambulation by debridement and placement of grafts or local pedicle skin flaps.

23. Microsurgical free tissue transfer can be performed:
    A. On atherosclerotic vessels.
    B. In patients with diabetes who have calcified vessels.
    C. As a simultaneous procedure with revascularization (bypass).
    D. To an in situ saphenous vein bypass greater than 40 cm in length.
    E. All of the above.

24. Which of the following statements is/are true regarding combined distal revascularization and microsurgical free tissue transfer for limb salvage in peripheral arterial occlusive disease?
    A. Salvage is contingent only upon adequate arterial inflow.
    B. Postoperative arteriograms remain unchanged.
    C. A perfusion gradient between the transferred flap and the wound margins promotes neovascularization.
    D. Indirect revascularization results in healing ischemic ulcers but no relief of rest pain or claudication.
    E. Failure results in a higher level of amputation.

25. Which of the following is *not* an appropriate application for the Fogarty embolectomy catheter?
    A. Temporary vessel occlusion.
    B. Calibration of vessel lumen diameter.
    C. Dilatation of atherosclerotic lesion.
    D. Thrombectomy of AV fistula.
    E. Embolectomy of a femoral artery.

26. Which of the following is true regarding the Fogarty catheter embolectomy technique?
    A. The Fogarty embolectomy catheter is well suited for thrombectomy of the venous system.
    B. Wetting the tip of the syringe is useful when using the 2F embolectomy catheter.
    C. Administration of heparin solution is contraindicated due to bleeding complications at the groin incision.
    D. A 5-cc syringe is well suited for inflating the 3F embolectomy balloon.
    E. The balloon should be approximately 1.5 times the vessel diameter.

27. Which of the following is *not* an appropriate method for evaluating distal patency of the arterial tree following embolectomy?
    A. Presence of vigorous back bleeding.
    B. Arteriography.
    C. Use of a pulse amplitude monitor.
    D. Angioscopy.
    E. All of the above.

28. Which of the following patterns of arterial disease are ideally suited to the application of endarterectomy techniques?
    A. Orificial occlusive disease of the innominate artery with symptoms of distal embolization.
    B. Combined visceral and renal artery occlusive disease with severe "coral-reef" atherosclerosis of the aorta.
    C. Bilateral high-grade orificial renal artery stenoses in the presence of a large infrarenal aortic aneurysm.
    D. A 30-cm occlusion of the superficial femoral artery located just above the adductor hiatus.
    E. All of the above.

29. Which of the following is/are true regarding the biologic characteristics of atherosclerosis and the technique of endarterectomy?
    A. Because atherosclerosis is a systemic, diffuse disease, endarterectomy is unsuitable for disobliteration of localized segments of occlusive disease.
    B. Except for the carotid bifurcation, recurrent atherosclerotic disease occurs with such high frequency following endarterectomy that bypass grafting has proved to be much more durable.
    C. Atherosclerosis affects the intima and inner media of the arterial wall without affecting the structural integrity of the outer media and adventitia.

D. There is usually poor adherence between the diseased (intima and inner media) and undiseased (outer media and adventitia) layers of the arterial wall, allowing a cleavage plane to be readily established.
E. All of the above.

30. Appropriate concerns regarding the application of endarterectomy to aortic branch (visceral and renal artery) occlusive disease include:
A. Aneurysmal degeneration of the pararenal aorta is a contraindication to endarterectomy of this segment.
B. Symptomatic visceral artery occlusive disease typically involves more than one vessel, such that endarterectomy can rarely be performed within the tolerable ischemic time of the tissues involved.
C. Endarterectomy has been proved to be less durable than direct bypass grafting operations for these vessels.
D. Visceral and renal artery occlusive disease is typically too diffuse, such that satisfactory distal endpoints cannot be readily obtained during endarterectomy.
E. All of the above.

31. The likelihood of significant coronary artery disease in vascular surgery patients is related to the extent of peripheral vascular occlusive disease present. **True** or **false?**

32. Patients undergoing vascular reconstruction have the same risk of postoperative myocardial infarction as those undergoing nonvascular, noncardiac surgical procedures. **True** or **false?**

33. Due to the magnitude of the operation, a patient undergoing aortic reconstruction is at substantially higher risk of an adverse cardiac event than a patient undergoing infrainguinal reconstruction. **True** or **false?**

34. In the last two decades numerous studies have attempted to identify clinical risk factors most predictive of perioperative cardiac risk. The Goldman Cardiac Risk Index (CRI) is among those most frequently employed. Which of the variables listed are included in the Goldman CRI?
A. Recent myocardial infarction.
B. Congestive heart failure.
C. Age >70 years.
D. Angina pectoris.
E. Diabetes mellitus.

35. Holter monitoring has traditionally been employed to evaluate cardiac dysrhythmia, but recent studies indicate that it is a useful method to assess perioperative cardiac risk in patients undergoing noncardiac surgical procedures. Advantages of ambulatory ECG monitoring over other noninvasive methods include:
A. Wider availability.
B. Unaffected by underlying rhythm disturbances.
C. Relative lower cost.
D. Ability to differentiate ST segment changes secondary to ischemia from alternate causes such as left ventricular hypertrophy.
E. ST segment depression often followed by symptomatic chest pain.

36. Stress thallium imaging, performed under conditions of near-maximal coronary blood flow (exercise or injection of dipyridamole—Persantine®) is a noninvasive method that can detect heterogenous myocardial perfusion due to stenoses as small as 50%. The test is based on:
A. The ability of thallium to be taken up by viable myocytes.
B. The ability of thallium to enter nonviable myocytes.
C. The ability of dipyridamole to increase coronary flow and in effect produce a steal phenomenon, unmasking stenotic coronary vessels.
D. The ability of dipyridamole to dilate stenotic coronary arteries to allow uptake of thallium in viable myocardium not previously visualized.
E. The ability of dipyridamole to stimulate prostacyclin synthesis and promote increased thallium uptake.

37. The use of dipyridamole thallium scintigraphy (DTS) to assess perioperative cardiac risk appears most effective when applied selectively. Eagle has suggested that patients with ≤2 clinical markers benefit from DTS, whereas those with either 0 or ≥3 markers do not. Eagle clinical markers include:
A. Age >70 years.
B. Q waves on resting ECG.
C. Diabetes mellitus.
D. Angina pectoris.
E. Arrythmia requiring treatment.

38. Which of the following are current indications for homologous blood transfusions?
A. Hemoglobin of 10 g.
B. Cardiovascular instability following blood loss.
C. To enhance delivery of oxygen at tissue level in bleeding patients.
D. To prevent wound infection.
E. Acute blood loss of greater than 600 ml.

39. Current, practical alternatives to homologous blood transfusion include:
    A. Acute isovolemic hemodilution.
    B. Intraoperative autotransfusion.
    C. Artificial blood.
    D. Preoperative donation of autologous blood.
    E. Promotion of hemostasis.

40. Advantages of autotransfused blood are:
    A. Net blood loss is reduced.
    B. There is no autoimmunization.
    C. Blood quality is equal or superior to bank blood.
    D. It never contributes to a coagulopathy.
    E. It can be used with impunity in patients with sickle-cell disease.

41. Autologous predonated blood should *not* routinely be transfused without indication because of:
    A. High risk of viral transmission.
    B. Danger of bacterial growth and endotoxin production during storage.
    C. Clerical errors do occur.
    D. Acute, intravascular hemolysis has been reported.
    E. Yersinia enterocolitica.

42. Which of the following statements is/are true concerning angioscopic evaluation of in situ saphenous vein grafts?
    A. The sensitivity to detect residual valve cusps is considerably higher than arteriography.
    B. Angioscopy causes intimal injury that correlates with reduced graft patency.
    C. Most surgeons using angioscopy have found residual valve cusps in at least 10% of grafts.
    D. One liter of saline irrigation is usually required for adequate irrigation, which limits the application in some patients.
    E. Correction of all graft defects identified by angiography increases early graft patency.

43. Intraoperative evaluation after carotid endarterectomy has revealed that:
    A. Five to 10% of endarterectomies have residual technical defects that warrant surgical re-exploration.
    B. Continuous-wave Doppler evaluation is as sensitive and as specific as other modalities of intraoperative evaluation.
    C. Pulsed Doppler spectral analysis provides anatomic confirmation of suspected endarterectomy defects.
    D. B-mode ultrasound detects many minor intimal defects that do not require correction.
    E. Duplex ultrasound identifies endarterectomy defects, but their size does *not* correlate with subsequent restenosis.

44. Which of the following statements are true concerning intraoperative evaluation of technical adequacy?
    A. Mesenteric and renal reconstructions are best evaluated by intraoperative arteriography.
    B. Intraoperative evaluation of balloon catheter embolectomy/thrombectomy is unnecessary if good back bleeding is obtained and distal pulses are restored.
    C. Continuous-wave Doppler pencil probes are best used as screening devices to guide the selective use of more sophisticated imaging techniques.
    D. Duplex scanning has not been sufficiently accurate to evaluate renal reconstruction intraoperatively.
    E. Angioscopy has been successfully used to evaluate grafts, endarterectomy segments, and thrombectomy sites in both the lower extremity and iliac arteries.

45. During routine follow-up, duplex ultrasound shows a femorodistal in situ graft to have narrowing at the distal anastomosis. The velocity at the anastomosis is 240 cm/s compared to 85 cm/s in the body of the graft 2 cm proximal to the anastomosis. The resting ABI is 0.90, which is unchanged from the improvement measured soon after bypass and well above the prebypass ABI of 0.50. Percutaneous transluminal angioplasty is attempted in order to dilate the stricture. The patency classification of this bypass graft is:
    A. Primary patency.
    B. Assisted primary patency.
    C. Secondary patency.
    D. Failure.
    E. B and C.
    F. A and B.

46. Refer to the case presentation in question 45. The PTA procedure performed at the distal anastomosis did not substantially relieve the stricture. Duplex measures of velocity remain 200 cm/s at the anastomosis compared to 95 cm/s proximal to the anastomosis. The resting ABI is 0.85. The decision is made to revise the distal anastomosis. Following revision the patency classification of the graft is:
    A. Primary patency.
    B. Assisted primary patency.
    C. Secondary patency.
    D. Failure.
    E. B and C.
    F. A and B.

47. In this same patient, after revision of the distal anastomosis the graft thromboses. Lytic therapy is performed with resultant opening of the graft. The patency classification for this graft is:
    A. Primary patency.
    B. Assisted primary patency.

C. Secondary patency.
D. Failure.
E. B and C.
F. A and B.

48. Although the ABI in this patient is again 0.90, improved from 0.60 prior to lytic therapy, a kink in the proximal anastomosis was determined to be the reason for graft failure. Elective revision of the proximal anastomosis is performed. The patency classification of this graft is now:

A. Primary patency.
B. Assisted primary patency.
C. Secondary patency.
D. Failure.
E. B and C.
F. A and B.

49. The patient has been placed in a skilled nursing facility because of a stroke, but as part of ongoing QA, a report is obtained which states that the patient is asymptomatic, although his ABI is 0.65. The patency classification for this graft is:

A. Primary patency.
B. Assisted primary patency.
C. Secondary patency.
D. Failure.
E. B and C.
F. A and B.

4

Answers

1. The answer is **E** (Rutherford, 4th ed., pp. 311–312).

The endothelium contributes to the procoagulant and anticoagulant properties of blood. Prostacyclin (PGI_2) is a vasodilator and an inhibitor of platelet aggregation. Thrombomodulin is an endothelial cell membrane receptor for thrombin. Von Willebrand's factor, produced and stored in the endothelium, is necessary for platelet binding to the subendothelial matrix. Factor V promotes the formation of the prothrombinase complex leading to the production of thrombin. Endothelial-derived relaxing factor, antithrombin III, heparan sulfate, protein S, urokinase, tissue plasminogen activator, plasminogen activator inhibitor-1, and thromboplastin are also produced by the endothelial cell.

2. The answer is **B** (Rutherford 4th ed., pp. 316–317).

Dermal gangrene of the breast, thigh, or buttocks is a rare complication of warfarin therapy. It is related to the hypercoagulable state caused by the warfarin-induced decrease in protein C. Protein C is an inhibitor of activated factors V and VIII and potentiates fibrinolytic activity. Other complications of warfarin therapy include bleeding, dermatitis, alopecia, fever, nausea, diarrhea, and hypersensitivity reactions. Osteoporosis is a complication of long-term heparin therapy that occurs in less than 1% of patients. Heparin therapy is associated with other complications, which include bleeding (10–20%), heparin-induced thrombocytopenia syndrome (4–5%), sensitivity reactions (2–5%), and alopecia (less than 1%). Dextran is associated with allergic reactions in approximately 1% of patients and anaphylactic responses in less than 0.1% of patients. The allergic/anaphylactic reactions can be prevented by the preinfusion with short-chain dextrans. Other complications of dextran therapy include hemorrhage, volume overload, and pulmonary insufficiency.

3. The answer is **B** (Rutherford, 4th ed., pp. 314–316).

Four to 5% of patients receiving heparin develop heparin-associated antiplatelet antibodies. The development of the heparin-induced thrombocytopenia syndrome is independent of the type, dose, or route (including heparin-coated catheters) of heparin administration. The heparin-induced thrombocytopenia syndrome should be suspected in patients that are receiving any form of heparin who have a platelet count of less than 100,000/ml or a falling platelet count, increasing resistance to heparin anticoagulation, or have developed thrombohemorrhagic complications. Prompt diagnosis of the heparin-induced thrombocytopenia (HIT) syndrome with discontinuation of heparin administration reduces the mortality and morbidity from 23% and 61%, respectively, to 12% and 22.5%. Once the diagnosis is suspected, the first step is the discontinuation of all heparin administrations. The development of HIT is independent of the type, dose, or route of administration of heparin. Platelet function is then inhibited on a daily basis with aspirin 325 mg by mouth or 600 mg per rectum. Confirmation of the diagnosis is made by an increasing platelet count with the discontinuation of heparin and by a positive platelet aggregometry or 14C-serotonin release study. Platelet transfusions are usually not necessary.

4. The answer is **E** (Rutherford, 4th ed., pp. 324–325).

In large vessels, viscosity is the most important factor influencing blood flow, after pressure and vessel diameter. Each of the factors mentioned influences blood viscosity. While the magnitude of influence of platelet and leukocyte aggregation is small compared to that of fibrinogen level and hematocrit, each of these factors is important in the microcirculation. When platelets and/or leukocytes are present in excess, as occurs in thrombocytosis and leukemias, viscosity increases.

5. The answer is **E** (Rutherford, 4th ed., pp. 324–325).

Multiple studies of patients with peripheral arterial disease have repeatedly confirmed the presence of multiple abnormal factors influencing blood viscosity, all in the direction of abnormally high viscosity. All of the choices are correct.

6. The answer is **D** (Rutherford, 4th ed., pp. 324, 327–328).

Blinded, placebo-controlled randomized studies performed in Europe and in the United States have repeatedly confirmed that pentoxifylline treatment results in improved treadmill walking distance in treated patients. The magnitude of the improvement is modest, however, and some patients with statistically significant improvements in walking distance report no change in walking in their daily lives. Pentoxifylline appears to exert its effect in the microcirculation, and repeated studies have failed to show any effect on ankle brachial pressure index or on total limb blood flow. Side effects are rare and require discontinuation of the drug in only 3–5% of patients.

7. The answer is **D** (Rutherford, 4th ed., pp. 328–329).

An important finding that has emerged from all randomized treatment trials to date of drugs intended for chronic ischemic rest pain and ischemic ulcers is that of a significant (25–40%) rate of improvement in the placebo-treated groups. Despite the fact that most surgeons are accustomed to regarding these symptoms as indicating limb-threatening ischemia, which inevitably results in limb loss if not corrected, the weight of the objective evidence shows that spontaneous improvement is a frequent event occurring in a substantial minority of patients. To date, no drug, prostaglandin or otherwise, has been conclusively shown in a randomized trial to result in an improved rate of limb salvage in such patients.

8. The answer is **E** (Rutherford, 4th ed., pp. 336–337).

Inhibitors of fibrinolysis are composed of two main groups: proteins that exhibit antiactivator activity (e.g., plasminogen activator inhibitor) and proteins that exhibit antiplasmin activity (e.g., α_2-antiplasmin, α_2-macroglobulin, protease nexin, and aprotinin). Plasminogen activator inhibitor blocks the fibrinolytic system at the activator level. Insulin appears to be a major physiologic regulator of plasminogen activator inhibitor. Antiplasmins exert their inhibition by blocking plasmin once and wherever it is formed. They are most active in plasma. Some specific inhibitors (e.g., protease nexin) are secreted by human fibroblasts. The third group of fibrinolytic inhibitors exert their antifibrinolytic effect by blocking the binding of plasmin to fibrin. These include ε-aminocaproic and tranexamic acid. Both of these agents produce conformational changes in the plasminogen molecule that *increase* its affinity to fibrin. Sufficient amounts of the antifibrinolytic agents, however, will block the lysine-binding sites of plasminogen and thus exert their antifibrinolytic effect.

9. The answers are **D, E** (Rutherford, 4th ed., pp. 339–340).

Urokinase is a naturally occurring plasminogen activator derived from human renal cell culture. No neutralizing antibodies are known. Urokinase does not contain lysine-binding sites, which helps explain its lack of affinity for fibrin. It directly converts plasminogen to plasmin, whereas streptokinase must combine with plasminogen to form an activator complex. Once urokinase is administered, it is rapidly removed from circulation by hepatic clearance. Half-life is estimated to be about 14 minutes.

10. The answers are **B, C** (Rutherford, 4th ed., pp. 343–344, 348–349).

Treatment of a hemorrhagic complication during thrombolytic therapy depends on the severity and the progress made during lytic therapy. When a significant hemorrhagic complication occurs, the drug should be immediately discontinued and the hemostatic defect corrected by administration of fresh-frozen plasma or cryoprecipitate. Administration of ε-aminocaproic acid or tranexamic acid, specifically aimed at blocking the fibrinolytic effect, can be associated with significant thrombotic complications, in view of the underlying indication for the lytic therapy. Thus, in most instances, antifibrinolytic agents are not indicated.

11. The answer is **E** (Rutherford, 4th ed., pp. 344, 349).

Pulmonary emboli may occur during both intra-arterial and intravenous lytic therapy. They occur with an incidence comparable to heparin therapy, on the order of 1–4%. A potential mechanism for this complication in the presence of an ischemic extremity is decreased venous flow with clot formation, partial lysis, dislodgement, and embolization. Treatment options include stopping lytic therapy and administering heparin or switching to systemic doses of intravenous lytic therapy. Although placement of a vena cava filter may be indicated in selected patients, in most instances, treatment with either lytic or heparin therapy is satisfactory.

12. The answer is **C** (Rutherford, 4th ed., p. 340).

Tissue plasminogen activator is a direct plasminogen activator, exhibiting mostly *endogenous* fibrinolytic activity, because it has high affinity for fibrin-bound plasminogen. *Exogenous* fibrinolysis involves plasmin formed in circulation, which then attacks the fibrin clot. Because t-PA works mostly within the thrombus, it is somewhat protected from antiplasmins. However, clinical studies of recombinant t-PA to date have not shown a decrease in hemorrhagic complications, despite its fibrin-selective properties. In fact, a slightly higher incidence of intracranial bleeding has been suggested. t-PA has been shown to bind and be activated on platelet surfaces. Due to this binding property, platelets may direct the action of t-PA on their surface, leading to rapid cleavage of platelet receptors and loss of platelet binding to von Willebrand factor. There is no intrinsic fibrinolytic activity of tissue plasminogen activator in the absence of plasminogen. Thus, plasminogen is necessary to exert the lytic effect.

13. The answers are **A, D, E** (Rutherford, 4th ed., pp. 352–365).

PTA is more successful when lesions are short, concentric, nonostial, single, and stenotic instead of occlusive.

14. The answers are **A, B, C, D** (Rutherford, 4th ed., pp. 369–375).

All of the above listed potential benefits of atherectomy devices over angioplasty procedures are true except that there has not been, to date, demonstrable *long-term* benefits. Because of added costs, larger sheath requirements, and relatively high frequency of complications compared to PTA, atherectomy should be reserved for PTA failures.

15. The answer is **B** (Rutherford, 4th ed., pp. 375–379).

The Palmaz Intraluminal Stent is the only stent thus far approved for peripheral arterial use in the United States, although others are regularly used in some European countries.

16. The answer is **C** (Rutherford, 4th ed., pp. 379–390).

Stents have proved to be important adjuncts in management of malignant SVC syndrome. Patency almost always parallels the patient's life expectancy. Stents have improved percutaneous management of iliac angioplasty for treatment of PTA-induced dissections, refractory eccentric lesions, and elastic recoil. Stents have enhanced percutaneous treatment of chronic iliac occlusions. They have improved *immediate* results in ostial lesions of the renal arteries and lesions of superficial femoral arteries, particularly in occlusions and PTA-induced dissection. Long-term patency does not appear to be improved in renal and superficial femoral arteries when compared to angioplasty alone.

17. The answers are **A, C, D** (Rutherford, 4th ed., pp. 402–403).

End-to-end anastomoses are conceptually the simplest and historically were the first performed in man. However, the first experimental vessel anastomosis was a side-to-side portocaval anastomosis performed in dogs by Nicolai Eck in 1877. It is the mandatory anastomosis for repair of aneurysms, but end-to-side anastomoses are more common for arterial bypass surgery. When performed as a perpendicular anastomosis in small vessels, end-to-end is prone to narrowing and secondary thrombosis, particularly if continuous suture technique is employed, because of a "purse-string effect." Because there are few other alternatives to an end-to-end technique in penetrating trauma, it should be performed in a fashion that avoids narrowing, e.g., using interrupted sutures, a triangulation technique, expanding the anastomotic line before tying the sutures, and/or beveling the ends to produce a larger, oblique suture line.

18. The answers are **B, D** (Rutherford, 4th ed., pp. 403–405).

End-to-side anastomosis is ideal for bypass grafts but not for interposition grafts where they would require more length and exposure and leave adjacent blind-ended cul de sacs. Acute-angled anastomoses are best, usually between 30 and 45°. Such an angle will usually produce an opening that is *twice* the diameter of the donor vessel, which is ideal. The recipient vessel is normally as large or larger. While matching *diameters* of the graft and outflow vessel is a sound principle, the anastomotic opening, being oblique and with an acute angle of entry, should be much bigger. One should start the anastomosis at the most inaccessible point on its circumference. Ordinarily, this is at the "heel" in acute-entry anastomoses but may be at the posterior midline in more perpendicular anastomoses where there is limited mobility. In repairing thoracoabdominal aneurysms, the visceral arteries are actually implanted end-to-side, even though performed like a lateral (side-to-side) anastomosis.

19. The answer is **D** (Rutherford, 4th ed., pp. 395–398).

Silk sutures are biodegradable and disintegrate with time, but they are quite acceptable for autogenous tissue anastomoses, which heal before the silk loses its strength. However, prosthetic anastomoses don't heal in the same fashion and depend indefinitely on the suture material for their integrity. Using silk in this setting was responsible for many if not most anastomotic aneurysms until the mid-1960s when the practice was discontinued. *Polyethylene* monofilament sutures were observed to "fracture" in time and created problems when used to place artificial heart valves. Braided dacron suture, coated to improve handling properties, then became popular until newer *polypropylene* monofilament suture proved durable. In the past, interrupted sutures were always used for anastomoses in children to allow for commensurate growth, but now synthetic absorbable monofilament suture with a suitably long half-life (e.g., polydiaxanone) allows continuous suture techniques to be employed. "Equal depth and travel" is a good rule in performing continuous anastomoses, although this is not always possible, particularly in aneurysm surgery. "Inside out on the artery, outside in on the graft" is the correct method for performing an anastomosis because penetrating arteriosclerotic arteries outside in might lift up an intimal plaque without penetrating it, thereby leading to intimal flaps, dissection, and thrombosis when flow is restored.

20. The answer is **C** (Rutherford, 4th ed., pp. 405–407).

The recipient anastomotic site should be selected by dissection under optical magnification in a zone where there is flexible, normal vessel wall outside the area of injury or disease. In a situation where damaged vessels must be resected back to normal vital tissue in which the vascular pedicle of the transfer is not long enough to reach the donor vessel easily, interposition vein grafts may be necessary. Synthetic bypass grafts cannot be used because of an unacceptable rate of thrombosis. Side branches of arteries or veins must be carefully ligated and coagulated at a distance removed from the main vessel.

21. The answer is **E** (Rutherford, 4th ed., p. 407).

Although the risk of arterial thrombosis may be reduced with the use of many vasodilating and antiplatelet agents, little effect has been achieved on venous patency. Unlike macrovascular surgery, heparin has limited usefulness and, in fact, can add to the risk of bleeding at sites of extensive dissection in flap donor areas and can cause obstruction of the microanastomoses by small hematomas at the transfer site. No prospective randomized double-blind studies have shown any benefit to postoperative anticoagulation by any pharmacologic agents. However, aspirin is routinely administered pre- and postoperatively for its antiplatelet effect. Postoperative low-molecular-weight Dextran is favored by some surgeons.

22. The answers are **D, E** (Rutherford, 4th ed., pp. 407–408).

Distal revascularization followed by free tissue transfer for coverage of ulcerative and necrotic lower-extremity defects can produce healed wounds and successful ambulation in diabetic patients. Conventional therapy consisting of skin grafts or local pedicle flaps are contraindicated in this setting due to lack of adequate recipient vessels and to local factors, including neuropathy and exposed tendon or bone (with or without infection). Even with aggressive revascularization by inframalleolar bypass, up to 20–40% of patients will ultimately come to amputation because of failure to heal advanced, ischemic, or infected ulcerations. Extensive tissue loss secondary to gangrene in diabetic patients traditionally has precluded salvage by conventional techniques despite the ability to bypass infrapopliteal occlusive disease. Many such patients progress to amputation despite arterial reconstruction because of large heel or ankle ulcers with exposed and infected tendon or bone. Most of these extremities can be saved if treated by distal revascularization and subsequent microvascular free tissue transfer.

23. The answer is **E** (Rutherford, 4th ed., pp. 408–409).

Microsurgical anastomosis may be completed to either a native artery, distal to a reversed or in situ saphenous vein graft, or to an autogenous vein graft itself if no native artery is available. Vein grafts up to 40 cm in length have been successfully used in free flap transfer, and length does not appear to correlate with patency. The steal phenomenon has not been documented in free flap transfer because average flow rates of 2–10 ml/minute are determined by the vascular bed of the flap and are inconsequential relative to the potential recipient vessel inflow. The presence of diabetes does not adversely affect patency.

24. The answer is **C** (Rutherford, 4th ed., pp. 407–410).

Combining arterial bypass with microvascular free tissue, or free tissue transfer alone when arterial inflow is marginal, can result in salvage of ischemic limbs. The pathophysiologic basis for this has been explained by the concept of the nutrient flap. Postoperative arteriograms of patients with severely atherosclerotic limbs who have undergone free tissue transfer demonstrate local proliferation and progressive development of new capillary networks. This treatment is effective not only in the absence of patent leg arteries but even in the absence of a patent plantar arch. It is hypothesized that this enhanced neovascularization is promoted by a perfusion gradient between the flap and the wound margin. Patients undergoing such treatment not only heal their wounds but report resolution of their rest pain and claudication as well. Neovascularization can be confirmed by postoperative arteriography. This observation suggests that perhaps a free flap alone may serve as a sole outflow source for a bypass graft in those patients with otherwise unacceptable runoff.

25. The answer is **C** (Rutherford, 4th ed., pp. 410–411).

The Fogarty embolectomy catheter employs an elastomeric balloon that, as illustrated in Figure 23–18, conforms to the environment in which it is placed. This feature makes it well suited to any application that requires conforming to the interior of the vessel, such as vessel occlusion or forming a seal within the vessel to facilitate removal of acute thrombus. Elastomeric balloons also increase in diameter according to the volume of fluid infused into the balloon, making them well suited to calibration of vessel lumen diameter. The conforming nature of the balloon is not well suited for dilatation, since the balloon will expand in the region of least resistance, which is not necessarily at the site of the atherosclerotic lesion.

26. The answer is **B** (Rutherford, 4th ed., pp. 411–413).

The stiff tip of the embolectomy catheter is well suited for passage through the clot, but is not designed to negotiate safely the valves of the venous system. As an alternative, the Fogarty venous thrombectomy catheter has a soft, flexible tip that will pass through the valves without disrupting them. Wetting the tip of a gas-filled 2F balloon can prevent leakage of the gas at the junction of the hub and syringe. Administration of heparin is used routinely to reduce the risk of thrombosis during embolectomy. It is very difficult to adjust the balloon diameter of a 3F embolectomy balloon with a 5-cc syringe. Use of a 1-cc or 3-cc syringe allows much better control of the balloon size during embolectomy. Use of excessively large balloons predisposes to subsequent myointimal hyperplasia in arteries by creating endothelial injuries.

27. The answer is **A** (Rutherford, 4th ed., pp. 411–413).

The presence of vigorous back bleeding is not a good indicator of distal patency because the clot can be discontinuous. Arteriography and piezoelectric pulse amplitude monitoring are, however, useful methods of evaluating distal patency.

28. The answers are **A, B, C** (Rutherford, 4th ed., pp. 414–419).

Direct innominate endarterectomy through median sternotomy exposure remains an extremely effective technique for managing occlusive disease of this artery, particularly in the presence of embolic symptoms. The procedure is facilitated by the use of a Wylie J-clamp, which allows the entire orifice of the innominate artery and adjacent aorta to be incorporated within it, while maintaining cerebral perfusion through the left common carotid artery. A "bovine arch" anomaly, in which both innominate and left common carotid arteries arise from the same aortic branch, precludes this possibility. The technique is one of open endarterectomy through a longitudinal innominate bifurcation; vein patch closure is not necessary. Transaortic endarterectomy is now the preferred technique for managing orificial occlusive disease of the visceral and renal arteries in many centers. It involves removing the atherosclerotic plaque from the aorta from which these branch lesions arise. The branch disease can be removed by extraction endarterectomy from within the aorta, or if necessary by addition of a branch arteriotomy to directly manage the distal endpoint. In either case, full exposure of the aorta and its branches by (left-to-right) medial visceral rotation allows sufficient control for effective endarterectomy through a longitudinal aortotomy. Transaortic renal artery endarterectomy may also be performed through the open cuff of the transected aorta at the time of infrarenal aortic prosthetic reconstruction. When aortic grafting is performed for aneurysmal disease, the dilating (degeneration) is usually limited to the infrarenal aorta, and the endarterectomized aortic stump provides adequate structural integrity to allow direct anastamosis of the prosthetic graft. Vein bypass is preferred for long lesions of the SFA. Short-segment (less than 15-cm) occlusive lesions of the superficial femoral artery remain effectively treated by endarterectomy, using either semiclosed techniques facilitated by stripping devices, or by open techniques with vein patch closure. Endarterectomy is ideal for lesions confined to the thigh, particularly when infection is of concern or there is no autologous vein available for bypass procedures.

29. The answers are **C, D** (Rutherford, 4th ed., pp. 414–419).

Atherosclerosis is a systemic disease that becomes clinically manifest through localized segments of stenosis or occlusion. These localized segments of occlusive atherosclerosis facilitate application of endarterectomy techniques. Recurrent atherosclerosis is actually quite unusual following endarterectomy and does not appear to be any more common in one location than another. Recurrent stenosis following endarterectomy is more often due to intimal hyperplasia. Both causes of recurrent stenosis are uncommon following endarterectomy, and this technique has proved highly durable in a wide variety of anatomic locations: in some sites, endarterectomy has proved more durable than bypass grafts of any type. Two of the features of atherosclerosis that permit endarterectomy to be feasible are listed in answers C and D. An additional feature of great importance is that occlusive disease of aortic branch arteries, such as the innominate, visceral, and renal arteries, is usually orificial in location, permitting endarterectomy. Endarterectomy of the aortoiliac or superficial femoral arteries is not limited by the biologic nature of the disease but by the time it takes to perform the technique correctly in comparison to bypass operations. Long-segment endarterectomy is limited by a high rate of recurrent stenosis caused by intimal hyperplasia. Development of effective treatments to limit intimal hyperplasia in the future may increase the role of endarterectomy procedures in lower-extremity revascularization.

30. The answer is **A** (Rutherford, 4th ed., pp. 414–419).

Transaortic endarterectomy of the visceral and renal branch arteries is currently one of the most important applications of endarterectomy excepting the carotid bifurcation. Adequate exposure is critical and is best obtained by a medial visceral rotation, along with dissection of an adequate portion of the branch arteries of interest. After aortic cross-clamping, a longitudinal aortotomy provides full exposure of the aortic branch artery orifices, and open endarterectomy can be rapidly performed under direct vision. This encompasses the circumference of the involved aorta and is extended to include the orifices of the affected branches. The orificial nature of disease in these arteries is typical (it actually represents an extension of aortic atherosclerosis), making satisfactory endpoints relatively easy to obtain. Because the endarterectomy actually encompasses the aorta, any evidence of aneurysmal dilation makes endarterectomy contraindicated. While it is true that symptomatic visceral artery disease typically requires disobliteration of both celiac and superior mesenteric arteries, this is readily accomplished by transaortic endarterectomy of both vessels, which can be performed well within the ischemia time tolerated by the viscera. In an extended experience with this technique at the University of California, San Francisco, and increasingly at other institutions, transaortic endarterectomy for visceral and/or renal artery occlusive disease has proved to be a safe and durable operation.

31. The answer is **false** (Rutherford, 4th ed., pp. 420–423).

In patients with peripheral vascular disease the incidence of *severe* CAD (30%, documented angiographically) is independent of the extent of peripheral arterial occlusive disease. The accuracy of clinical detection of CAD is often handicapped by the limitations in activity imposed by peripheral vascular disease. The Cleveland Clinic series demonstrated that in patients scheduled for elective vascular procedures, *normal* coronary arteriograms were present in only 4% of patients with and 14% of patients without clinically suspected CAD. Coronary artery bypass grafting (CABG) was performed in 70/250 (28%) patients with infrarenal AAA, 63/295 (21%) with cerebrovascular disease, and 70/381 (18%) with lower-extremity vascular insufficiency prior to the planned vascular reconstruction. Of these 216 patients identified with surgically correctable CAD who subsequently underwent coronary artery bypass, 72% were alive at 5 years postoperatively. In contrast, only 15/35 (43%) patients considered candidates but who never received CABG and 12/54 (22%) patients with severe, uncorrectable CAD remained alive at 5 years.

32. The answer is **false** (Rutherford, 4th ed., pp. 421–423).

The incidence of myocardial infarction (MI) after noncardiac surgery ranges from 0 to 0.7%, but the incidence increases substantially to 2 to 6.4% in patients undergoing elective *vascular reconstruction*, and nearly one half of these are fatal. Retrospective reviews generally report perioperative MI rates of about 3%, and more intensive prospective surveillance detection rates as high as 10 to 15%. Unless cardiac enzymes and ECGs are routinely obtained, postoperative MI is substantially underestimated. The observation that 50 to 90% of postoperative ischemic events detected by ambulatory ECG monitoring (Holter) are silent supports this contention.

33. The answer is **false** (Rutherford, 4th ed., p. 424).

The anatomic location of the planned vascular operation has little bearing on postoperative cardiac morbidity. The reported incidence of myocardial infarction following vascular surgery is fairly consistent regardless of the type of procedure performed, ranging from 2 to 6%. In a recent prospective comparison of patients undergoing infrainguinal reconstruction, the number of postoperative cardiac events (cardiac death, myocardial infarction, unstable angina, congestive heart failure, ventricular tachycardia) was similar to patients undergoing major abdominal procedures. Further, 57% of patients undergoing infrainguinal operations had documented ischemia by ambulatory ECG monitoring compared to 31% of patients undergoing aortic reconstruction ($p = 0.005$).

34. The answers are **A, B, C** (Rutherford, 4th ed., pp. 424–426).

Goldman and associates were among the first investigators to demonstrate that estimates of perioperative cardiac risk could be derived from information available in a careful history and physical exam. Of the clinical variables examined, (1) recent myocardial infarction and (2) congestive heart failure were the strongest predictors of adverse cardiac outcome; additional factors identified included (in order of decreasing importance): (3) abnormal rhythm; (4) >5 premature ventricular contractions per minute; (5) intra-abdominal, intrathoracic, or aortic surgery; (6) age >70 years; (7) significant aortic valvular stenosis; (8) emergency operation; and (9) poor general medical condition. Conspicuously absent as significant predictors of perioperative cardiac morbidity either by univariate or multivariate analysis are angina or diabetes.

35. The answers are **A, C** (Rutherford, 4th ed., pp. 426–428).

In studies of patients undergoing noncardiac surgery, Mangano found that 28% of patients had documented preoperative ischemia by Holter, and the incidence of ischemia nearly doubled in the postoperative period. Most (>75%) ischemic episodes are clinically silent. Advantages of ambulatory ECG monitoring over other noninvasive methods to determine cardiac risk, like dipyridamole thallium scintigraphy, include its wider availability and lower cost. Disadvantages include: 10% or more of patients have underlying ECG abnormalities that limit or preclude the interpretation of ST-segment depression; and ECG patterns like left ventricular hypertrophy may lead to false positive evidence of ST-segment depression that is not due to CAD.

36. The answers are **A, C** (Rutherford, 4th ed., p. 429).

Thallium[201] is taken up by myocardial cells in proportion to blood flow. Intravenous dipyridamole dilates coronary vessels, thus increasing flow to myocardium supplied by nonstenotic vessels. Dipyridamole acts by inhibiting myocardial cellular reuptake and endothelial transport of endogenously produced adenosine, a potent coronary vasodilator. As adenosine accumulates in the interstitium, coronary vasodilation ensues. The administration of dipyridamole, through its adenosine effect, results in an increase in coronary flow by two- to threefold. However, myocardium supplied by stenotic vessels has poor uptake (+ defect) on early scintigraphic scan. In effect, intravenous dipyridamole produces a *steal* phenomenon because nonstenotic arteries enjoy enhanced flow whereas stenotic arteries cannot vasodilate. Later this defect will resolve if viable myocardium is present, suggesting an area of myocardium potentially at risk during periods of increased stress; late uptake of thallium[201] in areas of myocardium initially underperfused is termed *redistribution*. In contrast, a persistent defect on thallium scan suggests an area of prior myocardial infarction and, therefore, myocardium already irreversibly injured (myocardial scarring).

37. The answers are **A, B, C, D, E** (Rutherford, 4th ed., pp. 429–431).

The selective use of preoperative DTS in vascular surgery patients has been investigated by Eagle. In the initial study, five clinical markers (age >70, Q waves, DM, angina, or arrhythmia requiring medication) identified in a retrospective analysis of 61 patients scheduled for vascular surgery predicted perioperative cardiac morbidity. These clinical variables were then applied prospectively to 50 consecutive patients undergoing vascular surgery. Only 3% of those who had no clinical indicators sustained an adverse postoperative cardiac event. In this low-risk group 52 DTSs were performed; 9 revealed reversible defects, and only 1 patient had an adverse ischemic event (angina). In contrast, 29% of patients with one or more clinical predictors suffered an adverse cardiac event, and a reversible defect was present in 33/59 (56%) patients. In a subsequent study, Eagle and colleagues corroborated their initial findings and were further able to identify an intermediate-risk group in whom DTS was most useful. Again in the low-risk group (0 clinical predictors) a 3% postoperative cardiac event rate was noted. Patients considered intermediate risk (1–2 clinical predictors) and high risk ($\geq$ 3 clinical predictors) had cardiac event rates of 33% and 50%, respectively. Performance of DTS in the intermediate-risk group demonstrated that in patients with normal thallium scans the event rate (3.2%) approximated that of the low-risk group, whereas 30% of those with thallium redistribution suffered postoperative cardiac morbidity. Therefore, DTS appears to add little to the preoperative evaluation of the low and high groups because accurate cardiac risk assessment is possible by clinical criteria alone. The identification of an intermediate-risk group by clinical criteria allows the selective application of DTS and permits additional stratification.

38. The answers are **B, C, E** (Rutherford, 4th ed., pp. 436–437).

The time-honored indication for blood transfusion in patients with a hemoglobin of 10 g or hematocrit of 30% is arbitrary and outdated. With current strict indications for transfusion, the basis for transfusion is clinical assessment that is related to delivery of oxygen at tissue level (e.g., cardiovascular instability, decreased pO_2, decreased cardiac output). Perfusion and oxygenation of tissues is usually well tolerated with hematocrits between 20 and 24%. Furthermore, no study has shown conclusively that moderate anemia increases wound infection or impairs recuperation.

39. The answers are **A, B, D, E** (Rutherford, 4th ed., pp. 437–439, 440–441).

Acute isovolemic hemodilution is widely practiced. Up to 20% of the patient's blood volume may be safely removed and given back at the completion of surgery. Blood loss at surgery has a lower hematocrit and is more easily replaced. Intraoperative autotransfusion has many advantages and is becoming the standard of care in major vascular surgery. Artificial blood is still essentially experimental and is realistically about two to three years from being a practical alternative. Preoperative donation is a very logical and practical alternative in elective vascular surgery, but it is underutilized. Promotion of hemostasis by good surgical technique or by medications or hemostatic agents should be every surgeon's goal, especially efforts to avoid a coagulopathy.

40. The answers are **A, B, C** (Rutherford, 4th ed., pp. 437–439).

Autotransfusion has many advantages, including net blood loss reduction, no risk of autoimmunization, disease transmission, or problems with incompatibility. In addition to the ready and rapid availability of autotransfused blood, it has been shown in many studies to be physiologically, biochemically, and morphologically superior or equal to bank blood. The autotransfusion technique removes clotting factors and platelets; therefore, a dilutional coagulopathy may occur if a replacement protocol is not used. Sickle-cell disease is a relative contraindication to autotransfusion techniques, as are sepsis contamination and cancer dissemination.

41. The answers are **B, C, D, E** (Rutherford, 4th ed., pp. 442–444).

Although the risks of viral transmission with predonated autologous blood are nil, errors and bacterial contamination can take place. The patient may have an acute infection at the time of donation, and during storage bacterial growth and endotoxin production may occur. Fatal cases of septic shock secondary to Yersinia enterocolitica have been reported after patients have received their own predonated blood. Also, acute intravascular hemolysis has been reported following infusion of inadequately deglycerolized previously frozen red blood cells. While the criteria for transfusion are not as strict as with homologous blood, blood should not be administered just because the patient requests it.

42. The answers are **A, C** (Rutherford, 4th ed., pp. 449–450).

Angioscopy has been proved to be a very sensitive method for intraoperative detection of defects in saphenous vein grafts. In studies directly comparing arteriography with angioscopy, arteriography was much less sensitive (22–67%) than angioscopy for detecting residual valve cusps of in situ grafts. This implies that many residual valve cusps are being left unlysed by surgeons using arteriography alone to evaluate these grafts. Since the early failure rate of grafts evaluated by arteriography is not high, this suggests that not all residual valve cusps detected by angioscopy will cause early graft failure. In fact, most studies using angioscopy have experienced approximately the same early graft failure rate (5–10%) as those employing conventional arteriography. Thus, it has not yet been demonstrated that the correction of all defects detected by angioscopy will improve graft patency. Whereas it is true that angioscopy has been shown experimentally to cause intimal injury, this has occurred after multiple passes with a relatively large-diameter scope. The use of small-diameter angioscopes clinically has not been shown to have any adverse effect on in situ saphenous vein graft patency. Even the most experienced investigators using angioscopy for the evaluation of in situ vein grafts have found that 10% of their grafts contained residual valve cusps after blind valve lysis, including their most recent experience. Most studies have reported residual valve cusps in an even higher percentage of patients. Saline irrigation is required for adequate visualization during angioscopy, but this can usually be limited to 500 ml. Furthermore, if anticipated as part of the overall operative fluid replacement, it can be used in nearly all patients.

43. The answers are **A, D** (Rutherford, 4th ed., pp. 451–453).

Large series of published reports concerning intraoperative evaluation of carotid endarterectomy have demonstrated that an average of 12% had residual defects, including 6.5% in the common or internal carotid artery. Similarly, 5.7% of carotid endarterectomy patients will have significant residual defects found postoperatively by duplex scanning. Most authors who have employed some form of intraoperative evaluation have found that from 5 to 10% of their carotid endarterectomies have significant residual technical defects that warrant surgical correction. Since the perioperative stroke rate is usually much lower, it is clear that many of these defects will not cause immediate stroke. However, in a study at UCSF using duplex ultrasound, the subsequent restenosis rate correlated well with the size of residual defects identified by duplex scanning (but left uncorrected after carotid endarterectomy). A variety of modalities are available to evaluate carotid endarterectomy sites intraoperatively, and each has advantages and disadvantages. The continuous-wave Doppler pencil probe is relatively sensitive in experienced hands, but not specific, since 30–70% of areas with increased frequency cannot be confirmed as defects by arteriography or exploration. Conversely, B-mode ultrasound detects many small defects, but unless these cause a stenosis ≥30% of the diameter or an intimal flap ≥3 mm long, these do not require correction based on subsequent evaluation of patients in whom these "minor" defects were not repaired. Pulsed Doppler spectral analysis provides a more objective assessment of velocity/frequency changes than does continuous-wave Doppler alone. However, it does not provide any anatomic confirmation of a potential defect, which has led most investigators to recommend this as a screening method for the selective application of arteriography or duplex scanning. Although the routine use of intraoperative evaluation after carotid endarterectomy will occasionally lead to an unnecessary re-exploration, most surgeons agree that this does not increase morbidity. In order to maintain acceptably low morbidity rates, most surgeons would benefit from the use of one or more of these techniques.

44. The answers are **C, E** (Rutherford, 4th ed., pp. 449–450, 453–455).

The intraoperative evaluation of renal and visceral reconstructions is more difficult due to the deep and somewhat inaccessible position of these arteries within the abdomen. Arteriography has not been optimal for this evaluation because it is difficult to obtain good x-ray penetration of the abdominal cavity with portal x-ray generators; it is difficult to obtain rapid injection of sufficient contrast in the high-flow aorta; and contrast may aggravate renal insufficiency present in many patients currently undergoing renal revascularization. Because of these problems with arteriography, duplex scanning has been evaluated and found to be quite accurate for the intraoperative assessment of renal and mesenteric reconstructions. One large study of renal revascularization found it to be 98% accurate for detecting significant defects based on follow-up duplex scanning. Angioscopy has now been used in most anatomic arterial beds to evaluate potential defects intraoperatively. Although it has been most widely applied for the evaluation of lower-extremity vein grafts, it has also been found to be very sensitive to detect residual thrombus after thrombectomy and to evaluate intimal flaps at endarterectomy sites. Furthermore, it can be used in arterial segments such as the iliac arteries, even if proximal surgical control of the inflow has not been obtained, by the use of balloon occlusion catheters passed proximally from a more distal site of surgical exposure. This technique appears to be very sensitive for the detection of intraoperative defects, although experience is required to ascertain which small defects then require operative repair. Although many surgeons do not routinely evaluate the extremities after balloon catheter embolectomy, collected reviews have shown that the incidence of residual thrombus or undetected balloon catheter injuries is high. Thus, the application of intraoperative arteriography or angioscopy has been recommended to reduce the need for subsequent intervention and to improve the completeness of thrombus extraction. Unfortunately, the palpation of distal pulses and the extent of arterial back bleeding at an embolectomy site does not exclude balloon catheter injuries or residual thrombus. Experience with continuous-wave Doppler pencil probes has shown these to be very useful intraoperatively since they are inexpensive and readily available. They provide a sensitive method for detecting potential graft defects, but unfortunately they do not provide anatomic confirmation and are less specific than other modalities. Accordingly, most surgeons use them as a screening procedure, to guide the use of more sophisticated techniques, such as duplex scanning or arteriography.

45. The answer is **E** (Rutherford, 4th ed., pp. 457–463).

Even if an intervention is performed to preserve patency, the graft is considered to be no longer primarily patent. The graft in this example is now classified as a secondary patency and a primary failure. However, because the outcome of grafts that thrombose is markedly different from those that are revised prior to thrombosis, the additional category of assisted primary patency may be reported. This is *not* a pure primary patency and should not be reported as such.

46. The answer is **E** (Rutherford, 4th ed., pp. 457–463).

This graft remains secondarily patent, and because it had not thrombosed prior to the revision of the distal anastomosis, it may also be classified as having assisted primary patency. It does not matter whether the secondary or assisted primary patency is maintained by percutaneous or operative means; what is important is that invasive intervention occurred.

47. The answer is **C** (Rutherford, 4th ed., pp. 457–463).

This graft has restored patency, which is identified as secondary patency. Once a graft fails, by definition it loses primary patency.

48. The answer is **D** (Rutherford, 4th ed., pp. 457–463).

Despite the elective nature of the revision, this graft has had *both* anastomoses revised and must be considered a "redo" following graft failure.

49. The answer is **D** (Rutherford, 4th ed., pp. 457–463).

Although asymptomatic in his current restricted lifestyle, this patient's graft has failed hemodynamically. The preoperative ABI for this reconstruction was 0.60, and the current ABI has fallen to within 0.10 of the preoperative value.

5

Vascular Grafts

1. The preferred conduit for renal arterial reconstruction in children is:
   A. PTFE.
   B. Hypogastric artery.
   C. Dacron.
   D. Saphenous vein.
   E. All of the above.

2. The following vessels are considered acceptable for use as an arterial autograft:
   A. Hypogastric artery.
   B. Occluded superficial femoral artery.
   C. Occluded internal carotid artery.
   D. External iliac artery.
   E. All of the above.

3. Which of the following statements concerning arterial autographs is/are true?
   A. Arterial autographs exhibit normal healing in infected fields.
   B. Arterial autografts demonstrate proportional growth when utilized as a bypass conduit in children.
   C. Arterial autografts can be constructed using an occluded artery after an endarterectomy of the occluded segment has been performed.
   D. All of the above.
   E. None of the above.

4. Which of the following statements about venous anatomy is/are true?
   A. The greater saphenous vein, in the majority of individuals, comprises a continuous trunk arising anterior to the ankle and ending in the common femoral vein.
   B. The greater saphenous vein is absent in 4% of patients.
   C. The valves in the saphenous vein are tricuspid.
   D. The valve cusps are oriented perpendicular to the surface of the skin.
   E. The usual location of the saphenous vein in the leg is 1–2 cm anterior to the medial border of the tibia.

5. All of the following are protective of the autogenous vein during harvest and preparation *except*:
   A. Pressure used to distend the vein be limited to less than 300 mm Hg.
   B. Use of papaverine either prior to or after vein harvest.
   C. Avoidance of dilation of veins prior to insertion into the arterial system.
   D. Avoidance of traction on the vein when ligating side branches.
   E. Use of a continuous incision when harvesting arm veins.

6. Which of the following factors has an adverse effect on long-term vein graft function?
   A. Use of in situ technique.
   B. Use of reversed technique.
   C. Use of translocated veins.
   D. Small size of vein—less than 2 mm in diameter.
   E. Use of endoscopy to incise valve cusps during in situ construction.

7. In humans, the time required to achieve complete endothelialization of a prosthetic graft is:
   A. 1–2 weeks.
   B. 1 month.
   C. 6 months.
   D. 1 year.
   E. Never.

8. Prosthetic grafts constructed of knitted dacron:
   A. Are the graft of choice for repair of thoracoabdominal aortic aneurysms due to their superior handling qualities.
   B. Are likely to dilate 10–20% in diameter after chronic implantation.
   C. Cause less platelet activation than occurs with e-PTFE grafts.
   D. Have significantly improved patency in small-caliber conduits (6 cm in diameter) when precoated with collagen or albumin.
   E. Exhibit less host incorporation when fabricated with velour yarns.

9. Which of the following characteristics of e-PTFE grafts as compared to textile prosthetic vascular conduits is/are true?
   A. e-PTFE grafts have better tissue ingrowth than textile grafts.
   B. Bacterial adherence is less with e-PTFE grafts.

C. e-PTFE grafts exhibit less dilatation.
D. e-PTFE grafts cause less complement activation than dacron grafts.
E. e-PTFE grafts are more compliant than textile grafts.

10. Which of the following statements regarding human umbilical vein (HUV) allografts is/are true?
A. HUV grafts have a lower patency rate for below-knee femoropopliteal bypass than e-PTFE grafts.
B. HUV grafts are easier to thrombectomize than e-PTFE grafts.
C. About 50% of HUV grafts become aneurysmal in long-term follow-up.
D. HUV grafts have a lower propensity for infection than e-PTFE grafts.
E. HUV grafts are easier to implant than e-PTFE grafts.

11. Which of the following statements about vascular prosthetic grafts is/are true?
A. The thrombogenicity of a graft is closely related to blood flow velocity.
B. The principal advantage of crimping of textile grafts is improved long-term patency.
C. The addition of external support rings to a prosthetic graft significantly improves the late patency of bypass grafts to the below-knee popliteal or tibial arteries.
D. Seeded endothelial cells adhere readily to the luminal surface of e-PTFE grafts.
E. High porosity is an indispensable requirement for satisfactory long-term patency of prosthetic grafts.

5

Answers

1. The answer is **B** (Rutherford, 4th ed., pp. 475–476).

Renal artery reconstruction in the pediatric population requires a conduit that will demonstrate both durable patency and proportional growth over time. Prosthetic grafts are problematic with respect to growth. Autogenous tissue is preferred, and it appears that there is a lower incidence of aneurysmal degeneration over time when an arterial autograft is used compared with saphenous vein grafts. Therefore, the hypogastric artery is the preferred conduit for renal artery reconstruction in the pediatric-age group.

2. The answer is **E** (Rutherford, 4th ed., pp. 475–476).

Arterial segments harvested from a variety of locations are suitable for use as an arterial autograft. Primary consideration is given to the size match of the vessel being replaced (renal, carotid). The hypogastric artery is ideally suited for renal artery reconstruction because of the distal branching pattern in both of these vascular beds. The occluded superficial femoral artery may be disobliterated by an eversion endarterectomy to be used as a conduit, or a segment of it can be harvested, an endarterectomy performed, and the segment placed as a patch. Similarly, the occluded internal carotid artery may be utilized for patch closure when performing an external carotid endarterectomy. Finally, there may be occasion to employ a patent external iliac artery as a conduit, replacing it with a synthetic prosthesis.

3. The answer is **D** (Rutherford, 4th ed., pp. 476–481).

Arterial autografts have been shown to function and heal normally when placed into contaminated fields. This property has allowed them to be effectively used in the arterial reconstruction of critical vascular beds following the removal of infected synthetic bypass grafts. When arterial autografts have been used for renal artery reconstruction in children, long-term follow-up has shown excellent patency and proportional growth of the conduit relative to native arteries and that the vessel is resistant to aneurysmal degeneration. Following an eversion endarterectomy, a previously occluded superficial femoral artery may be used to replace segmental defects or as a patch graft for longitudinal closure of small-diameter arterial segments. This technique is particularly efficacious for extended profundaplasty and in the performance of an external carotid reconstruction in the presence of an occluded internal carotid artery.

4. The answer is **B** (Rutherford, 4th ed., p. 482).

In the majority of cases, the saphenous vein is *not* a continuous trunk starting anterior to the ankle and ending in the common femoral vein. In the 1986 study by Shah et al., in Albany, only 38% of venograms demonstrated a conventional saphenous vein coursing through the leg. Work by Veith in 1979 demonstrated that the saphenous vein can be absent in up to 4% of patients. Valves in the saphenous vein are bicuspid valves, which are oriented parallel to the surface of the skin. The usual location of the saphenous vein is 1–2 cm *posterior* to the medial border of the tibia.

5. The answer is **C** (Rutherford, 4th ed., pp. 485–486).

That excessive pressure used to distend the vein is detrimental has been shown by a variety of studies. Ideally, the pressure should be limited to the 300–400-mm Hg range. The use of papaverine either prior to or after vein harvest has been demonstrated in studies by LoGorfo and others in 1981 to be beneficial in terms of preservation of all cellular elements of the vein graft. There are no data to suggest that the avoidance of careful dilatation prior to insertion is beneficial. There are some data suggesting that gentle dilatation actually is beneficial to the saphenous veins. Certainly it aids in the technical construction of the anastomosis. Traction on veins should be avoided when ligating side branches to avoid compromise in the lumen of the vein. Finally, continuous incision is advocated for use of arm veins because these veins are thin walled and delicate. Staggered incisions require more manipulation of the vein in order to remove it, thus increasing the possibility of injury.

6. The answer is **D** (Rutherford, 4th ed., pp. 489–491).

Only the small size of the vein, generally less than 2 mm, is associated with very poor short- and long-term graft patency. None of the other factors has been conclusively shown to affect long-term graft function. There has been a dearth of prospective randomized studies comparing the in situ versus the reverse vein technique. Those studies that have been done, by and large, have not shown any significant difference. The surgeon should select the operation that he or she can do best.

7. The answer is **E** (Rutherford, 4th ed., pp. 511–513).

Whereas the luminal surface of prosthetic grafts implanted in various laboratory animal species does often ultimately become covered with a confluent layer of viable host endothelial cells, this process has not been demonstrated to occur in humans with any currently available prosthetic graft. In man, endothelialization is seen only within 1–2 cm of the ends of the graft from transanastomotic pannus ingrowth or occasionally in patchy focal areas within portions of the body of the graft. The observation of "incomplete healing" in man is an important limitation to function of small-caliber prosthetic grafts and the basis for interest in development of "endothelial cell seeding" of prostheses.

8. The answer is **B** (Rutherford, 4th ed., pp. 496–500).

Although the acknowledged better-handling characteristics of knitted dacron grafts are a desirable feature in certain arterial reconstructions, extensive procedures such as repair of thoracoabdominal aortic aneurysms are likely to be associated with considerable blood loss or coagulation disturbances. In such settings, relatively high-porosity knitted dacron grafts are likely to be associated with greater blood loss despite efforts to adequately preclot the prosthesis, making low-porosity woven grafts or grafts made impervious to transgraft bleeding by coating with albumin, collagen, or gelatin the choice of most surgeons for this application. Such biologically coated grafts do not have any documented advantage in terms of improved patency of small-vessel reconstruction, however. Fabrication of dacron grafts with velour yarns is done to improve the healing process and leads to improved cellular ingrowth and incorporation by adjacent host fibrous tissue. Several studies have demonstrated greater platelet deposition and complement activation on the flow surface of dacron grafts compared to e-PTFE grafts. A recognized characteristic of textile prostheses, especially knitted grafts, is a tendency to dimensional instability related to yarn slippage and other possible mechanical degenerative causes. Knitted grafts have been shown often to dilate 10–20% over alleged manufacturers' stated size with exposure to arterial pressure on declamping, with possible progressive dilation over time as determined by late follow-up CT scans. The clinical relevance of graft dilation has not been precisely determined.

9. The answers are **B, C, D** (Rutherford, 4th ed., pp. 500–503).

Although e-PTFE grafts are usually adequately incorporated or "healed" by surrounding host tissues, relatively little cellular ingrowth into the graft wall occurs. This is in contrast to what is observed in all but very low-porosity textile grafts and is likely due to the microporous nature of the e-PTFE material and the external reinforcing layer used in W. L. Gore grafts. Bacterial adherence has been shown to be less with e-PTFE grafts, likely due to their smoother surface as compared to the interstices of knitted or woven textile grafts. Many surgeons feel this may make e-PTFE grafts more resistant to infection. Other potential advantages of e-PTFE prostheses are greater structural stability and reduced platelet deposition and complement activation as compared to dacron grafts. e-PTFE grafts are less compliant than dacron grafts, and such anastomotic compliance mismatch appears to be an important limitation to the long-term patency of small-vessel reconstruction with e-PTFE grafts.

10. The answer is **C** (Rutherford, 4th ed., pp. 504–506).

Several prospective randomized studies have found better patency for infrageniculate popliteal or tibial bypass with HUV grafts as opposed to e-PTFE conduits, particularly in poor run-off situations. Whereas other studies have suggested no significant patency differences with the two prostheses, no study has suggested that HUV grafts perform *worse* in terms of patency. HUV grafts have some definite disadvantages, however. They are technically more difficult to implant, harder to thrombectomize if occlusion occurs due to their fragility, and more prone to infection than e-PTFE conduits. By far the principal liability is their tendency for biodegeneration. Many studies have documented a significant incidence of aneurysmal change 3–5 years following implantation, affecting approximately 50% of HUV grafts still patent at this long-term interval.

11. The answer is **A** (Rutherford, 4th ed., pp. 492–514).

Regardless of the thrombogenicity of a particular graft or clotting potential of an individual patient, the faster blood flows through a graft the less opportunity for fibrin deposition and platelet aggregation and adherence on its flow surface. The lower the thrombogenicity of a graft surface, the lower flow a graft can tolerate. The concept of thrombotic threshold velocity is important in the generally poor results of small-caliber prosthetic grafts and a major reason for the superiority of autogenous grafts in low-flow situations. Crimping of grafts is done to increase elasticity and flexibility and to improve handling characteristics. Studies have shown that crimping interferes with smooth laminar flow and often increases the thickness of the luminal fibrin layer that is deposited in a graft. Such adverse consequences of crimping are detrimental to patency of small-caliber prosthetic grafts. External support may be helpful in preventing compression of subcutaneous grafts but has not been shown to improve patency of small-caliber grafts below the knee in a randomized prospective study by Gupta et al in 1991. While endothelial seeding is an attractive hypothesis, considerable difficulty has been noted in achieving adequate adherence of seeded cells to the graft surface. Precoating grafts with fibronectin or similar agents may help increase cell retention, but this remains a practical limitation to the techniques at present. Satisfactory patency performance of microporous e-PTFE grafts and various biologically derived grafts that are nonporous has brought the once-accepted concept of high porosity into doubt as an absolute requirement for graft design.

6

Complications of Vascular Surgery

1. Which of the following common perioperative variables may cause an imbalance between myocardial oxygen supply and demand?
   A. Sinus tachycardia.
   B. Anemia.
   C. Systemic hypertension.
   D. Systemic hypotension.
   E. All of the above.

2. Which of the following statements is/are *false* about dipyridamole thallium scans?
   A. Dipyridamole (Persantin) is a potent coronary vasodilator.
   B. Redistribution of thallium indicates areas of myocardial ischemia.
   C. Fixed defects are more important than redistribution in predicting perioperative cardiac risk.
   D. Aminophylline and caffeine block the vasodilatory effect of dipyridamole and should be withheld for 48 hours before scanning.
   E. All of the above.

3. Which of the following statements is/are true about the intraoperative management of vascular patients with associated coronary artery disease?
   A. All inhalation anesthetics are myocardial depressants and therefore have little role in the patient with coronary artery disease.
   B. Epidural anesthesia is associated with fewer cardiac complications than general anesthesia in patients with coronary artery disease.
   C. Clamping of the aorta causes a rise in LVDEP and a decrease in coronary perfusion pressure.
   D. Unclamping of the aorta may cause a sudden decrease in the peripheral resistance resulting in diastolic hypotension and a decrease in coronary perfusion pressure.

4. Nonpulmonary causes of respiratory compromise affecting the central nervous system, the upper airway, or the mechanical aspects of breathing are important causes of respiratory complications in vascular surgical patients. **True** or **false?**

5. Preoperative assessment of the potential for respiratory complications in vascular surgical patients includes:
   A. A careful history and physical examination.
   B. Formal pulmonary function testing in all preoperative patients.
   C. A chest x-ray, room air arterial blood gas determinations, and simple bedside spirometry in patients greater than age 40 and undergoing a major vascular reconstruction.
   D. Routine consultation by a pulmonary medicine specialist.

6. Optimization of the perioperative factors that decrease pulmonary complications include:
   A. Careful planning of the incision and type of anesthesia.
   B. Preoperative detection and correction of deficits in hemoglobin, hematocrit, and nutritional status.
   C. Instruction in vigorous deep-breathing exercises and short-term training with an incentive spirometer and the use of bronchodilators and/or antibiotics in patients with bronchospasm or infection.
   D. IPPB (without medications).

7. In postoperative vascular surgical patients the adult respiratory distress syndrome (ARDS):
   A. Is easily distinguishable from cardiogenic pulmonary edema.
   B. Is precipitated by specific mediators that cause abnormal capillary permeability.
   C. Is usually associated with a high pulmonary wedge pressure.
   D. Is associated with shock, prolonged ischemia, multiple transfusions, and sustained hypothermia.

8. Which of the following preparations is/are *not* appropriate for prevention of contrast-induced acute renal dysfunction?
   A. Twelve-hour prearteriographic crystalloid loading.
   B. Administration of Furosemide 4 hours before arteriography to insure high urine flows.
   C. Intravenous Mannitol immediately following arteriography.
   D. Limitation of total contrast load to less than 2ml/kg.
   E. None of the above.

9. Which of the following mechanisms is presumed to be the *initiating* event of postischemic acute renal failure?
   A. Thrombosis of arterioles within Bowman's capsule.

B. Sloughing of efferent arterioles with proximal thrombosis.
C. Production of basement membrane edema within Bowman's capsule and resultant decrease in filtration.
D. Sloughing of proximal tubular cells with resultant obstruction of the tubular luman.
E. Increase in back diffusion of glomerular filtrate.

10. Myoglobinuria secondary to extensive muscle necrosis causes acute renal failure by which of the following mechanisms?
A. Direct toxicity on the tubular cells.
B. Formation of complex protein moieties that block the efferent arterioles of Bowman's capsule.
C. Occlusion of the intercapillary spaces within the efferent arterioles of Bowman's capsule.
D. Its direct vasoconstructive properties, which produce decreased filtration.
E. Precipitation and obstruction of the tubule.

11. In liver disease, bleeding is caused by:
A. Deficiencies in clotting factors.
B. Deficiencies in platelets.
C. Excessive clot lysis.
D. Anatomical lesions.
E. All of the above.

12. Inhibitors to coagulation:
A. Always should be investigated when unexplained hemorrhage occurs.
B. Always cause bleeding.
C. Never cause bleeding.
D. Can be caused by drugs.
E. Can appear suddenly and put the patient in jeopardy.

13. Hemophilia means a deficiency of:
A. Factor VIII.
B. Factor IX.
C. Platelets.
D. Fibrinogen.
E. Thrombin.

14. Cryoprecipitate, a derivative of plasma, contains:
A. Factor VIII.
B. Factor IX.
C. Factor I (fibrinogen).
D. Factor II (prothrombin).
E. Factor XII.

15. Desmopressin (DDAVP) is useful in restoring hemostasis to individuals with:
A. Von Willebrand's disease, classical type.
B. Mild hemophilia.
C. Uremia.
D. All of the above.
E. None of the above.

16. Causes of early graft thrombosis include which of the following?
A. Technical failure.
B. Poor patient selection (extensive and uncorrected disease beyond the bypassed segments).
C. Graft surface thrombogenicity.
D. Hypercoagulable state.
E. All of the above.

17. Currently, the "gold standard" intraoperative evaluation technique after completion of an infrainguinal bypass is:
A. Operative angiography.
B. Continuous-wave Doppler examination.
C. B-mode ultrasound scanning.
D. Fiberoptic angioscopy.
E. Magnetic resonance angiography.

18. Adjunctive measures that have shown benefit in some studies in maintaining graft patency include which of the following?
A. Aspirin and dipyridamole.
B. Coumadin.
C. Dextran-40.
D. Hemodilution.
E. Pentoxifylline.

19. The *most* important mechanism in the development of a prosthetic graft infection is:
A. Graft implantation under emergency conditions, i.e., ruptured AAA.
B. Bacterial adherence to graft surfaces during implantation.
C. Development of a postoperative wound hematoma.
D. Failure to administer preoperative antibiotics.

20. The microorganisms most responsible for prosthetic graft infections are:
A. Slime-producing *Staphylococcus epidermidis*.
B. Coagulase-negative *Staphylococcus aureus*.
C. Coagulase-positive *Staphylococcus aureus*.
D. *Pseudomonas aueroginosa* species.

21. The most definitive diagnostic method for identifying a graft-enteric erosion/fistula in a patient with upper gastrointestinal hemorrhage and an aortic graft is:
    A. Upper endoscopy.
    B. Indium-labeled leukocyte scan.
    C. Magnetic resonance imaging of the abdomen.
    D. Exploratory celiotomy.

22. The most appropriate treatment for an infected thoracic aorta dacron graft is:
    A. Staged ex-situ axillobifemoral bypass followed by total graft excision.
    B. Perigraft Betadine irrigation and lifetime antibiotic administration.
    C. In situ prosthetic graft replacement using PTFE.
    D. Allograft replacement of the infected graft.

23. An anastomotic aneurysm:
    A. Is the dilatation of an artery at an anastomotic site caused by the hood of a prosthetic graft in an end-to-side anastomosis.
    B. Contains adventitia and media, but lacks intima.
    C. Is a fibrous tissue sac bridging the space between artery and graft at a point of anastomotic disruption.
    D. All of the above.

24. The cause of anastomotic aneurysm is:
    A. Suture failure.
    B. Infection.
    C. Inadequate suture purchase.
    D. Arterial wall degeneration.
    E. Anastomotic stress (traction).
    F. All of the above.

25. An anastomotic aneurysm can best be managed by:
    A. Careful observation with surgical intervention restricted to those anastomotic aneurysms that reach 2.5 times the diameter of the parent artery.
    B. Placing a few "reefing" sutures at the site of obvious disruption.
    C. Detachment and redo of the entire anastomosis with the possibility of interposition of a short segment of additional graft.
    D. Ligation of the graft.

26. Aortoenteric fistula (AEF) is *most commonly* due to:
    A. Intrinsic bowel disease in a segment of bowel adjacent to an aortic prosthesis.
    B. Erosion of aortic prosthesis or an aortoprosthetic anastomosis into any hollow viscus that is not effectively separated from the aortic repair by a layer of healthy tissue.
    C. Occult injury to the duodenum at the time of aneurysm repair.
    D. Primary graft infection producing an abscess with subsequent erosion into the bowel.
    E. Untreated abdominal aortic aneurysm that erodes into the overlying third portion of the duodenum.

27. Gastrointestinal bleeding is:
    A. Always massive in patients with aortoenteric fistula (AEF).
    B. The most common presenting symptom of aortoenteric fistula, causing immediate exsanguination due to direct continuity between the aorta and bowel lumen.
    C. Most commonly caused by aortoenteric fistula in patients with aortic prostheses.
    D. Distinct in its presentation in aortoenteric fistula, which readily distinguishes it from other causes of gastrointestinal bleeding.
    E. Usually characterized by one or more "herald" bleeding episodes in AEF that do not produce immediate exsanguination but stop spontaneously, allowing at least a brief period for investigation.

28. The diagnosis of aortoenteric fistula is most efficaciously established by:
    A. A CT or MR scan followed by endoscopy.
    B. Initial investigation with barium contrast studies to demonstrate a compression defect in the distal duodenum.
    C. Immediate aortography to demonstrate appearance of contrast into the lumen of the bowel or the presence of an anastomotic aneurysm.
    D. Tagged white blood cell or nonspecific (e.g., gallium) radionuclide studies to demonstrate graft infection.
    E. Tagged red cell radionuclide studies to define the presence and level or erosion into the bowel.

29. Surgical therapy for aortoenteric fistula (AEF):
    A. Can be delayed to see if bleeding will recur because in some patients the lesion heals spontaneously.
    B. Always requires graft excision and extra anastomotic bypass to remove the bleeding site and infected prosthesis and restore limb circulation.
    C. Can be managed by closure of the bowel defect, excision of the original prosthesis, debridement of obvious necrotic and infected tissue, and in situ replacement with a new prosthesis if the retroperitoneal area is not grossly infected.
    D. Infrequently requires immediate limb revascularization after graft excision; this step can usually be delayed until it is apparent that collaterals are inadequate.
    E. Always requires aneurysm resection and extra-anatomic bypass for *primary* AEF.

30. Regarding the blood supply of peripheral nerves, the following statements are true *except:*
    A. Metabolic needs of large nerves are met by intraneural blood vessels (vasa nervorum), whereas those of small nerves are met by diffusion from surrounding tissues.
    B. Intraneural blood vessels usually enter nerve trunks at one specific point, frequently near the nerve origin.
    C. The abundant collateral circulation pattern of peripheral nerves explains why occlusion of one nutrient artery rarely produces injury.
    D. The pattern of epineural vessels is remarkably constant in peripheral nerves.
    E. Sympathetically mediated vasoconstriction may be important in the pathogenesis of reflex-sympathetic dystrophy and chronic pain.

31. Ischemia of peripheral nerves:
    A. Affects axoplasmic transport irreversibly after 6–8 hours.
    B. Releases potassium into the extracellular space, causing irreversible depolarization of cell membranes.
    C. Results in irreversible nerve injury before muscle injury, according to almost all investigators.
    D. Produces pathologic changes that correlate well with the severity of chronic ischemia from vascular disease.
    E. In general, affects myelinated nerve fibers more than nonmyelinated fibers, producing axonal degeneration, particularly in the center of nerves.

32. Ischemic neuropathy that is present after repair of acute arterial insufficiency:
    A. Results in sensory losses along well-defined dermatome patterns.
    B. Occurs predictably after 1–2 hours of acute arterial occlusion.
    C. Produces symptoms of burning and paresthetic pain, frequently worse with rest at night.
    D. In *motor* nerve conduction studies, causes decrease or absence of the compound muscle action potential.
    E. In *sensory* nerve conduction studies, causes decrease or absence of conduction velocity, but sensory potential amplitude is normal.

33. The following statement(s) is/are true concerning ischemic mononeuropathy due to atherosclerotic disease:
    A. Compression of the peroneal nerve most commonly occurs at the fibular head, whereas ischemic damage is most frequent at the midportion of the nerve.
    B. A compressive peroneal neuropathy produces local conduction–slowing and block at the fibular head—whereas an ischemic lesion reduces motor and sensory potential amplitudes with uniform conduction velocities.
    C. Femoral neuropathy is rarely caused by diabetes because aortoiliac inflow disease is a relatively uncommon pattern of vascular disease in diabetics.
    D. Femoral nerve lesions produce spastic paralysis of the thigh abductor muscles and numbness over the lateral aspect of the thigh and leg to the level of the malleolus.
    E. Clinical evaluation of a patient with lower limb dysfunction can often help distinguish a lesion of the lumbosacral plexus from one affecting the spinal cord or peripheral nerve, but electromyography is usually essential to confirm the diagnosis.

34. The most important etiologic factor in the development of edema after infrainguinal bypass for chronic ischemia is:
    A. Deep venous thrombosis.
    B. Reperfusion injury caused by free oxygen radicals.
    C. Swelling of the smooth muscle cells causing elevated compartment pressures.
    D. Loss of autoregulation of the arteriolar smooth muscle.
    E. Lymphatic interruption.

35. Symptomatic retroperitoneal lymphocele following aortofemoral bypass that recurs after percutaneous aspiration should be treated with:
    A. Observation, intravenous antibiotics.
    B. Establishing a closed irrigation-drainage system.
    C. Unroofing the lymphocele, oversewing the lymphatic leak, and covering the exposed graft by omentum.
    D. Repeated aspirations.
    E. Injection of sclerosant into the lymphocele.

36. Three weeks after repair of an abdominal aortic aneurysm, a 73-year-old male patient develops ascites. The diagnosis of chylous ascites is made if the analysis of the abdominal fluid obtained with paracentesis reveals:
    A. A specific gravity ≥1.012.
    B. A protein content ≤1 g/dl.
    C. A fat content ranging from 0.4 to 4 g/dl.
    D. Fat in the fluid that stains positively with Sudan stain.
    E. Amylase ≥100 IU/dl.

37. The cysterna chyli:
    A. Is located on the right side of the inferior vena cava.
    B. Is usually at the level of the fourth lumbar vertebra.
    C. Is present in almost all patients.
    D. Is formed by the right and left lumbar and the mesenteric lymphatic trunks.
    E. Is usually between the aorta and vena cava.

38. The main route of arterial blood supply to the penis includes all of the following *except:*
    A. Common iliac artery.
    B. Internal pudendal artery.
    C. Anterior division of the internal iliac artery.
    D. Posterior division of the internal iliac artery.

39. Penile erection requires all of the following *except*:
    A. Intact innervation of the penis.
    B. Penile smooth muscle constriction.
    C. A penile/brachial blood pressure index >0.6.
    D. Normal subtunical venule constriction.

40. Which of the following have been implicated as causes of impotence following aortoiliac revascularization? (1) Penile ischemia; (2) psychological problems; (3) nerve injury; (4) endocrine dysfunction.
    A. 1, 2, and 3.
    B. 1 and 3.
    C. 2 and 4.
    D. 4 only.
    E. All of the above.

41. Which of the following may increase the likelihood of iatrogenic sexual dysfunction following aortoiliac revascularization? (1) Left-sided aortic dissection; (2) end-to-end aortic anastomosis; (3) opening iliac artery aneurysms; (4) internal iliac artery ligation.
    A. 1, 2, and 3.
    B. 1 and 3.
    C. 2 and 4.
    D. 4 only.
    E. All of the above.

42. Treatment of iatrogenic impotence following aortoiliac revascularization may commonly include: (1) penile prosthesis; (2) lumbar sympathectomy; (3) penile revascularization; (4) hormonal therapy.
    A. 1, 2, and 3.
    B. 1 and 3.
    C. 2 and 4.
    D. 4 only.
    E. All of the above.

6

Answers

1. The answer is **E** (Rutherford, 4th ed., pp. 528–529).

All of the variables listed are commonly associated with an unfavorable alteration in the balance between myocardial oxygen supply and demand. The majority of coronary perfusion occurs during diastole, when the perfusion pressure across the coronary vascular bed is the greatest. Tachycardia decreases the duration of diastole, so there is less time for coronary perfusion. Tachycardia also increases myocardial oxygen requirements. A reduction in the oxygen-carrying capacity of the blood from anemia, or a reduction in the inspired oxygen fraction, makes less oxygen available to the myocardium. Hypertension produces an increase in myocardial oxygen requirements. Systemic hypotension decreases the perfusion gradient across the coronary vascular bed, thereby reducing oxygen delivery.

2. The answer is **C** (Rutherford, 4th ed., pp. 531–533).

Redistribution of thallium on a preoperative scan, particularly if present in the anatomic distribution of *multiple* coronary arteries, has been reported to accurately predict postoperative cardiac events, although this an area of controversy. In general, fixed defects represent areas of scarred myocardium and unless very extensive are not associated with increased cardiac risk. Some fixed defects seen on a 3-hour scan may represent very poorly perfused areas of myocardium, which may reperfuse after a second injection of thallium and a third scan.

3. The answers are **C, D** (Rutherford, 4th ed., pp. 534–535).

The fact that inhalation agents decrease heart rate, blood pressure, and myocardial oxygen consumption makes them useful agents in patients with coronary artery disease provided that diastolic blood pressure is maintained. Available prospective studies have failed to show that the incidence of cardiac complications is less with epidural than general anesthesia, although a large multicenter trial is currently under way. However, epidural anesthesia is advantageous in the patient with COPD and enhances postoperative pulmonary toilet. Both clamping and declamping of the aorta can produce diminished coronary perfusion, reduce myocardial oxygen delivery, and precipitate a myocardial injury. The use of vasodilators prior to clamping and volume loading prior to unclamping are important to maintain optimal coronary perfusion.

4. The answer is **true** (Rutherford, 4th ed., pp. 540–541).

Nonpulmonary causes of respiratory compromise occur frequently and are important to recognize because, in most instances, they are readily treatable. Moreover, when prompt recognition and treatment do not occur, they often rapidly cause respiratory failure. Nonparenchymal/nonpulmonary causes of respiratory compromise can be grouped into three major categories: (1) CNS, (2) mechanical, (3) upper airway. Excessive anesthesia, sedation, and/or narcotic administration, provision of excess oxygen to patients with COPD or other advanced chronic lung disorders, or retention of CO_2 from any mechanical cause can lead to CNS-mediated respiratory arrest. In such circumstances, pharmacologic reversal or temporary ventilator support is usually adequate treatment. Mechanical problems such as malplaced oral or nasotracheal tubes, pneumo- and hemothorax (and tension pneumothorax), gastrointestinal dilatation causing ventilatory compromise, or aspiration and abdominal tamponade from hemoperitoneum are usually readily recognized. Because these disorders can occur unexpectedly and progress rapidly, constant awareness of their potential is mandatory. The airway is particularly vulnerable during transfers from the operating room to the recovery room or from the recovery room to the surgical intensive care unit or when patients are en route to diagnostic studies. Observations for properly secured airway, proper positioning of orotracheal tubes, and attentiveness to chest wall motion and the presence of bilateral breast sounds should suffice in most cases.

5. The answers are **A, C** (Rutherford, 4th ed., pp. 538–540).

The identification of patients who are high risk for pulmonary complications is fundamental for minimizing their effect on postoperative outcome. Vascular patients require skillful clinical appraisal of potential pulmonary risk. This assessment includes a careful general medical history and physical examination, a chest x-ray, and when indicated, formal pulmonary function testing. Specific signs and symptoms are sought (Table 32-1, p. 539). Patients with limited exercise tolerance due to severe intermittent claudication may be particularly difficult to assess with respect to pulmonary compromise. Not every patient requires formal pulmonary function testing. However, if the planned procedure requires an upper abdominal, thoracic, or thoracoabdominal incision, the patient is older than 45 years, and/or there are any positive historical or physical findings, a chest x-ray and room air arterial blood gases should be obtained. In addition, in patients undergoing major vascular reconstruction, any positive finding in the general history or physical exam should motivate more detailed assessment. Bedside spirometry measures tidal volume, respiratory capacity, vital capacity, and maximum voluntary ventilation. Significant abnormalities in bedside spirometry mandate formal pulmonary function testing and should trigger preoperative referral to the anesthesia service. Routine consultation by a pulmonary medicine specialist is not required by all patients.

6. The answers are **A, B, C** (Rutherford, 4th ed., pp. 540–542).

Highly individualized operative planning is essential to minimize pulmonary risk in specific patients. The use of retroperitoneal versus transabdominal approaches, transverse rather than vertical incisions, and spinal/epidural anesthesia rather than general anesthesia are valuable techniques in patients with respiratory compromise. Clearly, the operation itself and the technical requirements for access are the principle determinants of surgical approach, and secure control of the airway may obviate any perceived benefit to spinal/epidural anesthesia. Optimal outcomes depend upon minimizing any and all adverse effects from the planned surgical procedure, the necessary anesthesia, and postoperative analgesics. Detection and preoperative correction of deficits in hemoglobin and nutritional status, as well as vigorous deep-breathing exercises through instruction and short-term training with an incentive spirometer, will lessen potentially serious postoperative pulmonary complications. In addition, patients with bronchospasm should be treated with bronchodilators; those with chronic bronchitis or infection require treatment with antibiotics. Aerosolized mucolytic agents and bronchodilators are considered useful in the postoperative period when atelectasis develops. Intermittent positive pressure breathing (IPPB) by itself is not useful.

7. The answers are **B, D** (Rutherford, 4th ed., p. 542).

Adult respiratory distress syndrome (ARDS) is a generic term that refers to a number of conditions which present as acute respiratory distress and resemble, in some ways, cardiogenic pulmonary edema. Distinguishing features include pulmonary capital wedge pressure, which is low or normal, and other important clinical and radiologic differences. The mechanism of this "low-pressure pulmonary edema" is an abnormally permeable capillary membrane precipitated by specific mediators. While the list of predisposing clinical factors contributing to ARDS in general patient populations is long, certain of these commonly occur in vascular patients. Systemic shock and prolonged ischemia of gut and/or skeletal muscle, vigorous fluid resuscitation, and multiple transfusions (as might occur with a ruptured aneurysm) are widely recognized as precipitating ARDS. Hypothermia may also play an important role in this syndrome.

8. The answer is **B** (Rutherford, 4th ed., pp. 550–551).

Dehydration is a major risk factor for acceleration of the risk of contrast-induced renal failure. Therefore, hydration, not diuresis, is important in prearteriogram preparation. In addition, limitations of total contrast load and the use of Manitol to maximize urine flow immediately after arteriography further diminish the risk of acute renal failure following arteriography. In addition to its osmotic effects, Mannitol has efficacy as a free radical scavenger. Use of nonionic contrast agents may also diminish postarteriography renal failure, although this has not been proved conclusively.

9. The answer is **D** (Rutherford, 4th ed., pp. 543–545, 547).

The postischemic form of acute renal failure is initiated through tubular luminal obstruction caused by sloughed tubular cells. The resultant tubular obstruction is postulated to first cause a transtubular back leak of glomerular filtration. Because obstruction of tubular flow also leads to an increase in the tubular luminal hydrostatic pressure, differential exists between the glomerular filtration. Then, because of the increased interstitial permeability of the tubular lining and the resultant increased interstitial oncotic pressure, further back diffusion of filtered water occurs.

10. The answers are **A, E** (Rutherford 4th ed., p. 547).

Myoglobinuria is an important cause of renal failure in patients undergoing revascularization of limbs with prolonged extreme ischemia. Circulating as a breakdown product of muscle necrosis, myoglobin is freely filtered by the glomerulus. Myoglobin exerts its toxicity through direct tubular cell injury and through precipitation and obstruction of the tubule. Precipitation is inversely related to the pH of urine—that is, greater precipitation occurs in the presence of low pH. Therefore, prevention of injury to the kidney is directed toward maximizing urine flow rate with intravenous crystalloid infusion and diuretics, and by the alkalinization of the urine.

11. The answer is **E** (Rutherford, 4th ed., pp. 563, 565).

All coagulation factors are synthesized entirely or in part by the liver. In complete liver failure, 8 liters of plasma would be required each day to compensate for lack of synthesis and consumption. Renal insufficiency often accompanies hepatic insufficiency, which limits the volume of fluid that can be infused. Moreover, the renal disorder often results in platelet dysfunction. In patients with liver disease, the normal activators and inhibitors of the fibrinolytic system may become unbalanced, and systemic fibrinolysis can occur, jeopardizing hemostasis by attacking functionally adequate hemostatic plugs. Finally, it is well to remember that most bleeding occurs because of anatomical lesions—in the gastrointestinal track, in the postoperative state, etc.

12. The answers are **A, D, E** (Rutherford, 4th ed., pp. 555–556, 565–566).

Whereas inhibitors to coagulation do not always cause bleeding, they should always be investigated in those patients who do have bleeding. Catastrophic bleeding can result if surgery is undertaken in a patient who has a circulating inhibitor to a specific coagulation factor. These inhibitors are seen most frequently in hemophiliacs, who have an incidence as high as 6–10%. The pathogenesis of these nonspecific inhibitors is not known. Hemophiliacs, the most severely affected and, hence, commonly transfused patients, acquire these antibodies more frequently, suggesting that the immune system is producing alloantibodies in response to the transfused antigens. Circulating inhibitors to coagulation occur in the clinical setting of malignancy, in women just after parturition, and as a result of an adverse drug reaction. The inhibitors can appear suddenly and result in major hemorrhage.

13. The answers are **A, B** (Rutherford, 4th ed., p. 564).

Hemophilia A is a deficiency of Factor VIII, and hemophilia B, a less common type, is a deficiency of Factor IX. The clinical manifestations of hemophilia result from failure to amplify the initiation of hemostasis: deep bruises into muscle, spontaneous bleeding into joints, and frequent rebleeding from deep cuts well after hemostasis has been secured. Hemophiliacs do not bleed or bruise after superficial cuts and trauma and bleed only from mucosal surfaces when there is significant trauma to the surface or there is an underlying lesion such as a tumor or ulcer. The ability to initiate coagulation is intact in patients with hemophilia, and this explains why patients with only mild to moderate disease can escape detection well into middle age or until significant trauma or bleeding during surgery uncovers the defect.

14. The answers are **A, C** (Rutherford, 4th ed., pp. 556–557).

When plasma is frozen and then thawed slowly, a 10–20-ml precipitate develops in the bottom of the plasma container. This precipitate, called cryoprecipitate, contains virtually all of the Factor VIII complex, fibrinogen, fibronectin, or cold insoluble globulin in the parent unit of plasma, as well as variable amounts of other coagulation factors. However, there are negligible amounts of Factors IX, XII, and II (prothrombin) in cryoprecipitate.

15. The answer is **D** (Rutherford, 4th ed., p. 563).

Desmopressin (DDAVP) is an analogue of antidiuretic hormone, which is used as a vasoconstrictor. DDAVP stimulates release of Factor VIII and von Willebrand Factor from endothelium. This can result in a two- to threefold increase in plasma levels of von Willebrand Factor. DDAVP infusions can be effective for treatment of acute bleeding episodes in patients with Type I von Willebrand disease, who have the capacity to produce all sizes of VWF multimers. It is ineffective in patients with Type III disease, who cannot produce any VWF, and in those with Type IIa, who do not form the larger multimers. In the presence of renal disease, DDAVP promotes elevated concentrations of noradrenaline in the circulating plasma approximately 1–4 hours after the infusion. Small increases in the concentration of noradrenaline improve platelet function, probably by sensitizing or activating the alpha adrenergic receptors of platelets. This effect of producing a tide of noradrenaline is independent of its effects of inducing the release of high molecular weight hemostatically active Factor VIII/VWF from the endothelial cells. Increased concentration of the high multimeric forms of Factor VIII/VWF released from endothelial cells by DDAVP and the increased noradrenaline concentration acts synergistically to improve initiation and primary hemostasis sufficient to overcome the impediment to initiation of coagulation in renal failure.

16. The answer is **E** (Rutherford, 4th ed., pp. 572–574).

Early postoperative graft thrombosis occurs 2–20% of the time, depending upon the location of the graft, the size of the arteries, the extent of disease, and the type of graft used. The likely etiology of graft thrombosis changes as the time from implantation increases. Early postoperative thrombosis is generally attributed to technical error or poor patient selection. Occlusions occurring after the first few days but within one month may be due to more subtle technical imperfections; persistent underlying disease either proximal or distal to the bypassed segment; surface thrombogenicity of the graft, which exceeds its thrombotic threshold; and/or an underlying hypercoagulable state that has not been identified or treated. Each of these potential etiologies is preferably addressed prior to the redo revascularization procedure and must be specifically evaluated when treating patients for acute postoperative thrombosis.

17. The answer is **A** (Rutherford, 4th ed., pp. 574–575).

It has been shown that up to 25% of early graft thrombosis can be avoided with proper intraoperative evaluation. Some method of intraoperative detection of technical errors should be part of the operative routine, particularly after infrainguinal arterial reconstruction. Currently, the most practical method of evaluating the bypass intraoperatively is completion arteriography, which will identify problematic lesions and allow for their immediate correction, thereby reducing the incidence of early graft failure by up to 25%. In selected centers, B-mode imaging and fiberoptic angioscopy have been shown to be reliable methods, but results have not been consistently good in all reports. Moreover, the technology is not uniformly available for intraoperative use. Auscultation of the graft, anastomoses, and vessels adjacent to each anastomosis with a continuous-wave Doppler is easily accomplished and is a rapid screening examination that indicates velocity changes suspicious for underlying lesions and should be part of the operative routine. However, as a single test, the continuous-wave Doppler is inadequate in most instances.

18. The answers are **A, B, C** (Rutherford, 4th ed., pp. 575–576).

The combination of aspirin and dipyridamole has been shown to reduce platelet deposition on prosthetic femoral-popliteal bypasses compared to placebo. Whether the same benefit would be observed from aspirin alone has not been studied. Long-term patency of coronary artery bypass grafts is improved by aspirin and dipyridamole, shown by prospective, randomized double-blind trials. Dextran-40, which is a drug that decreases viscosity, reduces platelet adhesiveness, and reduces Factor VIII activity, has also been shown in prospective clinical studies to extend early patency of lower-extremity bypass grafts, particularly in composite (prosthetic plus vein) grafts and in complex infrageniculate bypasses. Warfarin compounds have been shown to increase antithrombin III levels and are associated with better long-term patency compared to patients not treated with long-term anticoagulants. However, not all studies have shown efficacy, and the risk of hemorrhage is substantial. A multicenter trial of Coumadin treatment after infraingiunal bypass is currently under way, sponsored by the Department of Veterans Affairs. Hemodilution and pentoxifylline produce favorable rheologic effects, but their efficacy in preventing graft thrombosis has not been rigorously studied.

19. The answer is **B** (Rutherford, 4th ed., pp. 588–591).

The pathogenesis of prosthetic graft infection involves several fundamental steps, including bacterial adhesion, microcolony formation within a biofilm, and activation of host defenses. The initiating event is bacterial adherence to the graft surface. Without bacterial adherence, the infectious process cannot become established, and host defenses can eradicate the inoculum. Bacterial adherence depends on a number of factors, including the bacterial cell wall features, microorganism growth characteristics, and physical and chemical properties of the biomaterial. Staphylococcal species demonstrate increased adherence to vascular prostheses compared to gram-negative bacteria, largely due to cell wall exopolysaccharides with specific adhesion to biomaterial surface receptors. Slime-producing staphylococcal strains adhere in greater number than strains without this characteristic. In addition to promoting adherence, the slime biofilm produced by the microorganisms protects against host defenses and antibiotics.

20. The answer is **C** (Rutherford, 4th ed., pp. 591–592).

Although the frequency of late-appearing graft infections caused by coagulase-negative staphylococcal species has increased, coagulase-positive *S. aureus* is the most common pathogen in graft infections responsible for approximately one half of infections. *S. aureus* is the infecting organism in approximately 90% of infrainguinal and extra-anatomic prosthetic graft infections and two thirds of early (less than 4 months) aortic graft infections. *S. epidermidis* strains and gram-negative bacteria account for the majority of late-appearing graft infections, with the latter organisms involved in graft-enteric erosion or fistula. Pathogenic *S. aureus* strains produce hemolysis and toxins to leukoctyes, which result in a virulent infection with classic signs of fever, leukocytosis, and perigraft pus with soft tissue invasion and necrosis.

21. The answer is **D** (Rutherford, 4th ed., pp. 592–595).

Prompt diagnosis and treatment of prosthetic graft infections are essential to avoid complications. Clinical manifestations are varied and may be subtle, particularly for grafts confined to the abdomen or thorax. Operative exploration is the most accurate method to exclude infection of a vascular prosthesis and may be required when clinical suspicion of graft enteric erosion exists. In equivocal cases, vascular surgeons must prove that graft infection is not present. Endoscopy is an important diagnostic modality in patients with suspected secondary aortoenteric fistula. The entire upper gastrointestinal track should be inspected, including the third and fourth portions of the duodenum, which are the most common sites of graft enteric fistula. Patients with recent massive gastrointestinal hemorrhage should be examined by endoscopy in the operating room with preparation for operation should exsanguination from the fistula be induced. A negative examination does *not* exclude the possibility of an aortoduodenal fistula. White blood cell scans have variable utility in the diagnosis of graft infections. False negative studies in early graft infections are unusual, so exclusion of early graft infection is possible, but normal studies have been reported in late-appearing aortic graft infection complicated by graft enteric erosion. A positive scan is associated with a positive predictive value of 80%. Magnetic resonance imaging (MRI) is useful in differentiating between perigraft fluid collection versus inflammation of the perigraft tissues. MRI and CT scanning, however, share the common limitation that they cannot delineate a perigraft abscess from sterile perigraft fluid.

22. The answer is **C** (Rutherford, 4th ed., pp. 595–602).

In situ replacement of prosthetic grafts is controversial. It should be applied only in carefully selected patients. When infection involves the thoracic aorta, in situ replacement may be the only practical approach because there is no simple means of extra-anatomic bypass as there is with abdominal aortic graft infection. In situ allograft replacement is fraught with the risk of later degeneration of allografts and pseudoaneurysm formation. Local therapy with irrigation is not recommended.

23. The answer is **C** (Rutherford, 4th ed., p. 604).

An anastomotic aneurysm is produced by a partial or complete disruption of a graft-to-artery anastomosis. The disruption usually takes place slowly, such that the fibrous tissue bond between graft and artery stretches and dilates. It is this fibrous tissue sac, containing blood, that dilates and takes on an aneurysmal configuration. The wall of the sac is entirely fibrous tissue and lacks any of the layers found within an artery wall.

24. The answer is **F** (Rutherford, 4th ed., pp. 604–606).

In the past, the commonest cause of anastomotic aneurysm was suture failure. The practice in the early history of vascular surgery was to utilize silk suture material for performing an anastomosis. Since silk is a biologic material, it underwent degeneration and absorption by phagocytosis. Primary bonding between graft and artery does not occur, and therefore the integrity of an anastomosis is forever dependent upon the integrity of the suture line. With the introduction of modern permanent sutures, the incidence of anastomotic aneurysm has sharply dropped. Currently, the most common cause of anastomotic aneurysm is probably infection. However, any factor leading to potential discontinuity between graft and artery, such as inadequate suture purchase, undue stress or traction between the artery and the graft, or degeneration within the arterial wall itself can lead to anastomotic separation.

25. The answer is **C** (Rutherford, 4th ed., pp. 608–610).

Once an anastomotic aneurysm is discovered, it should be surgically repaired unless the patient is terminally ill. The anastomotic aneurysm will continue to enlarge and with delay in surgical correction it becomes more difficult to repair as well as increases the potential for complications. The correct method of repair of an anastomotic aneurysm includes exposure of the distal graft and proximal and distal artery at the site of the anastomosis. The anastomosis should be taken down completely and the aneurysm wall trimmed. If it appears that there has been shortening of the graft, it may be best to resect a segment of the graft and interpose a new segment to be certain that there is no undue traction upon the new anastomotic site. Resecting a section of old graft also permits the opportunity to send this for culture to make sure that a low-grade infection is not the cause of the aneurysm. A new anastomosis will permit proper suture purchase and will limit the potential for suture pull-through or repeat anastomotic disruption. Ligation of a patent graft will produce extremity ischemia.

26. The answer is **B** (Rutherford, 4th ed., pp. 611–612).

The most common etiology of aortoenteric fistula is erosion of an anastomosis or an uncovered graft directly into overlying bowel, usually the third or fourth portion of the duodenum. Primary aortoenteric fistula due to direct erosion of an aneurysm into this segment of the duodenum is much less frequently encountered. The influence of graft infection on subsequent aortoenteric fistula is not well characterized.

27. The answer is **E** (Rutherford, 4th ed., pp. 611–612).

Gastrointestinal bleeding, although frequently the initial symptom of aortoenteric fistula, is not *always* present and usually does not often proceed to *immediate* exsanguination. Characteristically, hemorrhage will stop spontaneously and recur one or more times over a period of hours or days—so-called herald bleeding—until exsanguination finally occurs. Characteristic symptoms of gastrointestinal bleeding from aortoenteric fistula are otherwise indistinguishable from other causes of gastrointestinal hemorrhage, although there should be a high index of suspicion that an aortoenteric fistula is present when GI bleeding occurs in *any* patient with an aortic graft. However, even in patients with aortic prostheses, gastrointestinal bleeding is still most commonly due to primary gastrointestinal conditions and not AEF or aortoenteric erosion.

28. The answer is **A** (Rutherford, 4th ed., pp. 612–616).

CT or MRI should be the primary diagnostic maneuver in patients suspected of having aortoenteric fistula. This can establish the diagnosis by demonstrating an anastomotic aneurysm in direct association with the bowel wall or bowel erosion, and/or it may demonstrate perigraft air or fluid, suggesting associated graft infection. Upper gastrointestinal endoscopy is the next most valuable study and should generally be carried out as soon as the CT or MRI is completed, unless the imaging study unequivocally establishes the diagnosis. Arteriography occasionally demonstrates an anastomotic aneurysm, but will rarely reveal extravasation of contrast into the bowel. Barium studies identify primary gastrointestinal pathology but do not distinguish bleeding from nonbleeding lesions. Moreover, barium within the bowel precludes later arteriography and may interfere with postoperative bowel function. Radionuclide studies are helpful when there is a continued suspicion that an aortoenteric fistula is present and all other studies are negative.

29. The answer is **C** (Rutherford, 4th ed., pp. 616–618).

As soon as the diagnosis of AEF is either established or strongly suspected by virtue of the clinical picture and preliminary diagnostic procedures, surgical intervention should be carried out promptly. There is usually sufficient time from the initial bleeding to subsequent massive bleeding to perform the necessary diagnostic studies in anticipation of laparotomy. Closure of the bowel defect and in situ revascularization is the treatment of choice for primary fistula owing to abdominal aortic aneurysm. This procedure also may be employed selectively for secondary fistulas when the associated graft infection is minimal and the fistula is confined to the proximal small bowel or duodenum. More extensive graft and retroperitoneal infection require excision of the prosthesis. Extra-anatomic bypass in patients requiring graft excision may be preferable as the initial step when the diagnosis is clear and the patient is stable, but will be the second step when these criteria are not present. Limb revascularization should be done immediately after graft excision unless there is good evidence that adequate collateral circulation is present. Undue delay in performing revascularization will result in a frequent occurrence of limb loss and increased mortality.

30. The answers are **B, D** (Rutherford, 4th ed., p. 620).

Intraneural blood vessels (vasa nervorum) supply the metabolic needs of large nerves, whereas diffusion from surrounding tissues provides nutrients for small nerves. The vasa nervorum arrive from nearby major arteries and enter nerve trunks at *multiple levels,* frequently near joints. The epineural arteries branch and then arteriolar and precapillary branches penetrate the perineurium to perfuse the endoneurium. There is a complete terminal network of capillaries through the perineurium that provides blood supply to nerves at some distance from the nutrient arteries. Peripheral nerves have abundant collateral blood vessels (which explains why occlusion of one nutrient artery rarely produces injury). Regional nutrient arteries have been ligated over considerable lengths of a nerve trunk without disturbing blood supply to the nerve or adversely affecting structure and function of nerve fibers. Extensive studies of the microvascularature of peripheral nerves have demonstrated that the organization of vasa nervorum is such that a total interruption of circulation in nerves is very unlikely unless very drastic interference with blood supply is produced. The pattern of epineural vessels *varies* in different nerves, and some nerves may be more susceptible than others to ischemia. Sympathetic nerve fibers innervate vessels in the epineurium and perineurium. High sympathetic tone may significantly reduce intraneural circulation. Sympathetically mediated vasoconstriction may be important in the pathogenesis of reflex sympathetic dystrophy and chronic pain.

31. The answers are **A, B, E** (Rutherford, 4th ed., pp. 620–621).

A short period of experimental ischemia results in disturbed function of nerves, which can recover if circulation is restored. Severe acute ischemia appears to result in decreased or abolished conduction of impulses. Thus, if ischemia is of short duration or is mild, function in peripheral nerves can be impaired in a transient manner. However, if ischemia is prolonged or severe, damage may be permanent. Exactly how these functional changes of nerve occur is unknown. Clearly, ischemia impairs the metabolic processes that maintain the ionic gradient necessary for impulse transmission. Fast axoplasmic transport also depends on adequate blood supply. The transport of material in the axon is impaired by ischemia at the same time as conduction is impaired, suggesting that both depend on the same sources of energy. The block of fast axoplasmic transport becomes irreversible after 6–8 hours of ischemia. The permeability of endoneurial vessels during ischemia is impaired after 8–10 hours. Metabolic factors, including anoxia, hypercapnia, hyperkalemia, and acidosis, are probably important. Potassium in the extracellular space during anoxia may cause irreversible depolarization of cell membranes. There is controversy about the relative vulnerability of nerve and muscle to ischemia. Most older literature reports that muscle is more sensitive to ischemia than nerves. However, experimental results have been inconsistent, and Chervu et al. have recently shown that peripheral nerve is more susceptible to ischemia than skeletal muscle. Both muscle and nerves show significant pathologic changes after ischemia. A combination of segmental demyelination and axonal degeneration is found on pathologic section of nerve biopsies in patients with chronic arterial insufficiency. Both large fibers and small fibers are equally affected, but the severity of the pathologic changes do *not* correlate well with the severity of vascular disease. In experimental studies in animals, myelinated fibers are affected more by ischemia than unmyelinated fibers, producing axonal degeneration, particularly in the center of nerves.

32. The answers are **C, D** (Rutherford, 4th ed., pp. 621–622).

The clinical features of ischemic neuropathy following acute arterial insufficiency consist of several findings. One of the earliest symptoms is sensory loss noted by patients in the distalmost part of the area supplied by the ischemic nerve. Sensory losses in a stocking-glove pattern are often associated with distal muscle wasting and weakness and, sometimes, by late fibrosis and contracture. Although malpractice attorneys often ask expert witnesses to testify regarding an exact period of ischemia after which ischemic neuropathy is unavoidable, such a time period is quite variable depending on the degree of ischemia and the pre-existence of collateral circulation. In general, irreversible changes do occur after 6–8 hours, but even this figure is inexact. Typically, patients with ischemic neuropathy complain of pain that is burning and paresthetic in nature, frequently worse with rest and at night, and unaffected or relieved by walking. This is in marked contrast to the pain of claudication and is not consistent with ischemic rest pain either. Careful electrophysiologic studies can establish the diagnosis of ischemic neuropathy and define its severity. Usually, a unilateral axonal neuropathy involving distal nerves is present. Motor nerve conduction studies show a decrease or absence of the compound muscle action potential amplitude when the nerve is stimulated. Sensory nerve conduction studies show decreased or absent sensory potential amplitudes, whereas sensory conduction velocity, where recordable, is normal.

33. The answers are **B, E** (Rutherford, 4th ed., pp. 622–624).

The peroneal nerve diverges from the main vessels in the calf and is supplied in the region of the fibular head by small adjacent arteries. At the neck of the fibula, the major intraneural vessels occupy a superficial position that may expose them to damage from pressure. In the calf, the posterior tibial and peroneal nerve receive branches from the anterior and posterior tibial arteries. The intraneural arterial pattern in the buttock and thigh contain several arterial channels of fairly large caliber, whereas below the knee, one major vessel usually dominates. The peroneal nerve at the knee and perhaps the more distal portions of the peroneal and posterior tibial nerves may therefore be more liable to ischemic damage. Thus, while the nature of the vascular supply to the peroneal nerve at the fibular head predisposes it to ischemic damage, this is also the area where the nerve is prone to compression. Peroneal neuropathy presents with weakness of dorsal flexion and eversion of the ankle with preservation of inversion and plantar flexion, functions of the posterior calf muscles. The sensory deficit is confined to the dorsum of the foot. It is possible to confirm the diagnosis with nerve conduction studies that will demonstrate abnormality in peroneal function while all other nerve conduction is intact. It is usually possible to distinguish a compressive peroneal neuropathy, which produces a local area of conduction slowing and block at the fibular head, from an ischemic lesion, which is primarily axonal in nature and produces uniform conduction velocity throughout the length of the nerve and reduction in the motor and sensory potential amplitudes. Femoral neuropathy is a frequent complication of diabetes and is presumably due to abnormalities at the vasa nervorum. A femoral nerve lesion results in flaccid paralysis of the quadriceps muscle and absent knee jerk and loss of sensation over the anterior and medial thigh and inner aspect of the calf down to the level of the medial malleolus. Electrophysiologic studies show decreased or absent motor-evoked response from the quadriceps muscle when the femoral nerve is stimulated in the groin and an absent saphenous sensory potential at the ankle, together with fibrillation potentials and motor unit loss on needle electrode examination of the quadriceps muscle. Study of other nerves in the limb will be normal. Whether lumbosacral plexus lesions (rather than lower cord or cauda equina ischemia) result from occlusive vascular disease is not well documented. However, these lesions have been described after resection of an abdominal aortic aneurysm and aortobifemoral bypass grafting. Blood supply to the lumbosacral plexus is through five lumbar arteries from each side of the abdominal aorta, the deep circumflex iliac artery, a branch of the external iliac artery, and the iliolumbar and gluteal branches of the internal iliac artery. Clinical evaluation of the patient with unilateral lower limb dysfunction can often distinguish a lesion of the lumbosacral plexus from one affecting the spinal cord or a major peripheral nerve. Weakness involves proximal muscles as well as distal muscles. The limb is flaccid and areflexic with no response to plantar stimulation. This is in contrast to a spinal lesion, which produces a spastic hyper-reflexic limb with extensive plantar response and dissociated sensory loss. Electromyography is usually essential to confirm the diagnosis.

34. The answer is **E** (Rutherford, 4th ed., pp. 625–626).

Insufficiency of lymphatic transport plays the most important role in the development of postbypass edema. Lymphatic insufficiency develops for two main reasons. First, there is increased production of interstitial fluid following successful revascularization, which results in significant increase in the lymphatic load. More importantly, however, the transport capacity of the lymphatic system is reduced because of lymphatic injury and obstruction of major lymph channels. The incidence of deep venous thrombosis is not higher in those patients who develop postoperative edema compared to those without edema. Reperfusion injury is more significant in revascularization for acute ischemia than in patients who undergo infrainguinal bypass for chronic ischemia. Elevated compartment pressures are not typical in patients who develop postbypass edema. Loss of autoregulation of the arteriolar smooth muscle is a contributing factor in postbypass edema, but it plays a relatively minor role.

35. The answer is **C** (Rutherford, 4th ed., pp. 629–630).

Small asymptomatic retroperitoneal lymphoceles can be observed and followed with ultrasound or serial computed tomography. However, patients who develop abdominal pain or distention and an abdominal or flank mass should have needle aspiration of the lymphocele under computed tomography or ultrasound guidance. This maneuver is both diagnostic and therapeutic. Placement of an in-dwelling irrigation drainage system is associated with a high risk of infection. Therefore, if aspiration is unsuccessful, abdominal exploration, unroofing of the lymphocele, and oversewing or ligating the site of lymphatic injury is performed. Visualization of the site of the lymphatic injury can be facilitated by injecting 5 cc of lymphazurine dye into the ipsilateral foot subcutaneously between the first and third interdigital spaces. If the prosthetic graft is exposed, it should be covered by retroperitoneal tissue or omentum. Injection of sclerosant produces an excessive inflammatory reaction and is not recommended.

36. The answers are **A, C, D** (Rutherford, 4th ed., pp. 630–631).

The diagnosis of chylous ascites is confirmed by paracentesis that verifies the presence of chyle in the ascitic fluid. The chyle is an odorless, sterile, alkaline fluid that is milky in appearance. It has a specific gravity that is greater than 1.012. Its protein content is usually above 3 g/dl, and the fat content ranges from 0.4 to 4 g/dl. The fat in the fluid stains positively with Sudan stain. Amylase is not present in chyle.

37. The answers are **D, E** (Rutherford, 4th ed., p. 631).

To avoid injury to the cysterna chyli during operations on the upper abdominal aorta, it is important to know the usual location of this structure. The cysterna chyli is formed by the right and left lumbar and the mesenteric lymphatic trunks. It is usually located at the level of the second lumbar vertebra between the inferior vena cava and the abdominal aorta. In half of individuals a well-developed cysterna chyli is not present. The thoracic duct originates from the cysterna chyli and ascends upward and posterior to the aorta through the aortic hiatus in the diaphragm.

38. The answer is **D** (Rutherford, 4th ed., pp. 634–635).

The arterial supply to the penis is via the anterior division of the internal iliac artery, which gives rise to the internal pudendal artery. The dorsal penile artery, the deep penile artery, and the urethral artery arise from the internal pudendal artery.

39. The answer is **B** (Rutherford, 4th ed., p. 635).

Erection results from local genital stimulation or through central psychological stimuli. Either mechanism requires intact penile innervation. Erection is the result of penile smooth muscle *relaxation*, which causes filling of the lacunar spaces with blood as a result of dilatation of the cavernosal and helicine arteries. Increased pressure within the tunica albuginea causes subtunical venule constriction, resulting in blocked venous outflow, all of which leads to penile engorgement.

40. The answer is **A** (Rutherford, 4th ed., pp. 635–636).

Although penile ischemia and nerve injury are the most common reasons for postoperative sexual dysfunction, psychological problems associated with surgery can also occur. Endocrine causes have not been identified as a cause of iatrogenic sexual dysfunction following aortoiliac revascularization.

41. The answer is **E** (Rutherford, 4th ed., pp. 636–639).

Left aortic dissections and opening of iliac aneurysms (especially on the left side) can cause iatrogenic sexual dysfunction because the para-aortic and hypogastric nerve plexuses are in these locations. End-to-end aortic anastomoses can divert pelvic blood flow when retrograde flow from the groins is absent or impaired following aortofemoral bypass, as a result of bilateral external iliac artery occlusion. Internal iliac artery ligation can cause penile ischemia, especially when performed in the presence of ipsilateral external iliac artery occlusion or when ligation is performed bilaterally. Consideration should be given to internal iliac artery revascularization in these circumstances.

42. The answer is **B** (Rutherford, 4th ed., p. 639).

Because nerve injury and penile ischemia are the most common causes of iatrogenic sexual dysfunction following aortoiliac revascularization, it follows that the treatment for these etiologies (1 and 3 respectively) would be most successful for restoring potency. Lumbar sympathectomy is not a treatment for sexual dysfunction and when removing the lumbar ganglia bilaterally, retrograde ejaculation may occur. Endocrine dysfunction is not a cause of sexual dysfunction following aortoiliac revascularization.

7

Acute Arterial Ischemia

1. A 63-year-old man is admitted to the emergency room with a history of 6 hours of a cold and painful right foot. On examination he has normal pulses in the left leg, but there is only a weak femoral pulse on the right and no distal pulses. He has mild hypesthesia and some impairment of intrinsic motor function of the foot. The patient describes having had a recent myocardial infarction. Which of the following is/are preferable?

   A. Admission and observation.
   B. Heparinize the patient followed by fibrinolytic therapy.
   C. Heparinize the patient in preparation for an arteriogram and possible thrombolytic therapy.
   D. Administer 20,000 units of heparin intravenously, and schedule the patient for exploration and removal of suspected embolus.
   E. None of the above.

2. A 17-year-old man is admitted to the hospital after having been involved in an accident in which he was thrown from his motorcycle. He suffered fractures of the tibia and fibula of his left leg. At the time of admission there were no palpable pulses, the foot was cool and blue, and the lower limb was very swollen below the knee. The patient had a palpable femoral pulse on the side with the broken leg and normal pulses on the other side and no previous history of injury. The orthopedic surgeon requests your assistance in evaluating the possibility of vascular injury. Which of the following statements is/are most appropriate in the management of this patient?

   A. Measurements of ankle-brachial pressures; if the index is 0.9 or greater, there is no major arterial obstruction.
   B. Examination of the foot with continuous-wave Doppler; if arterial signals can be detected, severe ischemia is unlikely.
   C. If monophasic Doppler signals are present in the foot and the patient has perception of light touch and intrinsic motor function, orthopedic repair and reduction of the fractures can be performed. A vascular examination is then repeated in the operating room after external fixation of the bones has been obtained.
   D. During the course of the operation femoral arteriography with run-off films may be obtained. If patent vessels are observed and there is no evidence of intraluminal clots, it is likely that the recovery will be uneventful.
   E. If pedal pulses are not detectable and Doppler signals are not detectable at the ankle, the patient can be treated with fibrinolytic therapy after external fixation of the bones has been obtained.

3. A 25-year-old man is admitted to the emergency room after an automobile accident. He has no evidence of injuries of his extremities or abdomen. He is dyspneic and has contusions of the chest. A chest x-ray reveals that the mediastinum is slightly widened, approximately 10 cm in the second interspace in an upright chest film. This finding prompts a thoracic aortogram, which reveals a small false aneurysm of the subclavian artery just *distal* to the left vertebral artery. Which of the following is the best course of action?

   A. The artery should be repaired immediately through a median sternotomy.
   B. It is preferable to wait 8 weeks before attempting repair to allow the swelling to resolve and to reduce the chance of injury to the contiguous nerves.
   C. The artery should be repaired immediately after four vessel arteriograms document that the other vertebral is intact. The preferred approach would be through a left posterior-thoracotomy incision in the fifth interspace.
   D. The patient should be prepared for a thoracotomy as required, but the artery can be approached through the supraclavicular space with division of the clavicular head of the sternocleidomastoid muscle and removal of a portion of the clavicle if neccessary.
   E. None of the above.

4. A young man is admitted after having been shot in the neck. On arrival he was hypotensive and was taken immediately to the operating room because of a large hematoma and continued bleeding. Preoperatively the patient was moving all the extremities. The injuries included damage to the left internal jugular vein and transection of the left internal carotid artery, with brisk back bleeding. The procedure(s) of choice would be:

   A. Ligate both ends of the internal carotid artery.
   B. Reconstruct the internal carotid artery with the use of a dacron prosthetic graft.
   C. Ligate both ends of the internal carotid artery under the protection of systemic heparin followed by Warfarin anticoagulation.
   D. Reconstruct the internal carotid artery utilizing end-to-end anastomosis or an interposition graft of saphenous vein, followed by a completion arteriogram.
   E. Ligate both ends of the internal carotid artery and perform extracranial to intracranial bypass.

5. The most common site of acute obstruction by an arterial embolus is:

   A. The superficial femoral artery at the adductor canal.

B. The common femoral artery bifurcation.
C. The iliac artery bifurcation.
D. The popliteal artery bifurcation.
E. The brachial artery.

6. The most frequent site of origin of arterial emboli is:
A. The left atrium.
B. The left ventricle.
C. Diseased cardiac valves.
D. The thoracic aorta.
E. The abdominal aorta.

7. The most important determinant of the severity and ultimate outcome of an acute embolic arterial occlusion is:
A. Site of obstruction.
B. Duration of occlusion greater than 4–6 hours.
C. Size of the embolus.
D. Adequacy of collateral circulation.
E. Extent of secondary clot propagation.

8. Which of the following findings would be the one *most* reliable in establishing a diagnosis of a lower-extremity arterial embolus versus acute arterial thrombosis?
A. An abnormal EKG with prior myocardial infarction (MI).
B. The presence of full pulses in the opposite leg.
C. The presence of filling defect (clot) in both the profunda and popliteal arteries on arteriogram.
D. Arteriographic demonstration of abrupt occlusion of distal superficial femoral artery with minimal evidence of atherosclerosis elsewhere.
E. No prior history of claudication.

9. Which of the following statements concerning the management of an arterial embolus is/are true?
A. The addition of routine fasciotomy improves the results of surgical embolectomy.
B. Recent experience has shown thrombotic therapy to give results equivalent to catheter embolectomy.
C. The presence of good back bleeding is a reliable sign of successful distal embolectomy.
D. Long-term anticoagulation is unnecessary if a postoperative echocardiogram does not show cardiac thrombus.
E. The reported perioperative mortality of arterial embolectomy is approximately 15%.

10. Which of the following statements regarding atheroembolism is/are true?
A. It is easy to find cholesterol microemboli in amputated tissue after development of the blue toe syndrome.
B. Most episodes of atheroembolism are clinically silent.
C. The clinical presentation of atheroembolism correlates with the type of material embolized and its source.
D. The pathophysiology of microembolism causing amaurosis fugax is different from that of the blue toe syndrome.
E. All of the above.

11. Which of the following statements is/are true?
A. Cholesterol emboli lodge only in peripheral arterioles and capillaries.
B. Degenerative atherosclerosis of the ascending aorta is found in fewer than 5% of patients undergoing coronary bypass.
C. All patients with the blue toe syndrome have a palpable pulse in the affected extremity.
D. Frank digital gangrene usually occurs only after repeated episodes of atheroembolism.
E. None of the above.

12. Which of the following statements is/are true?
A. To heal atheroembolic lesions, the ankle systolic pressure must equal the arm pressure.
B. With severe atheroembolism, biopsy of the gastrocnemius muscle is the most accurate diagnostic test.
C. Work-up of atheroembolism includes duplex ultrasonography to evaluate the size of the popliteal arteries.
D. After atheroembolism has occurred, specific findings are present in the blood count (CBC), BUN, and creatinine.
E. Serum cholesterol levels correlate with cholesterol atheroembolism.

13. Which of the following is/are true?
A. Sympathectomy is no longer part of the treatment of atheroembolism.
B. Lesions causing microemboli from the level of the adductor canal always require formal femoral-popliteal bypass.
C. Over half of the patients suffering their first atheroembolic event will respond to antiplatelet therapy.
D. In disseminated atheroembolism, the kidneys are affected but the intestine is spared.
E. None of the above.

14. All of the following may contribute to development of gangrene after intra-arterial drug injection *except:*
A. The sedative effect of the drug allowing prolonged tourniquet time.
B. Local arterial injury.
C. Drug-induced vasodilation.
D. Drug excipients.
E. Venospasm.

15. The most common site of accidental intra-arterial drug injection is thought to be:
   A. The brachial artery.
   B. The femoral artery.
   C. The carotid artery.
   D. The pulmonary artery.
   E. The radial artery.

16. The following represent appropriate therapy for a mycotic femoral artery pseudoaneurysm after accidental drug injection at the common femoral artery bifurcation *except:*
   A. Resection of the common femoral artery bifurcation and direct revascularization with autologous saphenous vein.
   B. Resection of the common femoral artery bifurcation and extra-anatomic revascularization with prosthetic graft through the obturator canal.
   C. Resection of the common femoral artery bifurcation and extra-anatomic revascularization with autologous saphenous vein through the obturator canal.
   D. Resection of the common femoral artery bifurcation without reconstruction.
   E. Long-term intravenous antibiotics.

17. The following therapy is uniformly successful after accidental intra-arterial drug injection:
   A. Vasodilators.
   B. Streptokinase.
   C. Fasciotomy.
   D. Amputation.
   E. None of the above.

18. The puffy hand syndrome:
   A. Relates to acute intra-arterial drug injection.
   B. Relates to chronic lymphatic and venous obstruction.
   C. Relates to deep compartment infection.
   D. Is best treated with elevation and streptokinase.
   E. None of the above.

19. Traumatic dissection of the thoracic aorta at the isthmus may produce the acute coarctation syndrome. Salient features of this syndrome include:
   A. Superior vena cava syndrome.
   B. Hypertension in the arms and a difference in pulse amplitude between the upper and lower extremities.
   C. Dyspnea, coma, and hypotension.
   D. Interscapular systolic murmur, hoarseness, and pulse deficits.
   E. All of the above.

20. In consideration of the diagnosis of thoracic aortic rupture, the imaging technique with the greatest overall sensitivity and specificity is:
   A. Aortography.
   B. Contrast-enhanced CT scanning.
   C. Ultrasonography.
   D. Two-dimensional transesophageal echo.
   E. Chest x-ray.

21. Injuries to which segment of the abdominal aorta have the highest mortality rate?
   A. Supraceliac.
   B. Infraceliac-suprarenal.
   C. Infrarenal.
   D. Bifurcation.
   E. All of the above have equal mortality rates.

22. In general, isolated lacerations of the inferior vena cava are best repaired by:
   A. Lateral venorrhaphy.
   B. Resection and replacement with a spiral vein graft.
   C. Resection and replacement with an autogenous vein graft.
   D. Resection and replacement with a PTFE prosthetic graft.
   E. Ligation.

23. Which of the following statements regarding acute injuries of the internal carotid artery is/are true?
   A. Contralateral hemiparesis for more than 12 hours is a contraindication to repair of a penetrating wound of the internal carotid artery.
   B. Delayed repair of a laceration of the internal carotid artery is dangerous because of the possibility of causing conversion of a bland cerebral infarct into a hemorrhagic infarct.
   C. Patients with injuries of the carotid artery who are admitted with alterations in consciousness should not be operated upon until they become lucid.
   D. Occlusion of the internal carotid artery as a result of a stab wound should be treated nonoperatively.
   E. None of the above.

24. Patients who have sustained blunt trauma to the carotid artery from motor vehicle accidents may also have injuries of the head and neck. Which of the following statements is/are true?
   A. The clinical features suggestive of blunt trauma are straightforward and consist of contralateral hemiparesis or hemiplegia, difficulty speaking, and ataxia.
   B. Most patients who have injuries to the carotid artery caused by blunt trauma will have bruising, ecchymoses, swelling, or other signs of cervical trauma.
   C. Some patients with blunt trauma to the carotid artery may present with a Horner's syndrome or a transient attack of cerebral ischemia or perhaps only limb paresis.
   D. Hyperextension injuries of the neck usually pro-

duce discrete damage to the carotid artery at the level of the third cervical vertebra.

E. Patients who have had injuries to the carotid artery caused by blunt trauma almost always have signs of neurologic damage if a careful examination is performed.

25. A patient is admitted after having been in a motor vehicle accident in which he sustained steering wheel trauma to the chest. Which of the following statements is/are true?

A. Most patients who have injuries to the great vessels of the arch will have diminished pulses or reduced blood pressures in one or both arms and will usually have evidence of swelling in Burn's space or the supraclavicular space.
B. If the patient has a normal blood pressure and pulse in both upper extremities and no evidence of swelling in the neck and upper chest, an injury of one of the great vessels is extremely rare.
C. A mediastinum more than 6 cm wide in the second interspace in a clear upright chest radiograph is diagnostic of an injury to the aortic arch.
D. If a patient has suspected injuries of the aorta or the subclavian arteries, the preferred exposure is always through a median sternotomy.
E. None of the above.

26. Which of the following diagnostic procedures is *not* routinely used in assessing vascular injuries of the extremities?

A. Physical examination.
B. Angiography.
C. Duplex ultrasonography.
D. Angioscopy.
E. Doppler arterial pressure indexes.

27. Which of the following statements/is are true?

A. The use of arterial or venous shunts is discouraged in the management of vascular injuries of the extremities.
B. Stabilization of the bone should always precede vascular repair in order to protect the repair from movement at the fracture site.
C. Arterial repair should always be performed before venous repair or bone stabilization.
D. Venous reconstruction should precede arterial repair if the injured vein is the sole source of venous return.
E. Stabilizing fractures before vascular repair may block access to the injury.

28. Angiography:

A. Is no longer performed in asymptomatic patients with extremity injuries when proximity is the only indication.
B. Is currently recommended to plan the operative repair in all injuries requiring surgery, especially if distal ischemia is present.
C. Should be performed in every patient with an extremity vascular injury if primary amputation is contemplated.
D. If performed solely for proximity of a wound to a major vessel will reveal a vascular injury in more than 25% of cases.
E. None of the above.

29. Causalgia (or post-traumatic reflex sympathetic dystrophy):

A. Was first observed in soldiers injured in World War I.
B. Is derived from the Latin words for "causes pain."
C. Unless caused by overt nerve injury, is usually not associated with signs of autonomic imbalance.
D. Is usually associated with evidence of osseous involvement in all stages.
E. Ultimately will be associated with trophic skin changes in most cases

30. The treatment of causalgia pain:

A. Is conservative (nonoperative) in stage 1.
B. Is disappointing in stage 3.
C. Should be achieved by alcohol or phenol injection or radio frequency heat ablation if possible before resorting to surgery.
D. By surgical sympathectomy produces disappointing long-term results.
E. Is disappointing when encountered after lumbar discectomy.

31. Causalgia:

A. Can usually be diagnosed on clinical grounds.
B. May be mistaken for peripheral neuritis.
C. Changes its clinical characteristics over time.
D. Has an unpredictable response to sympathectomy.
E. Is effectively controlled by sympathomimetic drugs if the response to ganglion blockade is dramatic.

7

Answers

1. The answer is **D** (Rutherford, 4th ed., pp. 641–642, 645–646).

The most common cause of an acute intrinsic occlusion of a major axial artery is an embolus from the heart. This patient describes having had a recent myocardial infarct, which likely led to an intramural intracardiac thrombus. He presents with signs of impending limb loss. The sine qua non for maintaining limb viability is prompt restoration of arterial inflow. Although some authorities have suggested that heparinization alone is satisfactory, it is not the preferred treatment for major emboli in the iliofemoral and popliteal system. At the time of operation the clots are removed, and attention must be directed toward prevention of the reperfusion syndrome. The administration of Mannitol will establish an osmotic diuresis and thus reduce the chance of renal damage from myoglobinuria. Mannitol is also a scavenger of the toxic hydroxyl radical that may be released after ischemia-reperfusion. Heparinization must be continued, or recurrent embolization is likely to occur in up to one third of patients. If the source of the embolus cannot be identified and treated, recurrences are common. Thrombolytic therapy as a primary form of treatment is not suitable in this particular patient because he already has evidence of neuromuscular ischemia. Effective thrombolytic therapy may require 12–72 hours, which may result in irreparable damage to muscles and nerves.

2. The answers are **C, D** (Rutherford, 4th ed., pp. 643–645, 713–722).

Because of the bony and soft tissue deformity associated with blunt trauma and fractures, it often is difficult to correctly assess vascular supply to the foot. The adequacy of blood flow is usually based on the detection of distal extremity pulses or the presence of normal Doppler pressures. While it has been stated that an ankle-brachial index of 0.9 or greater is solid evidence that there is no major arterial injury, this is not true if the profunda femoral is injured or if one or two of the tibial arteries are injured. The pulse wave has a velocity of 12–13 m/second and may be transmitted through areas of soft clot or past an intimal flap, whereas the flow wave has a velocity of only 40–50 cm/second; these must be separated in the examiner's mind. If viability of the foot is not threatened and there is continued function of the neuromuscular structures, after the bones are stabilized with an external fixation device a re-evaluation may reveal normal pressures and pulses. If this is not true, then a femoral arteriogram performed with a single injection of 30 ml of a 60% contrast medium usually will be adequate to detect injuries to the tibial vessels. In some instances small tibial vessels and spasm may be seen on the arteriograms, but patency can be proved. Subsequently there will be a return of normal Doppler signals, pressures, and pulses.

3. The answer is **D** (Rutherford, 4th ed., pp. 710–712).

Injuries of the left subclavian artery that produce false aneurysms are unlikely to resolve spontaneously. In 1948, Schumacker described the natural history of post-traumatic false aneurysms and found that approximately 6% thrombosed spontaneously. Because spontaneous cure is unlikely, there is little reason to procrastinate and risk the development of thromboembolism or expansion and rupture of the false aneurysm. The proper surgical approach in this situation is through the supraclavicular incision, with the patient prepped and draped so a thoracotomy can be performed if necessary. Injuries of the second and third portions of the subclavian artery can almost always be repaired with this approach. It may be necessary to remove the medial half of the clavicle, depending upon how high the artery rises in the neck, but adequate exposure usually can be obtained without claviculectomy. Because it is necessary to divide the anterior scalene muscle and occasionally portions of the middle scalene muscle to obtain adequate exposure, the phrenic nerve and thoracic duct must be protected from injury. With an injury caused by blunt trauma it is unlikely that sufficient mobilization can be obtained for an adequate end-to-end anastomosis, and usually an interposition graft of autogenous tissue is favored. If that is unavailable, a short segment of a prosthetic graft can be used in these uncontaminated wounds.

4. The answer is **D** (Rutherford, 4th ed., pp. 705–709).

Although acute ligation of the internal carotid artery may be tolerated if the patient has a complete circle of Willis, careful arteriographic studies have demonstrated that the circle is intact, as depicted in anatomy books, in less than 50% of patients. Even under protection of systemic heparin, distal thromboembolism can occur. One can anticipate a significant stroke rate with acute ligation of this artery. With the presence of brisk back bleeding from the internal carotid artery, if it is feasible a direct end-to-end anastomosis can be performed. This should be followed by a completion arteriogram to detect technical defects and intracranial thromboembolism. Although prosthetic grafts may be used in uncontaminated wounds, autogenous tissue is preferable, and if the artery cannot be reapproximated without tension, an interposition graft of saphenous vein obtained from the groin is recommended. Extracranial to intracranial bypass should be considered only if direct internal carotid artery reconstruction is technically impossible.

5. The answer is **B** (Rutherford, 4th ed., pp. 650–651).

Approximately 70–80% of arterial emboli involve extremity vessels, with the lower extremity much more common than the upper extremity. Occlusion of the common femoral artery at its bifurcation is the most frequent in virtually all reported series, accounting for one third to one half of cases. Occlusion of the superficial femoral artery at the adductor canal would be more typical of acute thrombosis of a site of pre-existent chronic occlusive disease rather than an embolic event.

6. The answer is **A** (Rutherford, 4th ed., pp. 647–650).

The great majority of arterial emboli are formed in the heart. The most common cardiac abnormality is atrial fibrillation, which causes stasis and clot formation in the left atrium. While the cause of atrial fibrillation has shifted from rheumatic mitral valvular disease to arteriosclerotic heart disease, atrial fibrillation is associated with two thirds to three quarters of embolic events. The left ventricle is the next most common site of clot formation as a consequence of acute myocardial infarction or more remote infarction with possible ventricular aneurysm formation or areas of akenesis or congestive heart failure. Noncardiac sources of embolic clot, such as ulcerated atheromas or aneurysms of the thoracic or abdominal aorta, are documented in only about 5–10% of cases of emboli. Diseased cardiac valves or prosthetic heart valves are infrequent sources of macroemboli to major arteries.

7. The answer is **D** (Rutherford, 4th ed., pp. 651–652).

Although all of these factors influence the severity of ischemia resulting from embolic occlusion of a vessel, it is well established that the principal consideration is the amount of collateral circulation available in each instance. If sufficient collateral flow is present, there is no arbitrary "golden period" of tolerable ischemia. The size of the embolus will largely determine the site of occlusion at a particular arterial bifurcation. A larger embolus obstructing the aorta, iliac, or femoral bifurcation may render a greater extent of tissue potentially ischemic, but the physiologic impact and eventual outcome of the ischemic event is ultimately decided by the extent of available collateral flow to the limb. A smaller embolus occluding the popliteal bifurcation, for instance, may be more likely to result in limb loss if potential collateral networks are not present. Secondary propagation of clot is an important mechanism of worsening of ischemia following an embolus, potentially impairing the crucial determinant of available collateral blood flow. Hence, anticoagulation should be initiated immediately.

8. The answer is **C** (Rutherford, 4th ed., pp. 652–655).

Differentiation of an embolic cause of acute arterial occlusion from acute thrombosis of a diseased arterial segment is of prime importance, as the management of the two conditions is often considerably different. A prior MI by EKG would be common in patients with either condition in current practice. The presence of normal contralateral limb pulses and the absence of a prior history of claudication are helpful clues suggesting an embolus but not definitive. In difficult cases, arteriography may be quite helpful. Demonstration of occlusion of the superficial femoral artery in the region of the adductor canal would be much more likely due to thrombosis of diseased artery and a relatively uncommon site of embolic occlusion despite the relative absence of other atherosclerotic disease. The presence of multiple filling defects in separate arterial beds is almost certainly indicative of an embolic cause, representing either separate embolic events or a single embolus that has fragmented at a more proximal site. Careful examination of the filling defects may reveal a "meniscus" typical of emboli.

9. The answer is **E** (Rutherford, 4th ed., pp. 655–664).

Fasciotomy may be an important adjunct to embolectomy if severe ischemia has been present for a prolonged period (4–6 hours or more) or if significant swelling and increased compartmental pressures develop following revascularization. Its routine use, however, is not advocated in all cases of emboli, principally because of the increased hazards of infection or other wound problems in anticoagulated patients. Use of thrombolytic therapy may not be possible if severe ischemia requires more immediate relief and can have significant complications of its own. It may be considered for unusual cases difficult to manage by conventional surgical methods or as an adjunct to surgery for irretrievable distal clot, but prompt embolectomy remains the preferred procedure for most straightforward arterial emboli. Back bleeding does not necessarily mean no further distal clot is present, because it may result from arterial branches above a discontinuous residual distal clot. Completeness of embolectomy should be determined by restoration of distal pulses, intraoperative arteriography, or possibly angioscopy following embolectomy. Standard transthoracic echocardiography is often inaccurate in demonstrating intracardiac thrombus. Transesophageal echocardiogram may be more reliable, but emboli of presumed cardiac origin are best managed by lifelong anticoagulation with Warfarin to minimize the incidence of recurrent emboli unless the underlying cardiac condition itself can be corrected. Despite simplification of the operative procedure and improved perioperative management, the mortality of embolectomy remains high, from 10 to 20% even in modern series. This reflects the advanced age and severe associated cardiac problems commonly encountered in patients with arterial emboli.

10. The answer is **B** (Rutherford, 4th ed., pp. 669–673).

Within the last 40 years, the pathology of plaque degeneration has come to the attention of clinicians as a unifying mechanism for the production of profound cerebrovascular, visceral, cardiac, and limb ischemia. Atheroembolism is a clinical diagnosis: It is remarkably difficult to find the site of microembolic lodgement or cholesterol debris in peripheral tissues that are infarcted or debrided, even when a pathologist takes care to search for these findings in multiple tissue sections. The type of emboli causing the blue toe syndrome cannot be differentiated on clinical grounds, nor can the source be accurately predicted by the location embolized. It is clear from autopsy studies that the majority of microthromboembolism is silent. At autopsy, as many as 5% of patients will have some evidence for cholesterol embolism. Nevertheless, patients with a defined blue toe syndrome are a minority of the clinical experience of practitioners exclusively treating vascular disease. In a recent series, atheroembolism constituted a significant clinical problem in 0.03% of hospitalized patients. Amaurosis fugax is another example of transient embolism.

11. The answer is **D** (Rutherford, 4th ed., pp. 669–675).

Cholesterol crystal emboli have been found in the pulmonary capillary circulation. It appears that the smallest elements of this debris may pass through peripheral arteriolar-capillary shunts and thereby return in the venous circulation to lodge in the lung. Certainly cholesterol emboli are small enough to pass through large collateral vessels in limbs with chronic vascular occlusive disease. Therefore, a palpable pulse at the ankle may not necessarily be present in a patient with atheroembolism. Silent degeneration in the ascending aorta has been documented with intraoperative ultrasonography in approximately 20–25% of patients undergoing coronary bypass. A significant feature of atheroembolism is the appearance of lesions in crops, as if intermittent showers of debris occur. Collateral circulation in the affected beds is either undeveloped in the setting of this acute shower or destroyed by the emboli, accounting for the progressive nature of symptoms. Tissue is damaged with the first symptoms, but progression to gangrene usually occurs after repeated episodes of microembolism.

12. The answer is **C** (Rutherford, 4th ed., pp. 675–676).

Atheroembolic lesions will usually heal if the ankle pressure exceeds 100 torr as measured in compressible arteries or if the metatarsal level pulse volume tracings have a standard amplitude of 5 mm. Palpable pulses are not required. Patients with evidence of atheroembolism should also be studied with duplex ultrasonography in order to discover aneurysms, particularly in the abdominal aorta and femoral/popliteal segments. Muscle biopsy has received prominent attention in the literature pertaining to atheroembolism, and gastrocnemius muscle biopsies have confirmed atheroembolism in patients with suspicious clinical findings. However, this method has not found widespread use, and the overall accuracy of muscle biopsy has never been determined. There are no specific blood or laboratory tests that correlate with atheroembolism. Eosinophilia has been noted on blood smears and in urine. Renal function should be checked in patients with bilateral lesions. A deterioration of renal function may indicate a suprarenal source for emboli. There is no direct correlation of serum cholesterol and atheroembolism of cholesterol crystals.

13. The answer is **C** (Rutherford, 4th ed., pp. 675–676).

If the source of embolization is a highly stenotic lesion in the femoral or popliteal segments, localized endarterectomy with vein patch angioplasty has proved satisfactory. Sympathectomy may be useful for palliation of atheroembolic lesions. Not only is it an adjunct to direct surgical treatment of the offending arterial segment, but sympathectomy may be useful to control the pain of severe atheroembolic toe lesions in patients who otherwise cannot undergo direct repair of the embolic source or when correction does not improve distal perfusion. Sympathectomy is easily performed during aortic procedures; or postoperatively, it can be achieved through lumbar sympathetic blocks. In one study of the efficacy of aspirin for the treatment of atheroembolism, clinical improvement occurred in over 50% of patients so managed. Close follow-up is needed for these patients who are "medically managed" because repeated atheroembolism can lead to tissue loss. Nevertheless, after an appropriate work-up to define the source lesion, patients with their first episode of atheroembolism can be treated with aspirin, in a manner analgous to current management of moderate carotid disease. Disseminated atheroembolism occurs with disruption of plaques in the supravisceral aortic segments. Emboli are shed to the lower extremities, bowel, kidneys, and pelvic structures. Intestinal symptoms and signs from an atheroembolic shower can be confused with inflammatory bowel disease or ischemic colitis.

14. The answer is **C** (Rutherford 4th ed., pp. 678–682).

Gangrene is a common end result of ischemia following intra-arterial drug injection. While the exact timing of events leading to the development of gangrene remain unclear, delay in seeking medical attention is frequent. It is common for digital or even total extremity gangrene to be the presenting complaint. Vessel obstruction has been associated with drug excipients, drug crystals, endarteritis, and platelet aggregation. Prolonged tourniquet time in sedated drug users decreases venous flow and allows increased contact time between the drug toxins and the vascular endothelium. Direct local arterial injury is a contributing factor, especially in the case of inexperienced drug abusers. While the contribution of arterial constriction to the sequela intra-arterial drug injection remains controversial, drug-induced vasodilation does not contribute to the development of gangrene. Venospasm may play a more significant role in most cases.

15. The answer is **B** (Rutherford, 4th ed., pp. 678–680).

Because only the most severe complications of intra-arterial drug injections come to medical attention, it is impossible to calculate accurately the incidence of intra-arterial injections associated with drug abuse. Based on the experiences of several large urban medical centers, approximately three fourths of all admissions for accidental intra-arterial drug injection involve the lower extremity. Because the femoral artery is superficially located and an easy target for the drug abuser, it is the most likely site of injection. The brachial artery is the most common site of accidental injections in the upper extremity.

16. The answers are **D, E** (Rutherford 4th ed., pp. 679–680).

An infected pseudoaneurysm is a frequent complication following accidental drug injection at the common femoral artery bifurcation. There is a 33% risk of amputation when the common femoral artery bifurcation is resected without revascularization. Direct common femoral artery reconstruction should be performed using autologous saphenous vein whenever possible. An alternative is an extra-anatomic bypass through the obturator canal using either prosthetic graft or autologous saphenous vein. Nonoperative treatment with long-term intravenous antibiotics is not effective for established arterial wall infection.

17. The answer is **E** (Rutherford, 4th ed., pp. 682–683).

Acute ischemia following accidental intra-arterial drug injection constitutes a medical emergency. Therapy should involve multiple modalities and begin with immediate measures to relieve pain, prevent local limb and systemic hypothermia, and improve venous drainage by patient positioning. Arteriography should be performed early with the catheter positioned proximal to the suspected site of drug injection. The arteriogram catheter should be left in place for subsequent intra-arterial therapy. All of the interventions listed above have a role in short- or long-term treatment, but none is always successful.

18. The answer is **B** (Rutherford 4th ed., pp. 683–684).

Habitual use of superficial hand veins as drug injection sites eventually results in venous thrombosis. Superimposed lymphatic obstruction may occur secondary to recurrent infection and uptake of injected particulate debris. This results in the puffy hand syndrome (see Fig. 45–4). Operative management is usually not required. Elevation, antibiotics, and intravenous heparin may be indicated. Intractable edema may require management with fitted or pneumatic compression devices.

19. The answer is **E** (Rutherford, 4th ed., pp. 686–689).

Following blunt trauma, disruption of the thoracic aorta may occur at the isthmus. This is likely due to a combination of factors, including vertically directed forces, compression of the chest, horizontal decleration, and crush. The stress thus produced tears the relatively inelastic intima and media, resulting in dissection. A high index of suspicion is the most important factor in initiating a search for thoracic aortic disruption after trauma. Ascertaining the severity and mechanism of trauma is essential. Symptoms on admission are often related to associated injuries. The most common findings include chest pain (76%), dyspnea (56%), loss of consciousness or coma (37%), and hypotension (26%). Other less common signs are an interscapular systolic murmur and hoarseness. No single physical finding, or combination of findings, is diagnostic of acute thoracic aortic rupture. The acute coarctation syndrome (hypertension in the arms and a difference in the pulse amplitude between the upper and lower extremities) may be caused either by an intimal dissection or flap or by compression of the aortic lumen by a hematoma with relative renal hypopertusion that stimulates renin release. Alternatively, hypertension may be produced by the stimulation of receptors in or near the aortic isthmus. A systolic murmur over the precordium or posterior interscapular area may be noted and is probably due to the turbulence created as blood flows past the intimal flap. The percentage of patients in whom the complete acute aortic coarctation syndrome occurs is small. Likewise, acute superior vena cava syndrome is an occasional method of presentation (see Table 46–1, p. 687).

20. The answer is **A** (Rutherford, 4th ed., pp. 687–689).

Computerized tomography (CT) and transesophageal echo (TEE) have recently been suggested as potential modalities to establish the presence of thoracic aortic injuries. Concerns about CT relate to the fact that it may not be sensitive enough to detect aortic branch injuries. Further, the usual 8–10-mm sections may make satisfactory evaluation of the aorticopulmonary window difficult because of artifacts from volume averaging. A recent study found no adverse outcomes among 19 patients with normal CT scans who did not undergo angiography. A carefully controlled study comparing CT with angiography (in the same patient) will be required before the question of the true accuracy of CT scanning for this diagnosis can be answered. TEE has been reported as a diagnostic adjunct in patients with suspected thoracic aortic injury. The majority of reports do not compare TEE with angiography. A distinct disadvantage of TEE is that it requires a highly skilled operator and specialized equipment, which might not be available in most medical centers when the trauma patient arrives. Standard ultrasonography does not provide satisfactory detail, but intravascular ultrasound may be of use in the future. The accuracy of a standard chest x-ray to establish the diagnosis is poor, although it is a reasonable screening test when properly interpreted. Until additional information becomes available, aortography remains the imaging study of choice to establish the diagnosis.

21. The answer is **B** (Rutherford, 4th ed., pp. 696–702).

Injuries to the segment of the aorta between the renal arteries and the celiac axis have the highest mortality rate. Intraoperative exposure is extremely difficult because dense periaortic neural tissue surrounds the celiac axis, the superior mesenteric artery, and the pancreas. Injuries to the vena cava often accompany aortic injuries in this location. Exposure is best obtained by medial rotation of the viscera. When an injury of the inferior vena cava is suspected as well, a right rather than left gutter incision is preferable. The right colon, hepatic flexure, and duodenum are mobilized to the left.

22. The answer is **A** (Rutherford, 4th ed., pp. 701–703).

Most isolated lacerations of the inferior vena cava can be repaired by simple lateral venorrhaphy, taking care to prevent narrowing of the lumen. When the laceration extends to the posterior wall, repair can be accomplished through the lumen of the vena cava. Attempts at mobilization to permit posterior suture often extend the laceration further and exacerbate hemorrhage. Spiral vein grafts can be used when large segments of the vena cava are damaged or missing. They are very time consuming to construct and require prolonged occlusion of the vena cava, which may not be tolerated in hemodynamically unstable patients. Autogenous vein grafts are usually unsatisfactory substitutes for the vena cava because of their comparatively small size. In life-threatening situations, the vena cava may be ligated below the renal veins, but postoperative leg edema may be problematic.

23. The answer is **E** (Rutherford, 4th ed., pp. 705–709).

Although in the past it was believed that repair was contraindicated in patients who experienced carotid artery trauma and were admitted with alterations in consciousness because of the danger of converting a bland into a hemorrhagic infarct, recent studies have indicated that this is an unlikely event. Although many cerebral infarcts are accompanied by microhemorrhage, at the time of reperfusion most do not become grossly hemorrhagic. Moreover, it has been shown that in most patients with carotid artery trauma and continued pro-grade flow, even those with severe neurologic deficits, recovery of function is more likely if the artery is repaired than if it is left alone or ligated. In addition, there is some danger of delayed complications, such as false aneurysm or arteriovenous fistula if penetrating trauma to the internal carotid artery is not treated. Most experienced trauma surgeons recommend repair of *all* carotid artery injuries in suitable patients if it is technically feasible, and especially if there is continued patency of the artery.

24. The answer is **C** (Rutherford, 4th ed., pp. 705–709).

Blunt trauma to the carotid artery is almost always a difficult diagnosis to establish because fewer than half the patients will have telltale signs of injury to the superficial structures of the neck upon physical examination. Moreover, neurologic symptoms may be delayed. If the injury is severe, the patient will usually develop symptoms within 24 hours, but months or even years may pass before symptoms related to the artery manifest themselves. The diagnosis is made especially difficult in patients who have sustained hyperextension injuries in which the artery is stretched forcibly over the transverse process of C-2 and the body of C-1 because this stretching inflicts multiple medial and intimal tears that predispose to delayed thromboembolism. The diagnosis in most of these patients can be established only by careful biplane arteriography.

25. The answer is **E** (Rutherford, 4th ed., pp. 710–712).

Although the diagnosis of injuries to the great vessels as a result of blunt trauma can be difficult, most authorities believe that patients who have obscuration of the aortic knob, more than 8 cm widening of the mediastinum in the second interspace, an apical cap, depression of the left main stem bronchus, or medial deviation of an endotracheal tube or nasogastric tube are very likely to have significant vascular injuries in the mediastinum. Although in most instances this will be the result of venous bleeding, patients with these findings should have an aortogram with careful visualization of the great vessels to exclude major arterial injuries. Physical examination is important in these patients, but it has been demonstrated repeatedly that normal pulses may be present distal to an injured artery. The pulse wave is a pressure wave with velocities of 10–13 m/second and may be transmitted via small vessels and small collaterals, past intimal flaps, or even through limited soft clot. Moreover, tangential injuries of the great vessels may not alter blood flow or pulse pressures. The great vessels across the arch are most easily explored through a median sternotomy, with the exception of the descending aorta and the left subclavian, which are best approached through an anterior lateral left thoracotomy.

26. The answer is **D** (Rutherford, 4th ed., pp. 714–718).

Angiography remains the gold standard for the diagnosis of arterial injury. Less invasive studies have recently been employed, especially in patients suspected of having minimal injury or little likelihood of an injury requiring operative intervention. Duplex ultrasonography may become the preferred study to follow selected patients who are managed nonoperatively. In 1991, Meissner and colleagues reported their experience with 89 patients who sustained 93 injuries. In their series there were four false negative studies, but no major injuries were missed. They concluded that the study was cost effective and that it might serve as a reliable substitute for contrast angiography if occult injury is suspected. Angioscopy is a potential technique for evaluating arterial injury and may complement an equivocal angiogram or other noninvasive study. It is still under investigation for trauma and is not recommended for routine use at this time. Reliance on Doppler studies and arterial pressure indexes as part of the physical examination has added to its accuracy; however, minimal injuries such as intimal defects and small pseudoaneurysms still may not be detected. Recent series have reported a negative predictive value of 99% for an ABI of >0.90 and a sensitivity of 95% and specificity of 97% for major arterial injury if the ABI was <0.90.

27. The answers are **D, E** (Rutherford, 4th ed., pp. 720–721).

The appropriate sequence for arterial and venous reconstruction and the repair of skeletal injuries is important. If distal flow is maintained, the sequence of repair is a matter of personal preference. Arterial injuries causing distal ischemia or venous injuries causing venous hypertension require immediate restoration of blood flow. Flow can be temporarily restored by in-dwelling shunts if a delay in repair is required for attention to adjacent or remote injuries or harvesting of a vein graft. Venous reconstruction usually precedes arterial repair if the injured vein is the major or sole source of venous return. This provides better outflow and may enhance the success of arterial repair. The disadvantage of stabilizing fractures prior to vascular repair include delay in restoration of flow to ischemic tissue and possible interference with the vascular repair by the fixation device, which not only may block access to the injury but may also obscure the completed reconstruction on arteriography. Occasionally an extremity is so shortened or a fracture is so unstable that initial stabilization is mandatory. This situation is limited almost entirely to upper-extremity injuries.

28. The answer is **A** (Rutherford, 4th ed., pp. 718–719).

Whereas proximity of an injury to a major vessel used to be an indication for operative exploration, the large number of unnecessary procedures led most surgeons to rely on arteriography to rule out an injury. Recent interest has been focused on the incidence of injury that requires repair when proximity is the sole indication in the otherwise *completely asymptomatic patient.* Several studies have addressed this issue, and most conclude that proximity is no longer an indication for arteriography. In 1988, Reid et al. in a retrospective series of over 500 patients found an injury incidence of 3.6%, and only one half of those patients required a repair. Angiography should not be performed in patients with penetrating trauma and evidence of distal ischemia or threatened tissue viability. These patients should be operated upon expeditiously and intraoperative angiography obtained as required. Primary amputation on occasion is a necessary operation and is indicated with mangled extremities in which skeletal stabilization is not possible and/or the extremity is paralyzed and anesthetic. The attitude that vascular reconstruction is always indicated is inappropriate and may result in serious morbidity and even mortality in rare cases.

29. The answers are **D, E** (Rutherford, 4th ed., pp. 736–738).

Causalgia was mentioned by Paré (Napoleonic Wars) but clearly described by Weir-Mitchell following the U.S. Civil War. In fact, Mitchell's causalgia is one of its many synonyms. Causalgia is derived from two Greek words for "heat" and "pain" and literally means "burning pain." Autonomic imbalance is apparent early, with the affected part being characteristically dry, red, and warm in stage 1 and cold, clammy, mottled, and cyanotic in stage 2. Osseous involvement is apparent very early on from bone scans and begins to be apparent from the end of stage 1 on from x-rays. Without spontaneous remission or sympathectomy most patients will progress to stage 3, which is characterized by severe trophic skin changes and ankylosis of joints.

30. The answers are **A, B** (Rutherford, 4th ed., pp. 738–740).

Many early cases of causalgia can be relieved by repeated sympathetic blocks, physiotherapy, and non-narcotic drug therapy (phenytoin, amitriptyline, carbamazepine, or baclofen combined with nonsteroidal anti-inflammatory agents). If allowed to progress to the final trophic stage (3), reflex sympathetic dystrophy usually does not respond well to any therapy, including surgical sympathectomy. Chemical necrosis or thermal ablative techniques usually give incomplete or transient relief, and the inflammation and scarring they cause compromises subsequent surgical sympathectomy. If applied only to patients receiving dramatic relief from trial blocks, sympathectomy gives close to 90% long-term relief. Application in other cases (e.g., stage 3 disease, nerve pain of other etiology) may give initial relief but has poor long-term success. Using the same selection criterion (i.e., response to ganglion block), patients with residual causalgia pain following disc operations respond equally well.

31. The answers are **A, B, C** (Rutherford, 4th ed., pp. 737–740).

Because they both may have burning pain and neuropathy, peripheral neuritis and causalgia may be confused, but the latter is more rapid in onset, with a precipitating event (trauma) and usually has florid vasomotor changes and other obvious signs of autonomic imbalance (e.g., sweating). The autonomic imbalance, and the associated signs, undergo characteristic changes through the three classic stages of reflex sympathetic dystrophy—i.e., from the acute stage (dry, red, warm skin) to the dystrophic stage (cool, clammy, cyanotic, mottled skin) to the atrophic stage (shiny, pale, atrophic skin) Causalgia responds to sympathectomy in a predictable manner, directly reflecting its response to an anesthetic block of the appropriate ganglia. Sympatholytic, not sympathomimetic, agents *may* be effective against causalgia, but the degree of relief is rarely equal to that obtained by a sympathetic block.

8

Chronic Ischemia of the Lower Extremities

1. Which of the following parameters most reliably predicts prognosis for a patient with chronic lower-extremity ischemia with respect to the potential for limb loss?
   A. The ankle-brachial arterial systolic pressure ratio in the affected limb.
   B. The patient's description of *symptoms* of claudication, ischemic rest pain, or ischemic ulceration.
   C. The presence or absence of a decrease in ankle systolic pressure in response to treadmill walking.
   D. Patient age and sex.
   E. The magnitude of abnormality of atherosclerosis risk factors, including blood sugar, serum cholesterol, percentage of body fat, and amount of aerobic exercise.

2. Which of the following statements concerning long-term survival of patients with chronic lower-extremity ischemia is are/true?
   A. Long-term survival of patients with chronic lower-extremity ischemia is most closely related to the presence or absence of cigarette smoking.
   B. Long-term survival of patients with chronic lower-extremity ischemia is approximately the same as that found in age-matched controls without lower-extremity ischemia.
   C. Patients with chronic lower-extremity ischemia have markedly reduced long-term survival compared to age-matched controls, with the magnitude of the reduction directly related to the severity of the arterial disease as assessed by objective means.
   D. Patients with chronic lower-extremity ischemia have markedly reduced long-term survival compared to age-matched controls. The magnitude of the reduction in survival is most closely related to the severity of *symptoms* of coexisting coronary artery disease.
   E. Patients with chronic lower-extremity ischemia have markedly reduced long-term survival compared to age-matched controls. The magnitude of the reduction is most closely related to the presence or absence of coexisting malignancy.

3. Modification of which of the following risk factors has been shown to improve prognosis in patients with chronic lower-extremity ischemia?
   A. Elevated serum cholesterol.
   B. Absence of regular exercise.
   C. Obesity.
   D. Cigarette smoking.
   E. Diabetes mellitus.

4. Which of the following statements concerning the beneficial effects of walking exercise on symptoms of claudication is/are true?
   A. Walking exercise results in marked improvement in lower-extremity collateral flow, which results in improved walking distance.
   B. Walking exercise results in a decrease in the severity of arterial stenoses, producing increased ankle to brachial pressure ratios and improved walking distance.
   C. Walking exercise produces improved efficiency of muscular performance, characterized by increased extraction of oxygen from the available blood flow, resulting in improved walking distance.
   D. Walking exercise results in improved cardiac output, which increases muscle blood flow, resulting in improved walking distance.
   E. Walking exercise produces decreased body weight, resulting in improved walking distance.

5. Aortoiliac endarterectomy:
   A. Is technically easier than aortobifemoral bypass.
   B. Is most useful for disease ending at the iliac bifurcation.
   C. Should generally be extended to the femoral bifurcation.
   D. Is most useful for juxtarenal total aortic occlusion.
   E. Has poorer results in women than men.

6. An end-to-side proximal anastomosis for an aortobifemoral graft:
   A. Has better late patency as compared to grafts with an end-to-end proximal anastomosis in most published series.
   B. Provides inferior early hemodynamic improvement compared to an end-to-end graft.
   C. Has a lower incidence of embolic complications compared to end-to-end grafts.
   D. Is associated with an increased incidence of postoperative impotence as compared to an end-to-end anastomosis.
   E. Is preferred for patients with severe bilateral external iliac occlusive disease.

7. With respect to aortic graft reconstruction for aortoiliac occlusive disease, which of the following statements is/are true?
   A. Aortofemoral grafts have better long-term patency than aortoiliac grafts.

B. In patients with multilevel disease, routine profundaplasty improves the early hemodynamic result of aortofemoral grafts.
C. The addition of lumbar sympathectomy improves long-term graft patency in patients with poor runoff.
D. The most common late complication is an anastomotic aneurysm at the distal anastomosis.
E. For aortofemoral grafts, patency at 10 years can be expected to be 70–75%.

8. In a patient with combined aortoiliac and femoropopliteal occlusive disease demonstrated by preoperative arteriography, which of the following would be the best indicator of the need for a simultaneous distal bypass at the time of aortobifemoral grafting?

A. A severe profunda femoris origin stenosis.
B. A preoperative ankle-brachial index (ABI) of only 0.3.
C. Total occlusion of the entire length of the superficial femoral artery on arteriography.
D. Gangrenous toes.
E. Immediate intraoperative increase of ABI of only 0.2 in the operating room following proximal graft insertion.

9. Thrombosis of one limb of an aortobifemoral graft 3 years following implanation:

A. Is best treated by a femorofemoral graft.
B. Usually indicates the need for a distal bypass graft for successful correction.
C. Is most often caused by recurrent or progressive aortic disease at the proximal anastomosis.
D. Is best treated by insertion of a new aortobifemoral graft.
E. Can usually be managed by graft limb thrombectomy and profundaplasty.

10. Of the 2–7% early failure rate within 30 days of infrainguinal bypass, the most common cause of thrombosis is:

A. Antiphospholipid syndrome.
B. Antithrombin III deficiency.
C. Systemic hypotension.
D. Anastomotic suture line infection.
E. Technical defects.

11. Postoperative leg edema following infrainguinal revascularization results primarily from which of the following?

A. Residual hematoma.
B. Postsurgical interstitial edema.
C. Lymphatic interruption.
D. Venous occlusion.
E. Infection.

12. Which of the following most accurately represents the 5-year *overall* primary patency rates for femoropopliteal reconstruction with autogenous vein and PTFE?

	Vein	*PTFE*
A.	90%	30%
B	70%	40%
C.	50%	50%
D.	40%	60%
E.	40%	40%

13. Which of the following most accurately represents the 5-year *overall* primary patency rates associated with femorotibial reconstruction utilizing autogenous vein and PTFE?

	Vein	*PTFE*
A.	90%	35%
B.	80%	25%
C.	70%	15%
D.	60%	5%
E.	40%	20%

14. Which of the following statements regarding axillofemoral bypass, femorofemoral bypass and their combination, axillobifemoral bypass, is/are true?

A. There is no difference in the long-term patency rates for axillounifemoral and axillobifemoral bypass.
B. The peripheral resistance in the donor axillary artery is less following axillobifemoral than axillounifemoral bypass, causing higher flow rates.
C. Axillofemoral bypasses (unilateral or bilateral) have better long-term patencies when performed for indications *other* than atherosclerotic occlusive disease.
D. It is popular thinking but not proved that external support (rings) enhance the patency of these extra-anatomic bypasses.
E. Despite theoretical considerations, the angle of take off of the cross-over limb of an axillobifemoral has little, if any, bearing on patency.

15. Which of the following statements regarding femorofemoral (FF) bypass is/are true?

A. FF bypass was introduced after axillobifemoral bypass, having been developed to allow the latter to supply both lower extremities.
B. FF bypass has better patency than iliofemoral bypass.
C. FF bypass has a lower patency when performed in patients with superficial femoral occlusion than when the superficial femoral artery (SFA) is open.
D. FF bypass is the procedure of choice for unilateral aortobifemoral graft (AFBG) limb occlusion and carries a patency equivalent to *each* of these bypasses (AFBG and FF) when performed as primary procedures.
E. Stenosis of the donor iliac artery should *not* be treated by percutaneous transluminal angioplasty to allow FF bypass, because iliac restenosis will eventually threaten the bypass.

9

Upper-Extremity Vascular and Neurologic Disorders

1. Primary Raynaud's disease:
   A. Is synonymous with vasospastic Raynaud's syndrome.
   B. Is characterized by "fixed" obstruction of the digital arteries.
   C. Is often unilateral and may be isolated to one finger.
   D. May eventually be found to be associated with an autoimmune disease in some patients.
   E. Often causes painful fingertip ulcers.

2. Which of the following is/are not compatible with a diagnosis of *secondary* Raynaud's phenomenon?
   A. Finger blood pressure index of 0.90, but abnormal plethysmographic pulses at the fingertips when the hand is warmed.
   B. Finger blood pressure indexes of 0.60 in the right fourth and fifth fingers; pressures in the other fingers of both hands are normal.
   C. Pulses and blood pressures are normal in all fingers when the hand is warm, but pressures drop precipitously when the finger is cooled to 10° C.
   D. Nailfold capillary loops are enlarged, dilated, and distorted with areas of avascularity.
   E. A history of using vibratory tools.

3. Which of the following statements is/are correct?
   A. Exposure to cold consistently provokes a triphasic color change (white → blue → red) in the fingers of patients with cold sensitivity.
   B. A >20 mm Hg difference in brachial artery pressure is compatible with but not diagnostic of subclavian artery obstruction.
   C. Arteriolar constriction plays no role in cold sensitivity in patients with secondary Raynaud's phenomenon (obstructive Raynaud's syndrome).
   D. Disappearance of the palmar arch Doppler signal when the ulnar artery is compressed at the wrist indicates obstruction of the ulnar artery.
   E. Patients with scleroderma typically exhibit a *marked* decrease in digit pulse volume in response to sympathetic stimuli (deep breath, mental arithmetic) and a doubling of the pulse volume in response to reactive hyperemia.

4. Innominate artery lesions usually:
   A. Should be repaired prophylactically even when asymptomatic.
   B. Present with upper-extremity but not cerebrovascular symptoms.
   C. Present with neurologic symptoms of either anterior or posterior circulations, but may also present with ischemia of the upper extremity.
   D. Present with anterior circulation neurologic symptoms only.
   E. Produce upper-extremity major tissue loss.

5. Ascending aortoinnominate artery bypass grafting is:
   A. Less applicable to all patients than innominate artery endarterectomy and is therefore employed less than endarterectomy.
   B. Associated with excellent early results but with long-term relief in only 45–55% of patients.
   C. Best performed through a right thoracotomy.
   D. Associated with excellent early results and long-term relief in 85–95% of patients.
   E. Best performed through a median sternotomy.

6. Common carotid artery occlusive lesions are:
   A. Encountered three times more frequently than carotid bifurcation lesions.
   B. Usually treated with subclavian-carotid artery bypass grafting.
   C. Never symptomatic.
   D. Usually treated with retrograde endarterectomy performed through cervical incisions.
   E. Most commonly caused by Takayasu's disease.

7. Isolated subclavian artery occlusive lesions are:
   A. Usually encountered on the right side.
   B. Usually treated by carotid-subclavian artery bypass grafting or subclavian artery transposition.
   C. Usually treated by subclavian artery endarterectomy performed through a thoracotomy incision.
   D. Almost always associated with symptomatic subclavian-steal syndrome.
   E. One of the most common locations for atherosclerosis.

8. Brachial artery thrombosis following cardiac catheterization may result in:
   A. No symptoms.
   B. Symptoms of acute ischemia.
   C. Symptoms of chronic ischemia.
   D. Factitious hypertension.
   E. Pseudoaneurysm.

9. The brachial artery is a single vessel associated with a normal bifurcation in:
   A. 10% of cases.
   B. 50% of cases.
   C. 30% of cases.
   D. 80% of cases.
   E. 95% of cases.

10. The upper-extremity artery most frequently affected by embolic occlusion is:
   A. Subclavian artery.
   B. Axillary artery.
   C. Brachial artery.
   D. Radial artery.
   E. Ulnar artery.

11. A 68-year-old man presents with the acute onset of painful purple second and third digits of his left hand. A physical exam reveals normal brachial, radial, and ulnar pulses bilaterally. The distal phalanges of the second and third digits of the left hand are mottled and have poor capillary refill. The remaining digits on both hands are normal. The next step should be:
   A. Amputation of the affected fingers.
   B. Finger plethysmography, blood pressures, and immunology screen.
   C. Echocardiogram.
   D. Upper-extremity angiogram.
   E. None of the above.

12. A 28-year-old nonsmoking female computer programmer in San Francisco presents with a 5-year history of Raynaud's syndrome. She takes no medications. She has become concerned about her Raynaud's syndrome because she is considering a job in northern Michigan and is worried that the colder weather may be bad for her hands. The immunology screen is normal, finger photoplethysmographic wave forms and pressures are normal, and a cold challenge test is positive. She should be advised to:
   A. Not move to Michigan because the cold weather may lead to digital ulceration.
   B. Begin nifedipine if she does move to Michigan.
   C. Undergo thoracic sympathectomy if her symptoms worsen in cold weather.
   D. Wear gloves during cold weather, and if she becomes more symptomatic in cold weather to consider a trial of nifedipine.
   E. Undergo injection of intra-arterial reserpine.

13. Patients who present with Raynaud's syndrome, digital ulceration, and a connective tissue disease should be advised that:
   A. Multiple fingers will eventually require amputation.
   B. Once the ulcers heal they will not recur.
   C. While they may have recurrent ulcerations over the years, finger amputation is rarely required.
   D. Connective tissue diseases are easily cured with medication.
   E. Major limb amputation is inevitable.

14. Which of the following statements is/are true regarding the etiology of neurogenic thoracic outlet syndrome?
   A. In the majority of patients, a cervical rib is the cause of compression of the brachial plexus.
   B. The scalenus minimus muscle is present in about half of the patients and causes irritation of the C5 and C6 nerve roots, resulting in pain in the shoulder.
   C. Trauma to the neck precipitates symptoms by invoking an inflammatory response and fibrosis in the soft tissues around the brachial plexus.
   D. Histopathological studies of the anterior scalene muscle have revealed a predominance and hypertrophy of fast twitch, glycolytic fibers and have directed attention to the scalenes in symptom production.
   E. All of the above.

15. Which of the following statements is/are true in diagnosing neurogenic thoracic outlet syndrome (TOS)?
   A. The diagnosis can usually be made clinically based on history and physical examination alone.
   B. A positive Adson's test is the single most important physical finding in differentiating patients with TOS from those suffering from shoulder problems.
   C. A normal ulnar nerve conduction velocity and electromyography study will exclude the presence of TOS.
   D. Anteroposterior and lateral radiographs of the neck are mandatory for every patient.
   E. All of the above.

16. In surgical decompression of the brachial plexus in neurogenic thoracic outlet syndrome:
   A. In the absence of a cervical rib, the first thoracic rib is the main offending structure in brachial plexus compression and should be resected in every case.
   B. The main cause of recurrence after the classical transaxillary first rib resection is scarring around a residual posterior stump of the rib.
   C. The supraclavicular approach offers superior exposure of the scalene muscles and a better access to the posterior third of the first rib.
   D. Injury to the long thoracic nerve in supraclavicular operations is minimized by preserving the middle scalene muscle while performing anterior scalenectomy and brachial plexus neurolysis.
   E. None of the above.

17. Arterial complications of thoracic outlet compression:
    - **A.** Occur in approximately 15% of cases.
    - **B.** Present long after symptoms appear.
    - **C.** Occur more frequently from *incomplete* than from *complete* cervical ribs.
    - **D.** Can result from "whiplash" cervical injuries.
    - **E.** Are *not* caused by congenital abnormalities of the first thoracic rib.

18. The diagnosis of arterial disease caused by thoracic outlet syndrome:
    - **A.** Is rarely made at an early stage.
    - **B.** Should be suspected when Raynaud's syndrome or its equivalents occur.
    - **C.** Is suggested by predominantly ulnar artery emboli to the hands and digits.
    - **D.** Is often made early on because of microembolization.
    - **E.** May be difficult to establish when isolated subclavian artery occlusion occurs.

19. The *best* surgical management of the proximal arterial disorder in patients with arterial complications of thoracic outlet syndrome includes:
    - **A.** A transaxillary approach.
    - **B.** An anterolateral thoracic approach.
    - **C.** Removal of the entire clavicle.
    - **D.** A supraclavicular approach.
    - **E.** A supraclavicular approach combined with an infraclavicular incision.

20. Effort thrombosis of the axillary-subclavian vein (Paget-Schroetter syndrome) is caused by:
    - **A.** Sudden heavy lifting.
    - **B.** Sudden heavy lifting associated with an hypercoagulable state.
    - **C.** Compression of the axillary-subclavian vein in the thoracic outlet.
    - **D.** Overhead arm stress in people with lupus anticoagulant.
    - **E.** None of the above.

21. The most effective initial treatment for spontaneous axillary-subclavian vein thrombosis is:
    - **A.** Surgical thrombectomy followed by anticoagulation.
    - **B.** Heparin followed by long-term coumadin anticoagulation.
    - **C.** Intravenous streptokinase.
    - **D.** Catheter-directed local urokinase followed by anticoagulation.
    - **E.** Hirudin followed by long-term anticoagulation.

22. The role of surgical treatment in the Paget-Schroetter syndrome is to:
    - **A.** Decompress the thoracic outlet and relieve the constriction of the vein.
    - **B.** Create an arteriovenous fistula to maintain venous patency during the healing phase.
    - **C.** Reconstruct the narrow part of the vein with a patch angioplasty.
    - **D.** Bypass the compressed area by a jugular-subclavian anastamosis or interposition PTFE graft.
    - **E.** Reestablish lymphatic channels because the venous reconstruction is likely to fail.

23. Which of the following occurs if the stellate ganglion is excised?
    - **A.** Dilatation of the pupil.
    - **B.** Increased ipsilateral facial sweating.
    - **C.** Horner's syndrome.
    - **D.** Sensory loss in the T1 distribution.
    - **E.** Increased heart rate.

24. Which of the following are not accepted indications for dorsal sympathectomy?
    - **A.** Hyperhidrosis.
    - **B.** Angina pectoris.
    - **C.** Post-traumatic pain syndrome (causalgia).
    - **D.** Selected cases of upper-extremity digital ischemia.
    - **E.** Paget-Schroetter syndrome.

25. During a transaxillary thoracic sympathectomy, which of the following nerves is least likely to be injured?
    - **A.** Phrenic.
    - **B.** Long thoracic.
    - **C.** Intercostobrachial.
    - **D.** Nerve of Kuntz.
    - **E.** None of these nerves can be injured.

26. Which of the following statements is/are true regarding upper-extremity sympathectomy?
    - **A.** Relief of hyperhidrosis is usual after upper-extremity sympathectomy.
    - **B.** A dry hand in a patient with hyperhidrosis is more likely to be achieved with endoscopic thermocoagulation of the sympathetic chain than with transaxillary thoracic sympathectomy.
    - **C.** Extensive sympathetic denervation of the upper and lower extremities for hyperhidrosis should be avoided because orthostatic hypotension has been observed.
    - **D.** Patients are more likely to consent to contralateral sympathectomy if their original operation was done by open operation rather than endoscopically.
    - **E.** All of the above.

27. Which of the following occupations may cause Raynaud's phenomenon?
    A. Grinders.
    B. Machinists.
    C. Baseball catchers.
    D. Butchers.
    E. All of the above.

28. The most common site of injury to the artery in a patient with hypothenar hammer syndrome is:
    A. Brachial artery.
    B. Radial artery.
    C. Ulnar artery at the wrist.
    D. Terminal branch of the ulnar artery.
    E. Deep arch of the hand.

29. Exposure to polyvinylchloride can cause hand ischemia, and the characteristic findings are:
    A. Multiple arterial stenoses and occlusions of the digital arteries.
    B. Hypervascularity adjacent to areas of bony resorption.
    C. Aneurysm formation.
    D. Fever.
    E. All of the above.

30. The possible sites for arterial compression in thoracic outlet syndromes are:
    A. Anterior scalene muscle.
    B. Pectoris minor tendon.
    C. Humeral head.
    D. Cervical rib.
    E. All of the above.

9

Answers

1. The answers are **A, D** (Rutherford, 4th ed., pp. 918–920).

Primary Raynaud's disease and vasosopastic Raynaud's disease are synonymous and refer to the condition in which cold-induced episodic vasospasm occurs in patients with histologically normal digital arteries. In this condition, the digital arteries are hypersensitive to cold or alpha-adrenergic stimuli. Ischemia of the fingers is the result of concomitant construction of both the digital arteries and the terminal arterioles. When cold-induced episodic ischemia occurs in patients with constrictive lesions of the digital arteries ("fixed" obstruction), the condition is called secondary Raynaud's phenomenon or obstructive Raynaud's syndrome. (This terminology is preferable to the confusing designation Raynaud's *disease* versus Raynaud's *syndrome.)* Unlike secondary Raynaud's phenomenon, which may be limited to one hand and may be restricted to one or more fingers, primary Raynaud's disease is classically bilateral and symmetrical. Although skin changes and fingertip ulcers are common in patients with secondary Raynaud's phenomenon, these lesions are absent in patients with primary Raynaud's disease. Nonetheless, after many years some patients originally classified as having primary Raynaud's disease may develop manifestations of a connective tissue (autoimmune) disease such as scleroderma.

2. The answer is **C** (Rutherford, 4th ed., pp. 919–932).

Patients with secondary Raynaud's phenomenon have abnormal finger pressure or plethysmographic pulses (or both) even when their hands are warm. However, abnormal (obstructive, peaked) finger pulses may be the only objective hemodynamic finding in patients with secondary Raynaud's phenomenon whose digital arteries are not obstructed proximal to the site of cuff placement. Reduced pressures in the fourth and fifth fingers are typical of the hypothenar hammer syndrome, which is caused by trauma to the ulnar artery as it crosses the hook of the hamate in the palm of the hand. Vibratory trauma associated with the use of jackhammers, chain saws, etc., leads to palmar or digital artery obstruction and is a well-recognized cause of secondary Raynaud's phenomenon. A precipitous drop in finger blood pressure (often to zero) occurring in response to cooling of the hand or individual finger in a patient whose finger blood pressures and plethysmographic pulses are normal when his or her hands are warm is indicative of *primary* Raynaud's phenomenon. Abnormal nailfold capillary loops are found in 90% of patients with scleroderma and in many patients who later are diagnosed as having a connective tissue disease.

3. The answer is **B** (Rutherford, 4th ed., pp. 920–928).

It is often difficult in the laboratory environment to reproduce the triphasic color changes "typical" of Raynaud's phenomenon even in reliable patients with a good history of cold sensitivity. Many patients never experience the full sequence of color changes. To establish the presence of cold sensitivity, it is necessary to employ a cold-tolerance test. Simple tests follow the temperature recovery profile in fingers after a brief cold exposure. A delayed return (10–20 minutes) of fingertip temperature to pre-exposure levels is indicative of cold sensitivity. More elaborate tests measure changes in finger blood pressure as the fingers are cooled. A precipitous drop in pressure at 10–20° C is positive for cold sensitivity. A >20 mm Hg difference in brachial artery pressure is diagnostic of a stenosis or obstruction of any of the arterial segments proximal to the site of cuff placement, including the subclavian and axillary arteries on either side and the innominate artery on the right side. In patients with secondary Raynaud's phenomenon (who have "fixed" obstructions of the digital, palmar, or more proximal arteries), cold-induced constriction of the terminal arterioles is the mechanism responsible for episodic digital ischemia. Disappearance of the Doppler signal from the palmar arch when the ulnar artery is compressed indicates obstruction of the *radial* artery or an incomplete arch. When the palmar arch is intact and both the radial and ulnar arteries are patent, compression of either artery will have little effect on the audible Doppler signal. Responses to sympathetic stimuli and to reactive hyperemia are usually decreased in patients with scleroderma, owing to impaired sympathetic activity and to stiffening of microvascular walls.

4. The answer is **C** (Rutherford, 4th ed., pp. 935–937).

Asymptomatic innominate artery lesions are uncommon in surgical series. Although there are isolated reports of their concomitant repair with coronary artery bypass and their prophylactic repair in patients with extensive multiple-vessel arch disease, most authorities recommend reconstruction only for symptomatic disease. In the two most recent series, almost 80% of patients presented with neurologic symptoms, referable to either anterior or posterior cerebral circulations or both. In one series, 15% of the patients had symptoms of the right upper extremity, while in the other, 64% of patients had microembolization to or effort fatigue of that extremity. Major upper-extremity amputations are rarely required, but impairment of hand function and tissue loss can occur from emboli.

5. The answers are **D, E** (Rutherford, 4th ed., pp. 937–943).

Ascending aortoinnominate artery grafting is performed through a full-length median sternotomy incision, with the graft placed as far laterally on the ascending aorta as possible. Bypass grafting is applicable to all candidates for direct arch reconstructions, whereas innominate artery endarterectomy is offered only to those patients with atherosclerosis whose aortic arch and arch vessel anatomy and pathology permit. Excellent early results may be expected in approximately 95% of patients and excellent long-term results in 87–90% of patients.

6. The answer is **B** (Rutherford, 4th ed., pp. 943–947).

Common carotid artery occlusive lesions requiring operation account for only about 1–2% of the cases involving carotid or great vessel lesions. Symptomatic lesions should be repaired. Reconstruction by ipsilateral subclavian-carotid artery bypass grafting performed through supraclavicular and, if necessary, cervical incisions is most commonly employed. Fry et al. recently reported excellent results, with only one stroke and no deaths. Although Takayasu disease affects the common carotid artery, atherosclerosis remains the most frequent cause of occlusive disease.

7. The answers are **B, E** (Rutherford, 4th ed., pp. 947–951).

Isolated subclavian artery occlusive artery disease is one of the most common locations for atherosclerosis. Lesions are usually asymptomatic because of the rich arterial collateral network in the head, neck, and shoulder. Symptomatic lesions are associated with concomitant vertebral artery or carotid artery lesions in three quarters of the cases, although isolated lesions may cause atheroembolization. Clinical subclavian steal syndrome is rarely seen, especially in the absence of these concomitant lesions. The left subclavian artery is involved far more often than the right in atherosclerotic occlusive disease. Carotid-subclavian artery bypass with prosthetic grafts or subclavian artery transposition are the operations of choice for treatment of symptomatic patients. Subclavian artery endarterectomy performed through a thoracotomy was the procedure first performed for these lesions, but the mortality and morbidity associated with that operation and the advent of extrathoracic operations has relegated the original approach to infrequent application.

8. The answers are **A, B, C** (Rutherford, 4th ed., pp. 953–955).

Symptoms of ischemia following brachial artery thrombosis are related to the adequacy of collateral circulation. Arteries that contribute to this collateral bed include the deep brachial artery; superior and inferior ulnar collateral arteries; and the ulnar, radial, and interosseous recurrent arteries. In the presence of abundant collaterals and short segment occlusion, the limb may remain asymptomatic at rest and even with exercise. Thrombosis of a long segment of the artery will jeopardize collateral flow and result in acute symptoms requiring urgent or emergent surgical intervention. On the other hand, occlusion of a short segment may not produce significant acute ischemia, and symptoms may become apparent only after discharge with upper-extremity exercise. Because the right brachial artery is ordinarily used for these studies, most patients are rendered symptomatic in their dominant hand. A falsely *low* blood pressure may be measured after this disorder. While a pseudoaneurysm can occur after brachial artery puncture, *thrombosis* at the artery would not predispose to false aneurysm formation.

9. The answer is **D** (Rutherford, 4th ed., pp. 953–954).

The brachial artery extends from the lower border of the teres major to its bifurcation, which is normally adjacent to the head of the radius. It is a single vessel in approximately 80% of patients. An additional superficial brachial artery occurs in the remaining 20% of cases and begins at the upper brachial level and descends through the arm superficial to the median nerve. The superficial brachial artery consitutes a high radial artery in 10–15% of individuals and the ulnar artery in 2–3%.

10. The answer is **C** (Rutherford, 4th ed., p. 958).

The brachial artery is the upper-extremity vessel most frequently affected by embolic occlusion, being the location of embolus in approximately 60% of patients. Emboli tend to lodge just proximal to the origin of the deep brachial artery, at the origin of the superior ulnar collateral artery, or at the brachial bifurcation. The axillary (23%) and the subclavian arteries (12%) are less frequently involved. The radial and ulnar arteries are rarely the sites of cadiac embolic occlusion but are more frequently involved with emboli from a more proximal arterial source.

11. The answer is **B** (Rutherford, 4th ed., pp. 962–973).

The acute onset of severe digital ischemia is usually due to palmar and digital artery occlusive disease, which results from a systemic disease. Emboli are less common causes in this clinical setting. Patients who present with diffuse digital arterial disease generally have a systemic disorder such as a connective tissue disease, whereas patients with an isolated finding are more likely to have an embolic source. Finger plethysmography will determine if there is subclinical involvement of multiple digits (as indicated by decreased finger blood pressure and obstructive wave forms). The immunology screen should be obtained to determine if a systemic disease is present. If these tests demonstrate no systemic disease and no evidence of obstruction in any other digits, echocardiography and upper-extremity arteriography should be performed to rule out a proximal source of emboli.

12. The answer is **D** (Rutherford, 4th ed., pp. 961–973).

Significant digital ulcers are not seen in the absence of obstruction and thus would not be expected to occur in this patient. Thoracic sympathectomy does not provide more than 3 to 9 months of symptomatic relief in most patients with Raynaud's syndrome and is of extremely limited utility. Most patients who live in cool, damp climates such as San Francisco will not significantly worsen by moving to colder environments, so prophylactic medication is not necessary. Nifedipine may be useful if symptoms become severe. Reserpine for intravascular use is no longer available.

13. The answer is **C** (Rutherford, 4th ed., pp. 961–973).

Most patients with digital ulceration and Raynaud's syndrome secondary to a connective tissue disease have recurrent ulceration over the years. While fingertip debridement is occasionally required, formal finger amputation at the metacarpal-phalangeal joint is extremely rare. A few patients have only a single episode of ulceration, but that is the exception rather than the rule. Major limb amputation is rarely necessary.

14. The answer is **C** (Rutherford, 4th ed., pp. 976–980).

The exact etiology of neurogenic thoracic outlet syndrome is still debated, but it is generally agreed that the symptoms are a result of irritation or compression of the brachial plexus. Osseous elements, notably cervical ribs, are responsible in only a minority of cases. Most of the patients have soft tissue anomalies. The scalenus minimus arises from the transverse process of the C7 vertebra and inserts on the first rib behind the scalene tubercle or on the Sibson's fascia. It usually passes anterior to the C8 and T1 nerve roots and compresses them against the inner border of the first rib. These anatomical anomalies constitute a mechanical predisposition of brachial plexus compression, often precipitated by direct or indirect trauma to the neck. Studies of the scalene muscles using microscopy have indicated that trauma incites inflammation and fibrosis in the muscles, resulting in a chronically contracted state. Histochemical staining of the anterior scalene revealed predominance of slow twitch, oxidative (type I) fibers. The presence of fiber hypertrophy has not been confirmed.

15. The answers are **A, D** (Rutherford, 4th ed., pp. 980–983).

Differential diagnosis of neurogenic TOS includes spinal and shoulder pathology as well as nerve entrapment syndromes. The diagnosis can usually be made with a good history and a thorough physical examination. The most characteristic finding in these patients is the presence of supraclavicular tenderness. The classic Adson's maneuver is nonspecific and indicates only a compression of the subclavian artery. The elevated arm stress test (EAST) and the upper limb tension test are more reliable in demonstrating brachial plexus irritation. Plain radiographs of the neck should be obtained in every patient because cervical ribs, elongated C7 transverse process, or aberrations in the cervical spine can be easily detected. Many electrophysiologic studies, including ulnar nerve conduction velocity and electromyography, have been advocated but none have proved to be consistent and reliable. They are recommended in selected cases to rule out other neurologic conditions (e.g., carpal tunnel syndrome) but are not specific for diagnosing TOS.

16. The answer is **C** (Rutherford, 4th ed., pp. 983–991).

Although the classic transaxillary first rib resection is still widely carried out by many surgeons for treating neurogenic TOS, it has been increasingly recognized that the first rib does not pose actual mechanical compression to the brachial plexus. It serves a passive role for attachment of soft tissue structures. The recent trend is toward first rib preservation. The most frequent cause of recurrence after transaxillary rib resection is reattachment of the anterior scalene to the first rib bed. The supraclavicular approach offers superior exposure for the brachial plexus, facilitates scalenectomy, and allows better access to the neck of the first rib. The complete supraclavicular decompression should include resection of both the anterior and middle scalene muscles and neurolysis of the roots and trunks of the brachial plexus. The long thoracic nerve may be preserved from injury by resecting the middle scalene along a line inferior and parallel to the nerve.

17. The answers are **B, D** (Rutherford, 4th ed., pp. 992–995).

Arterial complications of thoracic outlet compression occur in less than 5% of operations performed for thoracic outlet syndrome (TOS). Longstanding compression of the subclavian artery may lead to major arterial lesions with thromboembolic complications and may, in turn, impair the function and even jeopardize the viability of the affected limb. There is usually a long delay before arterial lesions develop and symptoms appear. Congenital bony abnormalities are the most frequent cause of arterial compression. Complete, long cervical ribs are articulated or fused to a tubercle on the upper aspect of the first thoracic rib just behind the distal insertion of the anterior scalene muscle. Incomplete short cervical ribs do not directly reach the first thoracic rib, although they are commonly associated with a fibrous band that follows the same trajectory as a complete cervical rib. Incomplete cervical ribs, when symptomatic, usually cause nerve compression, whereas complete cervical ribs appear as the main causative factor of arterial compression and complications. In addition, congenital abnormalities of the first thoracic rib, while unusual, seem to be an even more frequent cause of arterial complications than those of cervical ribs. The most common abnormality is agenesis of the anterior part of the first rib. In these cases, the posterior part of the rib may be articulated with or fused to the second rib in the same way that a complete cervical rib articulates with the normal first thoracic rib. Finally, whiplash cervical injuries may also precipitate arterial compression by causing trauma and subsequent fibrosis of the scalene muscles. (See Question 14.)

18. The answers are **A, B, E** (Rutherford, 4th ed., pp. 992–996).

The diagnosis of arterial complications from thoracic outlet syndrome (TOS) is rarely made at an early stage before the appearance of thromboembolic complications. In most cases, the disease remains undiagnosed until thromboembolic complications occur. The most frequent early symptoms are due to embolic occlusions of the digital arteries or palmar arch. Raynaud's syndrome or its equivalents, including episodic pallor and/or cyanosis, paresthesias, coldness, pain, and cold sensitivity of the hands and digits, are commonly found at this stage of the disease. They must be recognized as vascular symptoms and their source properly managed before further showers of emboli or a larger embolus result in ischemic lesions of the fingertips or even frank gangrene of part or all of one or more digits. In general, the diagnosis of arterial embolism from thoracic outlet involvement of the subclavian artery is suggested by predominant distribution in the *radial* artery distribution of the hands and digits. Small emboli are especially frequent in the thumb and index finger, probably as a result of the straightforward pathway through the radial artery as opposed to that of the ulnar artery. Microembolization may last months or even years before major embolic complications occur. Acute ischemia due to proximal embolization is the most frequent complication. In a few cases of isolated subclavian artery occlusion, ischemia does not develop. Thus, it may be difficult to establish an unequivocal diagnosis in chronic occlusions because trauma, cardiogenic embolism, and even Takayasu's arteritis may produce this picture.

19. The answers are **D, E** (Rutherford, 4th ed., pp. 996–998).

An ideal surgical approach to the management of patients with arterial complications of thoracic outlet syndrome should allow simultaneous thoracic outlet decompression, treatment of the subclavian-axillary lesions, and upper dorsal sympathectomy, if indicated. The transaxillary approach is largely used for isolated rib resection in the presence of neurologic symptoms. An associated upper dorsal sympathectomy may be easily added; however, this approach does not offer a satisfactory exposure of the subclavian artery and is therefore contraindicated in the management of arterial complications. The same objections apply to the anterior lateral thoracic approach. In addition, a thoracic incision represents an unwarranted surgical procedure even in young or middle-aged patients. A transclavicular approach allows for wide exposure of the supraclavicular and axillary regions. Two approaches are available. The first involves transection of the mid-part of the clavicle, followed by osteosynthesis. However, this may lead to orthopedic complications such as malunion and/or hypertrophic callous of the clavicle. The second involves resection of the mid-part or medial two thirds of the clavicle. This is simpler and has a low incidence of cosmetic and functional impairment. However, the same surgical procedure can be performed without dividing the clavicle, using a supraclavicular approach. Thus, the only indication for clavicular resection are the rare cases of arterial complications for malunion and/or hypertrophic callus of the clavicle. The entire clavicle should not be removed. The supraclavicular approach offers complete exposure of the subclavian artery, cervical rib, and muscular or fibrous bands. This approach allows safe resection of the normal first rib, provided the subclavian artery and the brachial plexus are entirely dissected and protected from injury. Complete resection of the posterior part of the first rib is easily achieved. In addition, associated muscular fibrous abnormalities can be treated at this time. Occasionally, lesions extend to the more distal axillary artery. In these instances, additional exposure may be obtained through an infraclavicular incision, leaving the clavicle undisturbed.

20. The answer is **C** (Rutherford, 4th ed., pp. 999–1002).

The Paget-Schroetter syndrome is a consequence of repetitive compression of the axillary-subclavian vein between the subclavius tendon and the first rib—in individuals whose body habitus and anatomy predispose to such compression. The result is fibrosis, thickening, and eventually thrombosis. Heavy lifting may eventually result in hypertrophy of the scalene muscles, but venous compression is unusual, even in bodybuilders. Heavy lifting per se does not produce Paget-Schroetter syndrome. No hypercoagulable state has been consistently demonstrated in this disorder.

21. The answer is **D** (Rutherford, 4th ed., pp. 1002–1006).

Surgical thrombectomy has been followed by a high incidence of rethrombosis despite anticoagulation. Neither heparin nor systemic streptokinase have resulted in very successful recanalization of the vein compared with catheter-directed urokinase followed by a period of anticoagulation. Hirudin is a biologic antithrombin that holds great promise but is not currently available in the United States.

22. The answer is **A** (Rutherford, 4th ed., pp. 1002–1006).

After successful lytic therapy the residual compressive abnormality should be corrected to reduce the risk of rethrombosis and to relieve venous hypertension. Timing of surgery is the subject of some controversy, with some authorities recommending a 3-month interval of anticoagulation to allow healing of injured venous endothelium. Others favor less delay in surgical decompression. Lymphatic reconstruction is ineffective, unnecessary,and unachievable.

23. The answer is **C** (Rutherford, 4th ed., pp. 1008–1014).

There are conflicting aims in achieving complete sympathetic denervation of the upper extremity because Horner's syndrome will occur if the stellate ganglion is completely excised, and an inadequate sympathectomy will result if too little of the sympathetic chain is removed. Preganglionic fibers supply the upper limb and are derived from cells in the intermediolateral column of the gray matter of the spinal cord between its second and ninth segments. Most vasoconstrictor fibers supplying the arteries of the upper extremity emerge from the spinal cord in the ventral roots of the second and third thoracic nerves. The arteries in the upper extremity can be denervated by cutting the sympathetic trunk below the third thoracic ganglion and severing the rami communicantes of the second and third thoracic ganglia. The sympathetic nerve supply to the eccrine glands in the upper extremity may be similarly interrupted. It is necessary to divide the trunk below the fourth thoracic ganglion and divide its associated rami if the eccrine glands of the axilla are to be completely denervated. To produce sympathetic denervation of the upper extremity, it is unnecessary to excise any portion of the stellate ganglion or to divide the rami to the first thoracic ganglion.

24. The answers are **B, E** (Rutherford, 4th ed., pp. 1008–1014).

There is general agreement that a predictably good outcome will follow upper-extremity sympathectomy for hyperhidrosis. There is less agreement on the value of thoracic sympathectomy for post-traumatic pain syndromes and upper-extremity ischemia, but these are still accepted indications in selected cases. Historically, dorsal sympathectomy was performed in the management of some cases of angina pectoris, but it is no longer an accepted indication for the operation. Dorsal sympathectomy is not helpful after effort thrombosis of the upper extremity and may make symptoms worse.

25. The answer is **A** (Rutherford, 4th ed., pp. 1009–1014).

The intercostobrachial nerve is encountered early on in the axillary dissection and should be identified and preserved. The long thoracic nerve, supplying serratus anterior, is at risk, whereas the intercostal opening is extended posteriorly. The nerve of Kuntz is an intrathoracic nerve that passes from the second intercostal nerve to the T1 root and should be divided if encountered during thoracic sympathectomy. The phrenic nerve runs down from the lateral to the medial border of the scalenus anterior muscle and is therefore at risk during a supraclavicular sympathectomy but not with the transaxillary approach.

26. The answers are **A, C** (Rutherford, 4th ed., pp. 1011–1012).

The results of endoscopic or percutaneous upper-extremity sympathectomy are encouraging, and endoscopic sympathectomy is evolving as the preferred method for surgical control of hyperhidrosis. Relief of hyperhidrosis is usual after upper-extremity sympathectomy. In summarized results of the surgical management, success was achieved in 90% of 192 patients from three series treated endoscopically compared to 97% of 435 patients from six series undergoing cervical or transaxillary sympathectomy. The endoscopic sympathectomy was achieved by diathermy coagulation of the sympathetic chain, which may account for the lower incidence of success compared to excision of the sympathetic chain. Extensive sympathetic denervation of the upper and lower extremities for hyperhidrosis should be avoided because orthostatic hypotension has been observed. Patients are also more likely to accept bilateral procedures in contrast to open operation because about 20% of patients, having had successful unilateral sympathectomy, may not agree to have the other side operated upon because of the postoperative pain experienced during their initial operation.

27. The answer is **E** (Rutherford, 4th ed., pp. 1016–1024).

It is well known that repetitive trauma due either to the use of vibratory tools or impact to the hand may cause digital artery occlusion. Digital artery occlusion, therefore, may be seen in baseball catchers, butchers, and grinders. Machinists may use the hand as a hammer, and hence the term "hypothenar hammer syndrome" refers to injury to the ulnar artery.

28. The answer is **D** (Rutherford, 4th ed., pp. 1016–1024).

The anatomic location of the ulnar artery in the area of the hypothenar eminence places it in a vulnerable position. The terminal branches of the ulnar artery arise in a groove called Guyon's tunnel, bounded medially by the pisiform and hook of the hamate and dorsally by the transverse carpal ligament. Over a distance of 2 cm, the ulnar artery lies quite superficially in the palm, being covered only by skin, subcutaneous tissue, and the palmaris brevis muscle. When this area is repeatedly traumatized, damage to the ulnar artery can occur.

29. The answers are **A, B** (Rutherford, 4th ed., p. 1021).

Exposure to polyvinylchloride is a rare cause of hand ischemia. Arteriographic findings include multiple arterial stenoses and digital artery occlusion, along with nonspecific hypervascularity adjacent to areas of bony resorption. Aneurysm formation and fever do not commonly occur.

30. The answer is **D** (Rutherford, 4th ed., pp. 1022–1024).

In addition to the anterior scalene muscle, pectoris minor muscle tendon, and a cervical rib, humeral head compression of the axillary artery has recently been identified. Humeral head compression is often seen in baseball pitchers. Not only the axillary artery is compressed, but the circumflex artery, a major branch of the axillary artery, is also compressed by the humeral head, resulting in more severe ischemia.

10

Arterial Aneurysms

1 Which of the following statements is/are true regarding infrarenal aortic aneurysms?

A. The 5-year risk of aneurysm rupture increases linearly with increasing aneurysm size at the time of discovery.
B. The 5-year risk of aneurysm rupture increases dramatically with increasing aneurysm size at the time of discovery.
C. Aneurysms invariably expand with time, and rupture is inevitable unless repair is performed or death from another cause occurs.
D. Aneurysm expansion and rupture are unpredictable in individual patients.
E. Hypertension is a risk factor for accelerated expansion rates.

2. Which of the following factors are associated with an increased prevalence of abdominal aortic aneurysm in a given population?

A. Age greater than 40.
B. Evidence of peripheral vascular atherosclerotic disease.
C. Coronary artery disease.
D. Abdominal aortic aneurysm in a first-order relative.
E. All of the above.

3. In which of the following situations does the retroperitoneal approach have significant advantages for aneurysm repair?

A. Inflammatory aneurysm.
B. Previous history of intra-abdominal sepsis.
C. Presence of horseshoe kidney.
D. Abdominal aortic aneurysm associated with bilateral iliac artery involvement.
E. All of the above.

4. Which of the following statements is/are correct regarding the morbidity and mortality of abdominal aortic aneurysm repair?

A. Coronary artery disease is the leading cause of perioperative mortality.
B. Coronary artery disease is the leading cause of late mortality in patients who have undergone aneurysm repair.
C. The incidence of perioperative myocardial infarction in patients having *no* clinical evidence of coronary artery disease is approximately 7%.
D. Myocardial revascularization prior to aneurysm repair may reduce the risk of perioperative myocardial infarction.
E. All of the above.

5. The classic clinical triad of patients who present with ruptured abdominal aortic aneurysm include:

A. Cardiac arrest, abdominal mass, back pain.
B. Hypotension, abdominal distention, sudden onset of back pain.
C. Hypotension, pulsatile abdominal mass, sudden onset of abdominal or back pain.
D. Hypotension, peritonitis, abdominal pain.
E. Hypotension, anemia, back pain.

6. The most accurate test to diagnose retroperitoneal rupture of an abdominal aortic aneurysm is:

A. Physical examination.
B. Cross-table lateral abdominal roentgenogram.
C. Emergency B-mode ultrasonography.
D. Computed tomography.
E. Aortography.

7. The best preoperative predictors of death from a ruptured abdominal aortic aneurysm include:

A. Hypotension.
B. Pre-existing coronary artery disease.
C. Low-admission hematocrit.
D. Diabetes mellitus.
E. Preoperative cardiac arrest.

8. Which of the following is the *most frequently* encountered etiology of thoracoabdominal aortic aneurysmal disease?

A. Atherosclerosis.
B. Aortitis .
C. Medial degeneration.
D. Aortic dissection.
E. Trauma.

9. According to the classification of thoracoabdominal aortic aneurysms from type I to type IV, which one has the lowest incidence of spinal cord ischemia and neurologic dysfunction of the lower extremities following operative repair?

A. Type I.

B. Type II.
C. Type III.
D. Type IV.
E. Spinal cord ischemia occurs with equal frequency in all types.

10. What is the most valuable diagnostic tool in evaluating patients for thoracoabdominal aortic aneurysms?
A. Plain chest x-ray.
B. Plain abdominal x-ray.
C. Ultrasonography.
D. Computed tomography scan.
E. Aortography.

11. What is the *most* frequently encountered associated disease in patients with thoracoabdominal aortic aneurysms?
A. Aneurysm involving another aortic segment.
B. Cardiopulmonary disease.
C. Chronic renal disease.
D. Peripheral arterial occlusive disease.
E. Cerebrovascular disease.

12. A 65-year-old man presents to the emergency department at 2 A.M. complaining of two hours of severe substernal chest pain as well as numbness of the left leg. Past medical history is relevant only for hypertension, treated with an ACE inhibitor. Physical examination is remarkable for a BP of 210/120 in both arms and a cool, pulseless left leg. Portable upright CXR is normal, and an ECG shows diffuse, nonspecific ST-T wave changes. The most appropriate next step in this patient's management is:
A. Sublingual nitroglycerin, followed by intravenous infusion of nitroglycerin, and immediate transfer to the CCU for management of suspected acute myocardial infarction according to the R/O MI protocol.
B. Intravenous infusion of nitroglycerin, immediate administration of intravenous streptokinase (or rTPA) and heparin for suspected acute myocardial infarction, and transfer to the CCU.
C. Intravenous esmolol followed by nitroprusside to control hypertension and immediate transesophageal echocardiography (TEE).
D. Medical management and immediate vascular surgical consultation to evaluate the acute arterial ischemia of the left leg, which has complicated a probable myocardial infarction.
E. Immediate arteriography and initiation of intra-arterial thrombolytic therapy.

13. A 25-year-old patient with the Marfan syndrome presenting with chest pain is found to have an acute aortic dissection by transesophageal echocardiography. There is a large intimal tear in the distal ascending aorta, and the dissection extends into the abdominal aorta. Moderate aortic valve insufficiency is noted. The patient is hypertensive, the pulse pressure is wide, urine output is minimal, and the patient also complains of pain involving his right leg, which is pulseless and pale. The most appropriate next step in this patient's management is:
A. Emergency composite valve graft replacement of the aortic root with coronary reimplantation using cardiopulmonary bypass via a median sternotomy.
B. Aortography to delineate the distal vascular involvement with a view toward either abdominal aortic fenestration or other local revascularization procedure to alleviate the severe left leg ischemia and medical therapy for the dissection itself.
C. Infusion of urokinase into the right ileofemoral artery.
D. Nonadjunctive medical therapy (beta blockers and sodium nitroprusside) with operative intervention planned only if the limb ischemia does not improve with conservative management or if other complications develop.
E. Emergent replacement of the ascending aorta and resuspension of the aortic valve on cardiopulmonary bypass via a median sternotomy.

14. An otherwise healthy 55-year-old man presents with chest pain that began 12 hours previously. Physical examination is remarkable only for hypertension (190/110 in the right arm), diminished pulses in the left arm without severe limb ischemia, and a cool, pulseless, anesthetic right leg. The left femoral pulse is bounding. CXR demonstrates mediastinal widening with a left pleural effusion. TEE confirms an aortic dissection extending from the level of the left subclavian artery to the diaphragm. The proximal descending thoracic aorta is markedly enlarged due to localized dilatation of the aortic false lumen, with an overall dimension of 7 cm. There is no evidence of rupture. The most appropriate management plan for this patient involves:
A. Emergency thoracoabdominal aortic replacement.
B. Nonadjunctive medical therapy (antihypertensive and negative inotropic agents), reserving operation only if frank rupture or other major complications occur.
C. Medical therapy as above followed immediately by aortography and run-off arteriograms to assess the lower-extremity ischemia and to help plan a peripheral revascularization approach, e.g., a femerofemoral bypass graft.
D. Emergency replacement of the proximal descending thoracic aorta via a left thoracotomy.
E. Emergency right femoral artery embolectomy.

15. Which of the following represent frequent modes of presentation in patients with popliteal aneurysms?
A. Rupture of the aneurysm into the popliteal space.
B. Acute ischemia of the lower leg and foot.
C. Chronic thigh and calf claudication.
D. Acute popliteal venous thrombosis.
E. Asymptomatic finding of a prominent popliteal pulse.

16. Which of the following treatment modalities would be appropriate for an asymptomatic saccular popliteal aneurysm?
   A. Saphenous vein bypass, originating from the common femoral artery and terminating on the infragenicular popliteal artery distal to the aneurysm, with ligation of the popliteal artery just proximal to the anastomosis.
   B. Posterior exposure of the aneurysm, endoaneurysmorrhaphy, and end-to-end interposition of a large lesser saphenous vein between nondilated artery proximally and distally.
   C. Proximal and distal aneurysm ligation, with interposition of a short segment of polytetrafluoroethylene graft to restore arterial continuity.
   D. Proximal and distal aneurysm ligation, with interposition of a short segment of greater saphenous vein to restore continuity.
   E. Saphenous vein bypass, originating from the proximal superficial femoral artery and terminating on the distal posterior tibial artery, with ligation of the superficial femoral artery just beyond the proximal anastomosis.

17. Which of the following statements is/are true with regard to femoral artery anastomotic aneurysms?
   A. Infected aneurysms of aortofemoral anastomoses are most frequently associated with *Staphyloccus aureus, Staphyloccus epidermidis,* and *Escherichia coli.*
   B. Uninfected aneurysms of aortofemoral anastomoses commonly present several years after the original procedure.
   C. Anastomotic aneurysms represent "true" aneurysms of the femoral artery.
   D. Anastomotic aneurysms should be repaired only when their diameter exceeds 3.5 cm because complications are infrequent in smaller aneurysms.
   E. Anastomotic femoral aneurysms are associated with rupture and thrombosis and with limb-threatening complications in 20% of patients.

18. All of the following statements are true *except:*
   A. Asymptomatic atherosclerotic femoral artery aneurysms should be managed conservatively unless they are larger than 2 cm in diameter.
   B. Iatrogenic femoral aneurysms should be managed with operative repair if large, but conservative therapy with serial ultrasound examinations is indicated when the aneurysm is small.
   C. Risk factors for the development of femoral aneurysms following arteriographic procedures include systemic anticoagulation, the use of thrombolytic agents, large bore cannulation, and inadvertent puncture of the superficial femoral or profunda femoris vessels.
   D. Arteriography is an accurate means of delineating the diameter of a femoral aneurysm.
   E. Proximal control of the aortofemoral graft limb is usually unnecessary when treating an anastomotic femoral artery aneurysm.

19. All of the following are complications of subclavian aneurysms *except:*
   A. Ipsilateral gangrene of the fingertips.
   B. Left hemispheric stroke.
   C. Vertebral-basilar transient ischemic attacks.
   D. Upper-extremity pain and fatigue with exertion (effort fatigue).
   E. Right eye amaurosis fugax.

20. Which of the following statements regarding cervical ribs is *false*?
   A. Cervical ribs are bilateral in over 50% of affected individuals.
   B. Arterial complications most frequently affect the right upper extremity.
   C. Most cervical ribs do not require intervention.
   D. Cervical ribs are equally prevalent among males and females.
   E. Aneurysms associated with cervical ribs are due to compression and poststenotic dilation of the distal subclavian artery.

21. In a patient with a patent ulnar artery aneurysm and clinical and arteriographic evidence of distal embolization with profound digital ischemia, acceptable treatments include:
   A. Thrombolytic therapy.
   B. Aspirin.
   C. Warfarin.
   D. Aneurysmal resection.
   E. Cervicodorsal sympathectomy.

22. Splenic artery aneurysms are:
   A. More common than aneurysms of the hepatic and celiac arteries.
   B. More likely to affect women than men.
   C. Frequently saccular.
   D. At less risk for rupture if calcified.
   E. Associated with a 40% operative mortality if rupture occurs.

23. Hepatic artery aneurysms:
   A. Are intraparenchymal in 80% of cases.
   B. Are most commonly found in women.
   C. Rupture in an extremely small percentage of cases.
   D. Are usually asymptomatic.
   E. All of the above.

24. Gastroduodenal and pancreaticoduodenal artery aneurysms:
   A. Are often associated with pancreatitis.

B. Are typically symptomatic, presenting with abdominal pain or GI bleeding.
C. Best treated by intra-aneurysmal ligation of entering and exiting vessels.
D. May require pancreatic resection.
E. All of the above.

25. Mesenteric branch aneurysms involving the jejunal, ileal, and colic arteries:
A. Present with abdominal apoplexy more often than other splanchnic aneurysms.
B. Are more common in women than in men.
C. Are frequently due to acquired medial defects or an endarteritis.
D. Rarely rupture.
E. None of the above.

26. Post-traumatic infected femoral artery false aneurysms in active drug addicts are:
A. Optimally treated by excision and arterial reconstruction, placing a PTFE prosthesis in the bed of the resected aneurysm.
B. Treated by excision and arterial reconstruction placing an extra-anatomic PTFE prosthesis to avoid certain amputation.
C. Optimally treated by excision-ligation without arterial reconstruction when the aneurysm is limited to the profunda femoris artery.
D. Cured by antibiotic therapy with or without supplemental hyperbaric oxygen treatments.
E. Caused by septic emboli of cardiac valvular origin.

27. Classic mycotic aneurysms:
A. Were first described in a comprehensive manner by Sir William Osler in 1885.
B. By definition, refer to aneurysms arising as embolic complications of septic endocarditis.
C. Are invariably caused by fungal infections, as the term implies.
D. Have decreased in incidence in modern medical practice.
E. May occur in multiple sites in a single patient at one time.

28. Microbial arteritis with aneurysm formation:
A. Is best treated with an in situ prosthesis when both the supra and pararenal abdominal aorta are involved.
B. Is caused by septic emboli from bacterial endocarditis.
C. Will usually yield positive gram stains for bacteria on operative samples obtained from the aortic wall.
D. Is never appropriately treated with in situ grafting when the infrarenal aorta is involved.
E. Is usually caused by *Candida albicans*.

29. Ultrasound-guided compression of a pseudoaneurysm is acceptable therapy for all of the following *except:*
A. Femoral pseudoaneurysm following cardiac catheterization.
B. Brachial pseudoaneurysm following arterial puncture.
C. Anastomotic pseudoaneurysm.
D. Pseudoaneurysm following angiographic puncture of a prosthetic graft.
E. Infected pseudoaneurysm.

30. The component of a vascular anastomosis most important in preventing pseudoaneurysm formation is/are:
A. Mesenchymal tissue ingrowth.
B. Length of arteriotomy.
C. Type of arterial conduit utilized.
D. Type of suture material utilized.
E. "Purchase" of vessel wall.

31. An appropriate treatment strategy for an *infected* anastomotic femoral pseudoaneurysm is:
A. Triple vessel ligation only.
B. Excision and reconstruction with prosthetic material.
C. Excision and reconstruction with autogenous saphenous vein.
D. Muscle flap rotation only.
E. All of the above, depending on the organism.

32. Which of the following statements regarding the pathogenesis of anastomotic pseudoaneurysms is/are *false*?
A. Short end-to-side anastomoses may result in localized dilatation and increased tangential pressure according to LaPlace's law (T = Pr).
B. Because most graft materials are less compliant than native arteries, there is preferential dilatation of the artery, inducing disruptive stress on the anastomosis.
C. The most common organisms cultured from infected pseudoaneurysms are *Staphylococcus epidermidis* or other coagulase-negative staph species.
D. Micro-occlusive disease of the vasa vasorum is involved in the fibrous degeneration of host vessels proximal to the anastomosis.
E. End-to-side anastomoses are more prone to pseudoaneurysms than end-to-end anastomoses.

10

Answers

1. The answers are **B, D, E** (Rutherford, 4th ed., pp. 1035–1037).

Size is the most important predictor of infrarenal aortic aneurysm rupture. In general, the 5-year risk of rupture is low for aneurysms less than 5 cm but increases dramatically above this size. At the following sizes, *approximate* 5-year rupture rates are: 5 cm, 20–25%; 6 cm, 35%; 7 cm, 75%. Aneurysm surveillance with ultrasound has become an important part of the management of abdominal aortic aneurysm. As a general rule, aneurysms tend to expand with time, leading to eventual rupture unless they are repaired or death from another cause occurs. Expansion rates average about 0.5 cm per year. However, studies using ultrasound AAA surveillance demonstrate that individual patients exhibit unpredictable aneurysm expansion. Some aneurysms undergo minimal expansion, whereas others undergo progressive or intermittent expansion. Hypertension is one of the few variables uniformly identified as a risk factor for accelerated expansion. In some cases aneurysms remain stable and then undergo rapid expansion. Consequently, patients in whom repair is not performed should undergo frequent ultrasound imaging (every 6 months) in order to detect expansion to a size at which repair is indicated and to detect rapid expansion.

2. The answers are **B, C, D** (Rutherford, 4th ed., pp. 1032–1035).

Abdominal aortic aneurysm is predominantly a disease of elderly men. Age is an important risk factor for aneurysms, with the highest prevalence found in patients 65 and older. In populations chosen only on the basis of sex and age, aneurysms occur in approximately 5% of men between the ages of 65 and 79. The incidence is much lower in younger individuals. Although atherosclerosis is no longer thought to be the predominant pathophysiologic cause of abdominal aortic aneurysm, the presence of significant peripheral vascular disease (e.g., lower-extremity or carotid occlusive disease) and coronary artery disease are associated with increased prevalence of aneurysms. Genetic factors are apparently involved in the pathogenesis of some aneurysms, because the risk of developing an aneurysm is markedly increased in patients having a first-order relative with an aneurysm. Roughly one in five abdominal aortic aneurysms is familial. The incidence of aneurysms is lower in women compared to men having equivalent risk factors (e.g., age, family history).

3. The answers are **A, B, C** (Rutherford, 4th ed., pp. 1045–1049).

The retroperitoneal and transperitoneal exposures each have advantages favoring their use in certain circumstances; therefore, surgeons should be comfortable with both approaches. The retroperitoneal approach often allows easier exposure and repair of inflammatory aneurysms. Similarly, dense adhesions from previous intraperitoneal sepsis or multiple prior operations can be avoided with retroperitoneal exposure. This approach also facilitates the exposure and repair of aneurysms in the presence of a horseshoe kidney. Aberrant and accessory renal arteries commonly associated with horseshoe kidney are more easily identified with this approach. Right renal artery and right iliac artery exposures are limited with the retroperitoneal approach; therefore, transperitoneal exposure is preferable when disease of these vessels must also be repaired. Although many surgeons believe that the retroperitoneal repair causes less postoperative pulmonary dysfunction, this has not been established by randomized trials. Gastrointestinal function apparently returns more rapidly with the retroperitoneal approach; however, this has not reduced the length of hospitalization after aneurysm repair compared to the transperitoneal approach in all studies. In routine cases either approach may be used.

4. The answers are **A, B, D** (Rutherford, 4th ed., pp. 1037–1039, 1043–1044).

The risk of perioperative mortality associated with aneurysm repair is less than 5% in most recent studies (see Table 75–7). However, coronary artery disease remains the leading cause of perioperative mortality in these patients. In addition, it is also the most common cause of late death in patients who have undergone aneurysm repair. The incidence of significant (i.e., >50% stenosis) coronary disease is between 30 and 40% in these patients. However, most authorities do not recommend routine preoperative coronary angiography in patients having no evidence of coronary disease, given that the incidence of myocardial infarction in such patients is less than 2%. Although coronary revascularization reduces the risk of myocardial infarction with subsequent aneurysm repair, the mortality rate of coronary artery bypass must also be considered in such patients. Consequently, coronary revascularization should be performed only when indicated on its own merits. It must be noted, however, that no prospective or randomized study of coronary revascularization before vascular surgery has yet been performed.

5. The answer is **C** (Rutherford, 4th ed., pp. 1060–1062).

The classic clinical triad of a ruptured abdominal aortic aneurysm is abdominal or back pain of sudden onset, hypotension, and a pulsatile abdominal mass. Unfortunately, the complete triad is present in only approximately half the patients. Sudden onset of abdominal pain is the most common symptom, and in the Mayo Clinic series, reported in 1992, it was noted to be present in 82% of the patients. Approximately half the patients in this series had back pain. Patients with a perforated viscus also may present with shock and dramatic abdominal pain. However, signs of peritonitis with rigidity of the abdominal wall are striking features of perforation. In patients with acute mesenteric artery occlusion, pain is frequently out of proportion to the physical findings, and shock is late in appearance.

6. The answer is **D** (Rutherford, 4th ed., pp. 1060–1062).

Computed tomography is 77% sensitive for the presence of retroperitoneal blood and is 100% specific with an accuracy of 92%. Computed tomography, however, should be performed with caution and only in patients who have been and are hemodynamically stable. Supervision during computed tomography in patients suspected to have a ruptured abdominal aortic aneurysm should be very close, with preparations made to take the patient to the operating room immediately if necessary. Physical examination may reveal the presence of a pulsatile mass but will not necessarily confirm retroperitoneal hemorrhage. Aortography is not suitable to confirm the diagnosis of rupture, and it is an inaccurate test to confirm the presence of an abdominal aortic aneurysm. Emergency B-mode ultrasound imaging is a helpful test to confirm the presence of an aneurysm in patients who present with abdominal pain. In the Harborview experience, published in 1991, the abdominal aorta could be visualized in 95% of patients. The aneurysm was obscured by gas or fat in the remaining patients. As an alternative, though a much less accurate study, a cross-table lateral roentgenogram also may outline calcification in the wall of the aneurysm. However, it is helpful in the diagnosis in only about 60% of patients. *Neither* ultrasound nor plain abdominal films are suitable, however, to determine the presence or absence of rupture.

7. The answers are **A, C, E** (Rutherford, 4th ed., pp. 1065–1067).

Preoperative hypotension and low-admission hematocrit are significant predictors of death from ruptured abdominal aortic aneurysm. In the 1991 Harborview experience, age over 80 years, female gender, and preoperative cardiac arrest were additional preoperative predicting factors of high mortality. In the 1992 Mayo Clinic experience, significant preoperative predictors of death were a high APACHE II score, preoperative hypotension, low-admission hematocrit, and the presence of chronic obstructive pulmonary disease. Neither pre-existing coronary artery disease nor diabetes mellitus has been an accurate predictor of death in patients with ruptured aneurysm.

8. The answer is **C** (Rutherford, 4th ed., p. 1071).

All of the factors listed can be responsible for thoracoabdominal aortic aneurysms. All produce weakness and dilatation of the aortic wall, but the most frequently encountered etiologic factor is medical degeneration. This is followed by aortic dissection, atherosclerosis, aortitis, infection, and trauma in order of frequency.

9. The answer is **D** (Rutherford, 4th ed., pp.1071–1073, 1085–1086).

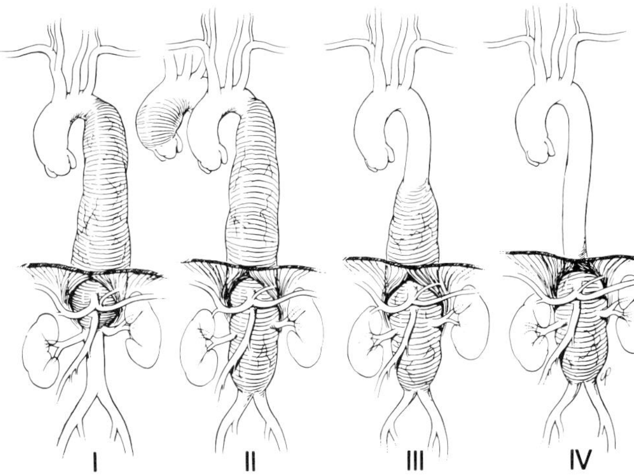

In patients with type I thoracoabdominal aneurysm, the aneurysmal changes involve most of the descending thoracic aorta and the upper abdominal aorta generally to the region of the celiac axis and superior mesenteric artery. In type II aneurysms most of the descending thoracic aorta is involved as well as most or all of the abdominal aorta. These aneurysms generally extend from the left subclavian artery down to the bifurcation and are at greatest risk for spinal cord ischemia. Those of type III involve only the distal descending thoracic aorta as well as varying segments of the abdominal aorta, including the visceral vessel origins. The aneurysms classified as type IV are located entirely in the abdominal aorta, generally extending from the diaphragm to the aortic bifurcation. Following thoracoabdominal aortic aneurysm surgery, the incidence of spinal cord ischemic injury is lowest in those with type IV involvement, because they usually begin below the accessory spinal artery.

10. The answer is **D** (Rutherford, 4th ed., pp. 1073–1075).

Plain chest roentgenograms may show widening of the cardiac silhouette, enlargement and tortuosity of the descending thoracic aorta, and calcifications confirming aortic aneurysmal disease. None of the above is consistently present and reliable. Likewise, abdominal x-rays are helpful in some patients but are not reliable. Ultrasonography may identify disease in the mid and lower abdomen, but the upper abdominal aorta and thorax are inaccessible. Even transthoracic and transesophageal echocardiography have limitations in evaluating the full extent of the thoracoabdominal aorta. Aortography is particularly valuable in identifying occlusive disease at the origin of branch vessels; however, in patients with intraluminal thrombus this modality frequently underestimates the extent of dilatation. Computed tomography scanning is precise regarding the diagnosis, location, and overall extent of aortic aneurysmal disease.

11. The answer is **A** (Rutherford, 4th ed., pp. 1075–1077).

Cardiopulmonary disease and chronic renal disease commonly accompany thoracoabdominal aortic aneurysms. But aortic aneurysmal disease involving another aortic segment is the *most* commonly associated condition and emphasizes the need for total aortic study and lifelong surveillance and treatment.

12. The answer is **C** (Rutherford, 4th ed., pp. 1090–1092).

Acute aortic dissection can masquerade as myocardial infarction (and many other illnesses) and should be suspected when more than one organ systems are simultaneously involved with an acute process. Misdiagnosis as myocardial infarction and treatment with thrombolytic agents can lead to disastrous consequences. Once the diagnosis of dissection is suspected, emergency transesophageal echocardiography can establish the diagnosis; today TEE is considered the diagnosis screening procedure of choice.

13. The answer is **A** (Rutherford, 4th ed., pp. 1092–1094).

The only accepted treatment of patients with acute type A aortic dissection (involvement of the ascending aorta) is surgical and consists of emergency replacement of the ascending aorta in order to prevent the most common cause of death, viz., intrapericardial rupture and tamponade. Although the aortic valve should generally be repaired (if possible), it should always be *replaced* in patients with the Marfan syndrome or annuloaortic ectasia to preclude subsequent aneurysmal dilatation of the sinuses of Valsalva and/or recurrent aortic valve insufficiency. Repair of the thoracic aortic problem alleviates the distal ischemia and usually obviates the need for peripheral revascularization procedures.

14. The answer is **D** (Rutherford, 4th ed., pp. 1092–1094).

The most optimal management of patients with acute type B aortic dissection remains controversial. Although the majority of physicians treat most patients with uncomplicated acute type B dissection medically and reserve operation for those who rupture or develop major complications, some selected patients (e.g., young individuals without other, severe coexisting medical disorders, those with a large localized false aneurysm or the Marfan syndrome) should be considered for early graft replacement of the descending thoracic aorta. Only the most severely damaged segment of the aorta should be replaced; more extensive replacement of the entire descending thoracic aorta or thoracoabdominal aorta in the acute phase should be avoided if possible to minimize the risk of paraplegia.

15. The answers are **B, E** (Rutherford, 4th ed., pp. 1103–1105).

Unlike abdominal aortic aneurysms, popliteal aneurysms are infrequently associated with rupture, which occurs in less than 3% of cases. Acute lower leg ischemia is the most common mode of presentation and generally results from thrombosis of the aneurysm. This thrombotic process may occur in a stepwise fashion, through sequential embolization to each tibial artery until the last of the outflow vessels becomes occluded. At this point, the outflow through the aneurysm is so severely diminished that retrograde thrombosis occurs, and the pulse in the aneurysm may eventually be lost. Alternatively, thrombosis of the aneurysm may occur as a primary event, with propagation of mural thrombus to a point where the lumen of the aneurysm is critically compromised. The leg may be less severely ischemic in the case of primary thrombosis, since the tibial arteries are free of embolism and may remain patent beyond the thrombosed aneurysm. Chronic calf claudication is commonly present in patients with popliteal aneurysms and develops as a result of the frequent association of popliteal dilatation with multiple diaphragm-like stenoses of the superficial femoral artery or advanced tibial thromboembolic occlusion. Thigh symptoms do not result from popliteal aneurysmal disease and are a sign of aortoiliac occlusive disease. Venous symptoms do occur with popliteal aneurysms as a result of local compression. However, venous phenomena are rare, presenting in less than 10% of popliteal aneurysm patients in most series. The increased awareness of popliteal aneurysmal disease, especially in patients with abdominal aortic aneurysms, has increased the proportion of patients presenting with asymptomatic disease. The majority of popliteal aneurysms are diagnosed prior to the development of symptoms, and aneurysms larger than 2 cm in diameter are best managed operatively.

16. The answers are **B, D** (Rutherford, 4th ed., pp. 1103–1107).

Saccular popliteal aneurysms are associated with compression of surrounding structures, specifically the tibial nerve and popliteal vein. Thus, therapy should be directed at arresting the expansion of the aneurysm, either with endoaneurysmorrhaphy or at least proximal and distal ligation. By contrast, symptoms from fusiform aneurysms are usually a result of thromboembolic phenomena, and the prevention of expansion is not at issue. Whereas a saphenous vein bypass from the common femoral artery to the infragenicular popliteal vessel would effectively bypass a saccular aneurysm, ligation of the popliteal artery distal to the aneurysm will not prevent continued enlargement of the process. Similarly, bypass to the posterior tibial artery with ligation of the superficial femoral artery will not prevent retrograde flow proximally to the aneurysm, and continued expansion may occur. The posterior exposure of the popliteal artery provides the opportunity to resect the aneurysm or perform an endoaneurysmorrhaphy, and a large lesser saphenous vein will allow one to utilize a single incision and preserve the greater saphenous vein for subsequent cardiac or peripheral vascular procedures. Irrespective of medial or posterior exposure, saphenous vein interposition with removal of the aneurysm sac from arterial continuity is the most appropriate method of repair. Prosthetic bypass grafts to the infragenicular popliteal artery are associated with poor durability and should be avoided whenever possible, especially in the case of an asymptomatic popliteal aneurysm.

17. The answers are **A, B, E** (Rutherford, 4th ed., pp. 1108–1110).

Anastomotic aneurysms presenting at the distal anastomosis of aortofemoral grafts are frequently secondary to infection when they develop soon after operation. *Staphylococcus aureus* and *Escherichia coli* are common pathogens in early anastomotic breakdown; *Staphylococcus epidermidis* may present later. Noninfected femoral aneurysms occur as a result of breakdown of the host tissue, suture, or graft material and characteristically occur 3 to 5 years following the initial procedure. Anastomotic aneurysms develop as a result of partial or complete disruption of the anastomosis, with leakage of blood into the perianastomotic tissue space. As such, anastomotic aneurysms are false aneurysms, without inclusion of the three layers of normal arterial wall. These aneurysms are prone to the complications of rupture and thrombosis, and 20% of patients develop limb-threatening complications if left untreated. For this reason, anastomotic aneurysms should be treated aggressively, with resection in all but the smallest, asymptomatic aneurysms less than 2 cm in diameter.

18. The answers are **D, E** (Rutherford, 4th ed., pp. 1108–1111).

Asymptomatic atherosclerotic femoral aneurysms rarely develop complications unless the size of the aneurysm is greater than 2–3 cm in diameter. Therefore, smaller, true femoral aneurysms should be managed conservatively. Likewise, smaller iatrogenic femoral aneurysms frequently undergo spontaneous thrombosis, and serial assessment with ultrasound examinations is an acceptable alternative to early operative repair. Risk factors for iatrogenic femoral aneurysms include systemic anticoagulation, the use of thrombolytic agents, large bore cannulation, inadvertent puncture of the superficial femoral or profunda femoris arteries, and obesity. Arteriography is never an accurate test to delineate the diameter of an aneurysm because of the presence of mural pannus, which prevents the arteriographic diameter from accurately representing the true diameter of the dilatation. The repair of an anastomotic femoral aneurysm can be technically demanding, with profuse hemorrhage if the false aneurysm sac is entered prior to achieving control of the graft limb, the proximal common femoral artery, and the profunda femoris artery. For this reason, the first step in the procedure is control of the graft limb, either at the shelving edge of the inguinal ligament or more proximally, through a separate retroperitoneal incision.

19. The answer is **B** (Rutherford, 4th ed., pp. 1112–1117).

All of the above complications stem from thromboembolic phenomena. Painful gangrene of the fingertips may be the presenting manifestation of a subclavian artery aneurysm that has shed microemboli to the hand and digital arteries. Microemboli may also travel to the vertebral-basilar circulations (may occur with right and left subclavian artery aneurysms) and to the right carotid territory (associated with right subclavian aneurysms), giving rise to vertebral-basilar and right hemispheric transient ischemic attacks and stroke. Right amaurosis fugax or retinal stroke may also occur. Cerebrovascular symptoms usually occur at the time of thrombosis of the aneurysm, with retrograde propagation of thrombus into the vertebral and/or right common carotid. Because of the origin of the left common carotid artery from the arch, left hemispheric symptoms do not occur. Thrombosis of subclavian artery aneurysms and embolic occlusion of the axillary and brachial arteries also give rise to upper-extremity fatiguability and pain with exertion (effort fatigue—the equivalent of intermittent claudication in the lower extremities).

20. The answer is **D** (Rutherford, 4th ed., pp. 1112–1117).

Cervical ribs are bilateral in 50–80% of cases and are more common in women. This latter fact accounts for the overwhelming female preponderance of arterial complications associated with cervical ribs reported in the literature. The vast majority of patients with cervical ribs are asymptomatic, have no arterial complications, and do not require intervention. Arterial complications occur because cervical ribs compress the subclavian artery against the tendinous portion of the scalenus anterior muscle at the point where the vessel crosses the first rib. Distal to this point, poststenotic dilation leads to aneurysmal change in the vessel, setting the stage for thromboembolic complications. Arterial complications most frequently occur in the right upper extremity because more frequent muscular activity in the dominant upper extremity leads to earlier and more pronounced changes in the artery on that side.

21. The answers are **A, D** (Rutherford, 4th ed., pp. 1119–1123).

Ideal treatment of a symtomatic ulnar artery aneurysm includes restoration of perfusion to the digital arteries and removal of the embolizing source. Thrombolytic therapy followed by aneurysm resection (with reanastomosis of the distal ulnar artery or vein graft replacement) is the correct choice. Long-term antithrombotic therapy with aspirin or warfarin might prevent recurrent embolic episodes but would do nothing acutely to improve digit perfusion. Cervicodorsal sympathectomy has been used in the past and might temporarily improve digit perfusion. However, the embolizing aneurysm would still be present, and recurrent ischemic episodes would result in digit loss.

22. The answers are **A, B, C** (Rutherford, 4th ed., pp. 1124–1128).

Splenic artery aneurysms are the most common splanchnic aneurysms, accounting for 60% of such lesions in most series. They demonstrate 4:1 female to male ratio and tend to occur at bifurcations of the distal vessel where they are typically saccular in configuration. Rupture has been reported to be just as likely when the aneurysm is calcified, occurs in a normotensive patient, or affects the elderly, as when these conditions are absent. Maternal mortality of aneurysm rupture during pregnancy is about 70%, and fetal mortality exceeds 75%. In nonpregnant patients, mortality after surgical treatment for aneurysm rupture is less than 25%.

23. The answer is **D** (Rutherford, 4th ed., pp. 1128–1130).

Hepatic artery aneurysms have an 80% likelihood of being extraparenchymal and occur twice as often in men as in women. Recent studies indicate a rupture rate of almost 20%, and the older literature reported a 44% rate of rupture. Hepatic artery aneurysms are usually asymptomatic, being initially noted as an incidental finding at operation or during unrelated diagnostic studies. However, symptomatic presentations are often catastrophic, producing hemorrhage into the biliary tree, GI tract, or peritoneal cavity.

24. The answer is **E** (Rutherford 4th ed., pp.1135–1137).

Gastroduodenal and pancreaticoduodenal artery aneurysms account for 1.5% and 2% of splanchnic artery aneurysms, respectively. They are frequently associated with pancreatitis (60% and 30%, respectively). Most present with abdominal pain, which may be related to associated pancreatitis, or with gastrointestinal bleeding. Because of the multiple feeding vessels supplying these aneurysms, intra-aneurysmal ligation of feeding branches is the preferred therapy, but drainage of pseudocysts or major pancreatic resection may be required in the case of inflammation-related pseudoaneurysms.

25. The answers are **A, C** (Rutherford, 4th ed., pp. 1133–1135).

Most mesenteric branch aneurysms are solitary and associated with acquired medial defects. Multiple aneurysms favor a diagnosis of endarteritis due to subacute bacterial endocarditis or a necrotizing vasculitis associated with a connective tissue disorder. There is no apparent sex predilection. Although rupture is uncommon, it is not rare, and these aneurysms are more likely to cause abdominal apoplexy than other splanchnic artery aneurysms.

26. The answer is **C** (Rutherford, 4th ed., pp. 1144–1151).

Whereas mycotic aneurysms can be caused by septic emboli of cardiac valvular origin, infected false aneurysms in drug addicts are caused by septic arterial injuries complicated by surrounding soft tissue sepsis and are considered post-traumatic. Although management of post-traumatic infected false aneurysms in drug addicts remains controversial, there is agreement that illicit drug users pay inadequate attention to antisepsis. When chronic drug users resort to habitual abuse of the groin, attempting femoral vein injections, repetitive arterial wall injuries occur. The vessel wall is further injured by infection following the introduction of microbial pathogens. Most chronic drug users return to a drug-related lifestyle and resume drug abuse even after prolonged hospitalization during which they were drug free. Thus, prosthetic grafts to reconstitute arterial continuity should be avoided in treating arterial infections in these patients because of a high rate of septic graft complications. Although some surgeons favor routine placement of extra-anatomic bypass in these patients to avoid amputation, others have noted that most patients with femoral artery excision will avoid amputation *without* arterial reconstruction. Although most of these patients will experience severe claudication initially, symptoms improve as collaterals develop. Patients with isolated femoral artery excision seldom require amputation or experience serious claudication when the common to superficial femoral artery axis is preserved. Although antibiotic therapy is a necessary adjunct to operative management, it will rarely produce cure. Hyperbaric oxygen therapy does not play a role in treatment. These patients require prompt surgical management.

27. The answers are **A, B, D, E** (Rutherford, 4th ed., pp. 1139–1142).

Although prior authors had associated endocarditis with arterial abscesses in the popliteal and superior mesenteric arteries, it was Osler in his Gulstonian lecture in 1885 who presented the first coherent understanding of mycotic aneurysms. Osler entitled his lecture "The Gulstonian Lecture on Malignant Endocarditis" and coined the term "mycotic aneurysm," which, by definition, refers to aneurysms arising as embolic complications of septic endocarditis. The gross pathologic appearance of the mycotic aneurysm resembles certain features of fungal colonies and led to the unfortunate misnomer "mycotic." In fact, most mycotic aneurysms are bacterial. Microbiology protocols to identify organisms and antibiotic regimens to target microorganisms coupled with modern imaging methods allow early identification and treatment of endocarditis. This has greatly reduced the incidence of mycotic aneurysms in modern medical practice. Mycotic aneurysms have been described in most named arteries and typically occur synchronously at multiple sites.

28. The answer is **A** (Rutherford, 4th ed., pp. 1142–1147).

Microbial arteritis is typically produced by hematogenous micro-organism inoculation of a diseased artery. The native arterial walls' structural defenses have been disrupted by the atherosclerotic process, and infection further disrupts the arterial wall, resulting in an eccentric *saccular* aneurysm. A distinction is made between this pathologic entity and a secondary infection of a pre-existing aneurysm, which occurs in a small number of patients. Many of these patients will have culture-positive samples from the aneurysm contents, with no evidence of clinical or invasive infection. Microbial arteritis, though uncommon, usually occurs in patients who do not have endocarditis, indicating a different pathogenesis than mycotic aneurysms. When the proximal abdominal aorta is involved, placement of an in situ prosthesis through the bed of the resected aneurysm is often the only practical solution that allows restoration of arterial flow to vital organs as well as to the pelvis and lower extremities. The traditional approach to treating arterial infections of the infrarenal aorta, which relies on extra-anatomic grafting for the restoration of arterial continuity, is impractical when the aorta is involved at the level of the visceral and renal arteries. When the septic process is less extensive and the pathogen less virulent, recent reports confirm that an in situ graft is appropriate when treating microbial arteritis of the infrarenal aorta. A complete list of pathogens causing microbial arteritis in descending order of frequency includes *Candida albicans*, but it appears near the bottom. *Salmonella* infection occurs most frequently. Retrospective clinical reports have shown that whereas operative gram stains are often negative, the culture results are positive. Accordingly, the operating surgeon must rely on other features of the clinical picture to plan and complete the operation rather than relying on operative gram stains.

29. The answers are **C, E** (Rutherford, 4th ed., pp. 1155–1161).

Ultrasound-guided compression of acute pseudoaneurysms is a relatively new accepted therapy for all of the clinical situations mentioned except anastomotic pseudoaneurysms, which are chronic in nature, and infected pseudoaneurysms. Compression treatment is most successful when applied shortly after the iatrogenic injury. Infected pseudoaneurysms must be treated by operative resection.

30. The answers are **D, E** (Rutherford, 4th ed., pp. 1153–1155).

The strength of an anastomosis and the union between graft and artery depend primarily on the durability and integrity of suture material. Mesenchymal tissue ingrowth alone is inadequate to provide required strength. In addition, inadequate incorporation ("purchase") of vessel wall in the anastomosis predisposes to anastomatic pseudoaneurysm. Before 1967, when silk suture material was widely used, up to 25% of all groin anastomoses resulted in pseudoaneurysm formation. More recently, the incidence has decreased to 1.7–2.6%, likely due to improvements in technique and more durable suture material.

31. The answer is **C** (Rutherford, 4th ed., p. 1159).

Patients treated with triple vessel ligation without reconstruction experience a 20% amputation rate and a 100% claudication rate (see question 26). In those reconstructed with prosthetic grafts, nearly all become infected and require removal. Those patients undergoing excision and saphenous vein graft reconstruction experience significantly lower rates of recurrent infection and acceptable long-term graft patency. Debridement without excision of the infected tissue is unacceptable treatment, even for infections caused by low-virulence organisms.

32. The answer is **A** (Rutherford, 4th ed., pp. 1154–1155).

Elongated end-to-side anastomoses have been implicated in the pathogenesis of iatrogenic pseudoaneurysms. All other statements are true.

11

Arteriovenous Communications and Congenital Vascular Malformations

1. Which of the following statements is/are correct regarding flow patterns associated with arteriovenous fistulas?
   A. If the fistula is small and the arterial collaterals are poorly developed, flow in the artery immediately distal to the fistula will be antegrade.
   B. If the fistula is small and the arterial collaterals are poorly developed, flow in the artery immediately distal to the fistula will be retrograde.
   C. If the fistula is large and the arterial collaterals are well developed, flow in the artery immediately distal to the fistula will be retrograde.
   D. If the fistula is large and the arterial collaterals are well developed, flow in the artery immediately distal to the fistula will be antegrade.
   E. Because of increased blood flow, blood pressure in the vein proximal to an arteriovenous fistula is greatly elevated, often approaching arterial levels.
   F. Although blood flow in the tissues peripheral to an arteriovenous fistula may be decreased, blood pressure is usually maintained at normal levels by arteriolar constriction.

2. Arterial pressure and blood flow in tissues distal to a *large chronic* arteriovenous fistula with well-developed collaterals will be *increased* by compression of which of the following vessels?
   A. Proximal artery.
   B. Distal artery.
   C. Collateral artery.
   D. Fistula.
   E. Proximal vein.

3. Which of the following statements regarding the systemic effects of chronic arteriovenous fistulas is/are true?
   A. Cardiac output is increased largely as a result of an increased heart rate.
   B. The increase in blood volume is the result of activation of sodium- and water-retaining mechanisms mediated through the renin-angiotensin-aldosterone mechanism.
   C. Systemic effects are independent of the location of the fistula.
   D. Total peripheral resistance is maintained at normal levels by an increase in systemic resistance and an increase in the cardiac output.
   E. A fall in central blood pressure is prevented by generalized peripheral vasoconstriction.

4. Which of the following is/are true regarding the diagnostic evaluation of congenital arteriovenous fistulas?
   A. They can usually be detected by arterial Doppler velocity signals.
   B. They produce venous Doppler signals characteristic of both obstruction and valve reflux.
   C. They can reliably be detected by arteriography.
   D. They produce characteristic lymphangiographic changes.
   E. Arteriography is required to determine their true anatomic extent.

5. A longstanding radiocephalic angioaccess fistula in a patient with mild hand ischemia will show which of the following findings on noninvasive testing?
   A. Decreased flow velocity in the ulnar artery.
   B. Reduced antegrade flow in the distal radial artery.
   C. Improved digital pressure with compression of the distal radial artery.
   D. Increased digital plethysmographic excursions when the brachial artery proximal to the fistula is compressed.
   E. Improved digital pressures and plethysmography by compression of the cephalic vein.

6. MRI is superior to arteriography for the initial evaluation of AV malformations in children because:
   A. It requires no sedation or anesthesia.
   B. It does not require injection of a contrast agent.
   C. It better visualizes venous malformations.
   D. It shows the anatomic extent of an AVM better than arteriography.
   E. It is less expensive because of lower facility and equipment costs.

7. A 20-year-old football player suffers a posterior dislocation of the knee. On examination he has an unstable knee and palpable pedal pulses. No immediate orthopedic operation is planned. As vascular consultant, you recommend:
   A. May be discharged home in a splint. Return if the foot changes color.
   B. Admit for angiography.
   C. Immediate operative exploration of the popliteal artery.
   D. Immediate heparinization to maintain arterial patency.
   E. Magnetic resonance imaging.

8. You are called regarding a 67-year-old man who returned to the ward after a two-hour left transbrachial cardiac catheterization. Although his left hand is cool and the brachial and wrist pulses are reported as difficult to feel, he has audible Doppler signals at the wrist. Your phone diagnosis is:
   A. Vasospasm.
   B. Brachial artery thrombosis.
   C. No significant arterial injury or thrombosis.
   D. Emboli from the catheter site to the hand.
   E. None of the above.

9. A 43-year-old farmer fractured his femur 14 months ago. In the past 5 months this leg has become increasingly larger. On examination he has full pulses and distention of his venous system. A hand-held Doppler records pulsatile common femoral vein flow. Your best diagnosis is:
   A. Lymphedema.
   B. Deep venous thrombosis.
   C. Compression of veins by a large false aneurysm.
   D. Arteriovenous fistula of the superficial femoral artery and vein.
   E. Chronic venous insufficiency.

10. While climbing a fence during a hike on a farm, your companion falls on a sharp stick, causing immediate, profuse bleeding. Examination reveals a 2-inch gash in the upper inner thigh with bright red blood pouring from the wound. You next:
   A. Apply immediate pressure.
   B. Construct and apply a crude tourniquet above the site of injury.
   C. Check for distal pulses.
   D. Cover with a blanket to maintain heat.
   E. Extend the laceration to expose the arterial injury.

11. The *major* factor related to the development of cardiac symptoms from an arteriovenous fistula is:
   A. The proximity of the fistula to the aortic valve.
   B. The duration of the fistula.
   C. The size of the fistula.
   D. The degree of venous hypertension created by the fistula.
   E. The specific artery giving rise to the fistula.

12. A fistula between an internal iliac artery and the iliac vein can be managed by:
   A. Occlusion of the internal iliac artery with a detachable balloon placed at the site of the fistula.
   B. Surgical ligation of the internal iliac artery above and below the site of the fistula.
   C. Suture closure through an incision in the iliac vein opposite the fistula.
   D. Ligation of the internal iliac artery above the fistula.
   E. Ligation of the common and the external iliac arteries above and below the fistula.

13. A chronic fistula between the superficial femoral artery and superficial femoral vein may include all the physical findings *except:*
   A. Ischemic ulcerations on the dorsum of the ipsilateral foot.
   B. A rise in the heart rate with compression of the common femoral artery.
   C. Varicosities of the lesser saphenous system.
   D. An audible bruit over the medial thigh.
   E. A palpable thrill in the medial thigh.

14. Congenital AVMs:
   A. Are genetically transmitted and found frequently in other family members.
   B. Require aggressive treatment in most cases.
   C. Are commonly associated with high output congestive failure.
   D. Commonly have complex arteriovenous connections.
   E. May show progression during menarche and pregnancy.

15. Hemangiomas tend to occur in infancy and are characterized by:
   A. Relentless growth and a poor prognosis.
   B. Marked proliferation of endothelial cells.
   C. High-output congestive failure when there is extensive hepatic involvement.
   D. Slow flow through large venous spaces.
   E. All of the above.

16. The characteristic features of Klippel-Trenaunay syndrome include:
   A. Extensive arteriovenous fistulas.
   B. Anomalous venous drainage of the lower extremity.
   C. Bilateral leg involvement.
   D. Poor response to surgical treatment in most cases.
   E. Spontaneous resolution in late childhood.

17. Embolization procedures for congenital AVMs:
   A. Are often curative.
   B. Accomplish the same occlusion of feeding arteries as surgical ligation.
   C. May be used to turn an unresectable lesion into one that can be resected.
   D. Employ deeply penetrating embolic agents in an effort to occlude the nidus of the lesion.
   E. All of the above.

11

Answers

1. The answers are **A, C** (Rutherford, 4th ed., pp. 1166–1174).

The direction of blood flow in the artery distal to an arteriovenous fistula depends on the ratio of the resistance of the fistula (R_F) to that of the artery proximal to the fistula (R_{PA}) and the ratio of the resistance of the peripheral vascular bed (R_{VB}) to that of the arterial collaterals (R_C). When R_F/R_{PA} exceeds R_{VB}/R_C, flow in the distal artery is antegrade (toward the periphery). This is most likely to occur when the fistula is small (high resistance) and the collaterals are poorly developed, a situation that produces little pressure drop across the proximal artery but a large pressure drop across the collaterals. As a result, pressure in the artery at the level of the fistula exceeds that distally where the collaterals enter the artery, causing flow in the distal artery to continue in the normal direction. When, on the other hand, R_F/R_{PA} is less than R_{VB}/R_C, flow in the distal artery is retrograde (toward the fistula). This is most likely to occur when the fistula is large (low resistance) and the collaterals are well developed, a situation that produces a relatively large pressure drop across the proximal artery but little pressure drop across the collaterals. As a result, pressure in the artery at the level of the fistula is less than that distally where the collaterals enter the artery, causing reversal of flow in the distal artery. Provided the proximal vein is not obstructed, venous pressure is ordinarily quite low (only a few millimeters Hg). The low outflow resistance and compliance of the veins accommodates the increased blood flow with little increase in pressure. Autoregulation (arteriolar dilatation) tends to maintain peripheral blood flow at near-normal levels. As a result, peripheral blood pressure is usually decreased distal to a large arteriovenous fistula.

2. The answers are **B, D, E** (Rutherford, 4th ed., pp. 1174–1175).

Compression of the proximal artery always decreases peripheral pressure and blood flow, regardless of the size of the fistula. Even when the fistula is small, this maneuver causes flow in the peripheral artery to reverse, causing some of the collateral flow originally destined for the periphery to be diverted into the fistula. When the fistula is large, compression of the proximal artery increases the reversed flow and augments the steal. When the fistula is large, compression of the distal artery eliminates reversed flow and allows more of the collateral inflow to reach the periphery. However, when the fistula is small and flow in the distal artery is antegrade, compression of the distal artery may decrease blood pressure and blood flow in the peripheral tissues. Compression of collateral arteries increases the total inflow resistance and always decreases peripheral perfusion. On the other hand, compressing the proximal vein increases outflow resistance from the fistula and usually increases the peripheral pressure, albeit by a relatively small amount. Isolated compression of the fistula restores the normal blood flow pattern. Compression of the fistula, together with the proximal and distal arteries and veins, eliminates the steal and may also augment peripheral blood flow provided the arterial and venous collaterals are well developed.

3. The answer is **B** (Rutherford, 4th ed., pp. 1174–1179).

Although the heart rate may be slightly elevated in patients with chronic arteriovenous fistulas, the increase in cardiac output is largely due to an increase in stroke volume. Activation of the renin-angiotensin-aldosterone mechanism is thought to be responsible for the expanded blood volume typical of patients with large chronic arteriovenous fistulas. Atrial natriuretic peptide may also play a role. Fistulas between large central arteries and veins (such as the aorta and vena cava) have a much more profound systemic effect than fistulas between small peripheral vessels, which have a relatively high resistance and divert less blood through the parasitic circuit. High-output cardiac failure is common with large central fistulas but rare when fistulas are located peripherally. Total peripheral resistance (the resistance "seen" by the left ventricle) is always reduced in patients with arteriovenous fistulas. Because the reciprocal of the total peripheral resistance is the sum of the reciprocals of the fistula resistance and the systemic resistance (the resistance of all the peripheral vascular beds), the total peripheral resistance is always less than that of the fistula itself. Vasoconstriction, therefore, is not only counterproductive in terms of tissue perfusion but also has a relatively minor effect on total peripheral resistance and can do little to maintain central blood pressure. Central blood pressure is maintained at near-normal levels by an increase in the cardiac output, which compensates for the decreased total peripheral resistance.

4. The answers are **A, B, D** (Rutherford, 4th ed., pp. 1192–1204).

Arteriovenous fistulas reduce regional peripheral resistance and increase flow, which eliminates end systolic flow reversal and increases end diastolic flow, changing the pattern of extremity arterial Doppler analog tracings (wave forms) to a high-flow, low-resistance pattern (i.e., more like a carotid than an extremity artery). Venous dilation produces valvular reflux detectable by Doppler exam. Pulsatile venous flow produces "continuous" signals synchronous with the cardiac cycle, rather than the usual "phasic" flow with respiration, which is also characteristic of proximal venous obstruction. Up to 30% of congenital arteriovenous fistulas are not seen on arteriography. These "microfistulous" AVMs may be detected by quantifying AV shunt flow by comparing pulmonary uptake on a gamma camera following proximal arterial and peripheral venous injections of 99Tc-labeled albumen microspheres. Increased arterial flow and venous hypertension both produce increased lymph flow and the lymphatic hypertrophy seen on lymphangiography. Rapid diversion of contrast into main channels may prevent other AVFs in a complex malformation from being visualized. The true anatomic extent is best determined by magnetic resonance imaging (MRI).

5. The answers are **C, E** (Rutherford 4th ed., pp. 1192–1193, 1204–1206).

Ulnar artery flow is *increased* in response to a radiocephalic fistula. Fistula flow at first slows in the distal radial artery but in longstanding fistulas it is reversed, potentially creating a "steal." Compressing the distal radial artery cuts down on the steal and improves digital perfusion pressures (see Figure 85–14). Compression of the proximal brachial artery will reduce fistula flow but further *decreases* distal perfusion. Compression of the venous outflow, like compressing the radial artery distal to the fistula or the fistula itself, improves distal perfusion as reflected by improved digital pressures and plethysmography.

6. The answers are **C, D** (Rutherford, 4th ed., pp. 1198–1203).

MRI may be achieved without anesthesia but not without sedation. Children don't usually voluntarily lie still. MRI can be performed without angiographic contrast media, but gadolinium is now usually used as an enhancing (contrast) agent for this purpose. Arteriography demonstrates draining veins, as does MRI, but MRI can distinguish venous malformations difficult to visualize by angiography unless special venographic techniques are used. MRI shows the anatomic extent better than arteriography because, in the latter, contrast may be seen to travel only through the larger communications and because it clearly distinguishes the different tissues (e.g., muscle, fat, bone) and their involvement with the AVM in multiple dimensions/views. The housing structure and equipment for MRI is more expensive than an angiography suite but has a much higher utilization rate. In addition, angiography costs more because of the greater involvement of skilled personnel in performing the invasive parts of the procedure and the use of sterile preps and disposable supplies (contrast, catheters, syringes, etc.).

7. The answer is **B** (Rutherford, 4th ed., pp. 1207–1211).

In this young man the popliteal artery may have been injured by the posteriorly displaced tibia. Intimal disruption may be present despite palpable pedal pulses. As time passes, the intima may become dissected or thrombus may form. Delayed arterial occlusion, often occurring at home, may doom a salvageable, functional extremity. Therefore, the patient cannot be discharged home. Although angiography is the current gold standard for ruling out arterial injury, duplex ultrasonography has been used in a similar role. Unfortunately, expertise with this technique is often not available in the wee hours of the morning when it might be best utilized. Serial observation in the hospital utilizing Doppler pressures is impractical in many orthopedic patients with extensive casts or splints. Immediate operation would not be indicated if no injury is indeed present. Immediate heparinization in a traumatized patient may be unnecessary and dangerous. MRI using special software to obtain magnetic resonance angiograms has potential to visualize arterial anatomy, but it does not produce images of adequate clarity at present.

8. The answer is **B** (Rutherford, 4th ed., pp. 1207–1211).

The absence of pulses at the wrist indicates there is a blockage between the more proximal palpable pulse and the absent distal pulse. The presence of Doppler signals indicates that there is some flow past the proximal occlusion and that the hand is viable, but this does not rule out a proximal brachial artery thrombosis. If sufficient collateral arterial supply exists about the elbow (as it most often does), Doppler signals, will be heard at the wrist, although they are not normal. Most nurses and physicians cannot differentiate normal from abnormal audible Doppler signals and are easily misled by the presence of these signals. Although significant arterial injury may not exist if, in fact, pulses are normal, this should not be your first reaction when called. Although he may have emboli from the catheter site to the hand, such small emboli would not alter pulses at the wrist. Vasospasm may occur in selected patients, but most vascular surgeons spell vasospasm *"c-l-o-t."*

9. The answer is **D** (Rutherford, 4th ed., pp. 1207–1211).

The superficial femoral vessels are located deep in the leg and cross directly behind the femur in the distal one third of the thigh. These vessels are not infrequently injured when the femur fractures in this location. Most probably a spicule of bone punctured both the artery and the vein, creating a relatively small A-V fistula. In the ensuing 14 months this fistula slowly increased in size, and flow from the high-pressure arterial system into the low-pressure venous system subsequently increased in volume and venous pressure. The leg enlarged secondary to this increased venous pressure. On examination this patient should have a bruit in the distal thigh and may have a palpable thrill at this location. The exact site of the fistula can be identified by duplex Doppler scanning or arteriography. Treatment is surgical. Lymphedema can occur after injury but should have occurred immediately postinjury and should improve over time. Deep venous thrombosis could have been present, but the presence of pulsatile, common femoral vein flow effectively rules out clot and strongly suggests A-V fistula. A large false aneurysm could compress veins and cause pulsatile common femoral vein flow, but this is distinctly unusual in the absence of other symptoms.

10. The answer is **A** (Rutherford, 4th ed., pp. 1207–1211).

Bleeding from any source is best controlled by direct pressure. Properly applied direct pressure will easily control venous bleeding and is also the best method for controlling arterial hemorrhage. Tourniquets are almost impossible to apply effectively. The amount of pressure exerted rarely exceeds arterial pressure. The pressure applied may injure nerves if the tourniquet is excessively maintained. If the pressure applied exceeds venous pressure but is less than arterial pressure, the tourniquet may actually increase venous bleeding. Furthermore, to apply a tourniquet in the upper thigh is difficult if not impossible. Although eventually you will want to check for distal pulses, and covering a patient in shock is useful to maintain heat, these are not immediate priorities. Surgical exposure of the arterial injury is contraindicated in the field.

11. The answer is **C** (Rutherford, 4th ed., pp. 1211–1213).

Although a small to moderate-size fistula that is left untreated for many years may lead to ventricular hypertrophy and congestive failure, the major factor that leads to cardiac failure is the size of the shunt, measured in terms of the percentage of cardiac output that passes through the fistula. The proximity of the fistula to the heart is not a significant factor. Venous hypertension is a function of the size of the fistula and the associated vein. As the venous system dilates, proximal venous hypertension may diminish, but valvular incompetence and venous insufficiency may increase. Although central arteries are more likely to produce fistulas that are hemodynamically significant, even peripheral fistulas can cause cardiac symptoms when they are large enough.

12. The answers are **A, B, C** (Rutherford, 4th ed., pp. 1213–1217).

Balloon closure of the fistula is very successful treatment for arteries that can be sacrificed. Ligation of the artery is equally successful. For both procedures it is important to exclude the fistula completely and not allow any collateral arterial blood flow access to the venous system. Transvenous repair is seldom performed, but occasionally may be helpful if the vein is dilated and scar in the area of the fistula obscures important structures such as a ureter. Proximal arterial ligation should be avoided at all times because it provides only temporary reduction in flow through the fistula and greatly hampers future definitive endovascular therapy.

13. The answer is **B** (Rutherford, 4th ed., pp. 1212–1213).

Most arteriovenous fistulas can be detected by physical examination. A palpable thrill and a continuous murmur are the hallmarks of the fistula. A chronic fistula may be associated with dilated distal veins and incompetent venous valves as a result of the increased venous pressure and flow. If the fistula is of large size, sufficient blood may be shunted away from the peripheral tissues to create ischemic changes, including ulceration. Tachycardia as a manifestation of increased cardiac output in response to the shunting of blood through the fistula is often noted. Compression of the fistula or the feeding artery should temporarily reduce the flow of blood through the fistula, reduce the cardiac output, and result in a *slowing* of the heart rate (Branham's sign).

14. The answers are **D, E** (Rutherford, 4th ed., pp. 1218–1221).

Except for a few rare syndromes such as Rendu-Osler-Weber syndrome, congenital AVMs tend to be isolated lesions with no pattern of genetic inheritance. Most congenital AVMs show slow growth commensurate with the growth rate of the individual and in the absence of specific symptoms or complications do not require aggressive treatment. It is quite uncommon for congenital AVMs, even when extensive, to be manifested by high-output congestive failure. This is presumably due to maintenance of peripheral vascular resistance by the complexity of the arteriovenous connections. In contrast, arteriovenous fistulas tend to be associated with larger shunts and potential congestive failure. In some cases congenital vascular malformations react to changes in the hormonal environment and show marked progression during menarche and pregnancy. Patients with extensive lesions should be warned of this possibility prior to their becoming pregnant.

15. The answers are **B, C** (Rutherford, 4th ed., pp. 1229–1231).

Hemangiomas are benign neoplasms of infancy that show a characteristic period of rapid proliferation during late infancy and early childhood, followed by spontaneous involution in almost every case. Overall, prognosis is excellent, and conservative management should be employed whenever possible. Pathologically, these are benign neoplasms as opposed to malformations and demonstrate marked proliferation of endothelial cells. True vascular malformations show no evidence of cellular proliferation. While most cutaneous hemangiomas present only cosmetic problems, extensive visceral involvement, particularly in the liver, is associated with congestive heart failure, which is often fatal. Treatment is directed both at the congestive failure and the underlying shunting within the liver. Large venous spaces characterize cavernous venous malformations, not hemangiomas. Venous malformations, like other vascular malformations, show slow growth with the individual and do not show spontaneous involution.

16. The answers are **B, D** (Rutherford, 4th ed., pp. 1228–1229).

Klippel-Trenaunay syndrome is a combination of anomalies primarily characterized by abnormal development of the venous drainage of extremity. The syndrome generally involves a single lower extremity, though upper-extremity involvement and bilateral extremity involvement can occur. Angiography demonstrates no significant arteriovenous shunting, while venography typically demonstrates a hypoplastic or absent deep venous system with venous drainage through anomalous superficial channels. For this reason, stripping and other surgical approaches to Klippel-Trenaunay syndrome often lead to worsening of the leg edema because the superficial channels may represent the primary route of venous drainage for the extremity. Whereas hemangiomas usually involute spontaneously, the anomalies in Klippel-Trenaunay syndrome do not improve over time.

17. The answers are **C, D** (Rutherford, 4th ed., pp. 1223–1228).

Congenital vascular malformations are extremely difficult to treat, and complete cures are uncommon, whether attempted surgically or by embolization. Embolization differs from the surgical approach in that an attempt is made to penetrate the nidus of the lesion rather than occluding feeding arteries proximally, as is accomplished with surgical ligation. This latter approach almost invariably leads to recurrence of the lesion, with resupply via complex patterns of collaterals. In some cases, embolization can be used preoperatively in order to reduce the vascularity of the lesion and render the lesion resectable.

12

Angioaccess

1. After the construction of a radio-basilic PTFE dialysis fistula, the entire upper extremity becomes severely edematous. Which of the following statements is/are true?
   A. A technical error or thrombosis at the venous anastomosis could be the cause of the edema.
   B. In the days immediately postoperative such swelling is common and will resolve.
   C. The patient likely had a history of a percutaneous dialysis catheter in the ipsilateral subclavian or internal jugular vein.
   D. The edema will resolve with ligation of the fistula.
   E. Subclavian vein stenosis is the probable cause.

2. Select from best choice to last the order of site selection for placement of a dialysis arteriovenous fistula:
   A. Common femoral artery to saphenous vein bridge fistula.
   B. Brachial artery to cephalic vein forearm loop bridge fistula.
   C. Radiocephalic (Brescia-Cimino) autologous arteriovenous fistula.
   D. Superficial femoral artery to saphenous vein bridge fistula.
   E. Distal radial artery to brachial vein bridge fistula.
   F. Axillary artery to contralateral axillary vein.
   G. Brachial artery to axillary vein bridge fistula.

3. Which of the following statements is/are true regarding vascular steal in the patient with a dialysis A-V fistula?
   A. The symptoms of vascular steal caused by a forearm fistula may mimic carpal tunnel syndrome.
   B. Claudication or ankle-brachial pressures less than 0.75 put the patient at risk for arterial insufficiency if a thigh A-V fistula is constructed.
   C. Ligation of the artery distal to the anastomosis will eliminate the steal and is the first line of treatment.
   D. In the side-to-side autologous (Brescia-Cimino) A-V fistula, reversal of flow in the radial artery distal to the anastomosis is required for steal, and flow reversal occurs in less than 10% of fistula constructions.
   E. All of the above.

4. Peritoneal dialysis can be utilized effectively in the acute setting for all of the conditions listed below *except*:
   A. Hypothermia.
   B. Hyperuricemia.
   C. Psoriasis.
   D. Hypokalemia.
   E. Congestive heart failure.

5. Absolute contraindications to long-term peritoneal dialysis include all of the following *except:*
   A. Recent abdominal surgery.
   B. Presence of a colostomy.
   C. Peritoneal fibrosis.
   D. Psychosis.
   E. Chronic obstructive pulmonary disease.

6. All of the following are true concerning peritonitis in those patients *except:*
   A. Diagnosis of peritonitis can be made by measuring the absolute white blood cell count of the effluent as well as the differential.
   B. The most common pathogen responsible for peritonitis in these patients is *Pseudomonas aeurigi-nosa*.
   C. A perforated viscus can present as polymicrobial peritonitis in these patients.
   D. The majority of patients can be treated at home with instillation of antibiotics through the catheter itself.
   E. If recurrent peritonitis occurs, the catheter should be removed because it is probably the source of the infection.

7. Advantages of silicone catheters when compared to polyethylene catheters include all of the following *except:*
   A. Decreased infection risk.
   B. Decreased thrombogenicity.
   C. Greater flexibility.
   D. Less expensive.
   E. Longer life expectancy.

8. Long-term venous access catheters placed in the inferior vena cava have a higher risk of which of the following when compared with superior vena cava placement?
   A. Infection.
   B. Vessel thrombosis.
   C. Dislodgement or catheter migration.
   D. Vascular injury.
   E. None of the above.

9. The most common long-term complication of permanent venous access devices is:
   A. Infection.
   B. Vessel thrombosis.
   C. Catheter occlusion or malfunction.
   D. Dislodgement or catheter migration.
   E. Vascular trauma or injury.

10. All of the following long-term venous access devices require periodic heparin flushes to maintain patency *except:*
    A. Broviac catheters.
    B. Hickman catheters.
    C. Groshong catheters.
    D. Implantable central venous access devices such as Port-a-cath.
    E. None of the above.

11. The difference between Broviac and Hickman catheters include all of the following *except:*
    A. Internal diameter.
    B. External diameter.
    C. Catheter wall thickness.
    D. The presence of a dacron cuff.
    E. None of the above.

12. Following a transfemoral coronary arteriogram and percutaneous coronary balloon angioplasty, a 60-year-old woman develops a slowly enlarging 4-cm femoral false aneurysm. You should:
    A. Apply a compressive bandage to the groin.
    B. Perform emergency surgical exploration.
    C. Perform an ultrasound for attempted ultrasound-guided compression closure.
    D. Perform angiographic embolization.
    E. None of the above.

13. Two hours after a transaxillary arteriogram, a 45-year-old man begins to complain of tingling and mild weakness of his hand. The axillary puncture site has mild ecchymosis and swelling but no palpable hematoma. The radial pulse is normal. You should:
    A. Reassure the patient and observe.
    B. Explore the axillary sheath if the radial pulse disappears.
    C. Order an electromyelogram and operate if it is abnormal.
    D. Explore and decompress the axillary sheath, artery, and nerves immediately.
    E. Begin intravenous heparin therapy.

14. After percutaneous placement of an intra-aortic balloon pump through the femoral artery, an unstable cardiac patient loses the ipsilateral pedal pulse and Doppler flow over the pedal vessels. Cardiac index is 1.8 L/m^2. Foot motion and sensation are decreased. You should consider doing all of the following *except:*
    A. Maximize cardiac output.
    B. Consider removing the balloon pump and moving it to the contralateral femoral artery.
    C. Apply nitroglycerin paste to the foot and a heating blanket to the lower extremity.
    D. Consider leaving the balloon pump in place and performing a femorofemoral cross-over graft to below the femoral insertion site of the balloon pump.
    E. Observe the leg if Doppler signals return and neurosensory examination is normal.

15. Following a transbrachial arteriogram, a 50-year-old construction worker is noted to have an underlying asymptomatic brachial artery occlusion. You should:
    A. Heparinize and observe.
    B. Repair the brachial artery if he complains of any ischemic symptoms in the future.
    C. Start intravenous thrombolytic therapy to lyse the thrombosis.
    D. Repair the brachial artery immediately under local anesthesia if the patient's condition is stable.
    E. None of the above.

12

Answers

1. The answers are **C, D, E** (Rutherford 4th ed., pp 1233–1237, 1242)

If swelling of the entire extremity occurs following fistula construction, then central vein stenosis is the likely cause. Central vein thrombosis/stenosis, in this setting, is most often secondary to central vein cannulation for dialysis access. Catheter-associated thrombosis/stenosis is reported as high as 50%, with most being occult. When venous return is increased by fistula construction, the stenosis becomes flow limiting, and venous hypertension and edema ensue. To avoid this complication, the subclavian vein should be evaluated preoperatively with duplex ultrasound or venogram in patients with a history of ipsilateral central vein cannulation. Thrombolytic therapy and percutaneous transluminal angioplasty (with and without use of intraluminal stents) have been successfully used to correct this problem; however, in most cases the A-V fistula must be ligated. Edema of the extremity proximal to the venous anastomosis (not including the upper arm) may be due to technical error, thrombosis, or intimal hyperplasia at the venous anastomosis. These diagnoses can be established with angiography and then corrected using endovascular or surgical techniques. Proximal venous hypertension is commonly due to an "arterialized" venous system proximal to the venous anastomosis and is corrected by ligating the venous tributary proximal to the end-to-side anastomosis.

2. The answers are **C, E, B, G, D, A, F** (Rutherford, 4th ed., pp. 1236–1241).

Careful site selection is essential for the construction of a successful fistula and to ensure that access sites are optimized for the life of the dialysis patient. The radiocephalic autogenous fistula is the first choice because it is the simplest to construct and has superior long-term patency and fewer associated complications compared to PTFE bridge fistulas. The guiding principles in site selection are distal constructions before proximal ones and upper-extremity constructions before lower-extremity ones. Proximal sites are preferred to maximize future access sites and to avoid potentially limb- or life-threatening complications (such as thrombosis, infection, or aneurysm) at the suture lines of large vessels such as the axillary or common femoral arteries. Though thigh A-V fistulas have superior patency rates because of the higher flow afforded by the larger vessels, they are less desirable because of increased incidence of infection, risk of distal arterial insufficiency, and limitations on patient mobility. In accord with the above principles, the superficial femoral artery is chosen over the common femoral for thigh constructions. In some patients conventional sites may be exhausted and axillary vein to axillary artery construction may be necessary.

3. The answers are **A, B** (Rutherford, 4th ed., p. 1242).

Symptomatic ischemia distal to autogenous or prosthetic fistulas is reported to occur in 3–7% of patients. Signs of vascular steal include pain, coldness, numbness, and occasionally motor dysfunction of the fingers and hand—the symptoms may mimic carpal tunnel syndrome. In the side-to-side Brescia-Cimino fistula, the venous connection acts as a low-resistance, low-pressure sink so that reversal of flow *always* occurs in the radial artery distal to the anastomosis. To avoid symptomatic steal, the collateral blood supply from the ulnar artery must be adequate. Thus, it is imperative that ulnar flow be assessed preoperatively using the Allen test. Patients with pre-existing arterial insufficiency of the lower extremities (as indicated by claudication and/or ankle-brachial pressure indexes less than 0.75) are at risk for limb-threatening vascular steal. Indeed, there are reports of lower-extremity amputations required to treat ischemic complications caused by ill-placed thigh A-V fistulas. In the Brescia-Cimino fistula, ligation of the radial artery distal to the anastomosis creates an effective end-to-side anastomosis and eliminates the steal. In this configuration, ligation is a common and relatively safe maneuver. In many configurations, artery ligation may increase the symptoms, and with large proximal vessels, such as the axillary and femoral arteries, ligation is contraindicated. Reduction of flow through the fistula by suture narrowing the anastomosis or by banding the prosthesis may correct the steal; however, these techniques are unreliable, and in most cases the fistula must be removed and lateral arteriorraphy performed.

4. The answer is **D** (Rutherford, 4th ed., pp. 1245–1246).

Peritoneal dialysis can be used when acute renal failure occurs to correct *hyperkalemia* (not *hypokalemia*), fluid overload, metabolic acidosis, electrolyte disorders, and congestive heart failure secondary to the fluid overload. Hyperuricemia associated with gouty nephropathy can be treated acutely with peritoneal dialysis, as can psoriasis and hypothermia.

5. The answer is **E** (Rutherford, 4th ed., pp. 1246–1248).

Major contraindications to chronic peritoneal dialysis include recent abdominal surgery due to drains and wounds, inflammatory bowel disease, and presence of extensive peritoneal fibrosis and patients who are immunosuppressed. Those patients with a significant neurological deficit, psychosis, and poor intellect, or those who are not motivated, also cannot be considered as candidates for peritoneal dialysis. Blind patients or those with crippling arthritis cannot perform their own peritoneal dialysis and must have a family member available to assist them or they cannot be considered for peritoneal dialysis. *Minor* contraindications include chronic obstructive pulmonary disease, diverticulosis, polycystic kidney disease, hyperlipidemia, obesity, lumbar back disease, and protein malnutrition.

6. The answer is **B** (Rutherford, 4th ed., pp. 1248–1250).

Peritonitis in patients on peritoneal dialysis is responsible for one third of the hospitalizations for these individuals. The most common reason for termination of peritoneal dialysis in patients is peritonitis (25–60% of cases). It is estimated that 15% of deaths in these patients are attributable to peritonitis. The diagnosis of peritonitis can be made by the presence of a cloudy effluent and abdominal discomfort. The white blood cell count increases to greater than 100/cc, and neutrophils predominate—>50%—rather than the typical monocyte. The most common pathogen is *Staphylococcus aureus* or coagulase-negative *Staphylococcus*. Polymicrobial flora retrieved from the peritoneal fluid should raise the possibility of a perforated viscus.

7. The answer is **D** (Rutherford, 4th ed., pp. 1254–1255).

Long-term success with central venous catheters of Teflon, polyethylene, and polyvinyl chloride has been limited by unacceptable rates of sepsis and thrombosis. Advances in catheter technology have made available silicone rubber catheters. Advantages of the silicone catheter include greater flexibility, decreased thrombogenicity, and decreased incidence of sepsis as compared to polyethylene catheters. Silicone catheters are more expensive but have a longer life expectancy than polyethylene catheters.

8. The answer is **B** (Rutherford, 4th ed., pp. 1255–1256).

Cannulation of the inferior vena cava can be successfully performed via the saphenous vein. Infection rates have been comparable to catheters placed in the superior vena cava (SVC); however, there appears to be an increased risk of iliofemoral thrombosis. In 1991, Williard et al. reported on 31 catheters placed infraumbilically in 26 patients and found a statistically significant difference in central vein thrombosis when compared with catheters placed in the SVC (13% vs. 1.5%, respectively).

9. The answer is **A** (Rutherford, 4th ed., p. 1257).

Infection is the most common long-term complication of permanent access devices, with rates reported as high as 30%. Whereas vessel thrombosis is relatively unusual, there is a substantial incidence of late stenosis and scarring.

10. The answer is **C** (Rutherford, 4th ed., p. 1255).

The Broviac and Hickman catheters require daily heparin flushes to avoid thrombosis. The Groshong catheter requires only weekly *saline* flushes when not in use. The implantable central venous access devices require flushing with heparinized saline after blood sampling or infusion. When not in use, the system requires flushing every 4 weeks.

11. The answer is **D** (Rutherford, 4th ed., p. 1255).

The Broviac catheter, introduced in 1973, is a silicone rubber right atrial catheter (internal/external diameter of 1.0 mm/2.2 mm) for prolonged parenteral alimentation. Hickman et al. modified the Broviac catheter, making it larger (internal/external diameter 1.6 mm/3.2 mm) and suitable for blood sampling and infusion of drugs, intravenous solutions, and blood products. Broviac and Hickman catheters are 90 cm long, are radiopaque, and have a dacron cuff 30 cm from the Luer lock at the external end. These catheters come with one, two, or three lumens and one or two dacron cuffs placed on the extravascular segment.

12. The answer is **C** (Rutherford, 4th ed., pp. 1255–1259).

Femoral pseudoaneurysms are currently the most common complication following transfemoral arteriograms, especially for coronary balloon angioplasty, thrombolytic therapy, or intervascular stenting. The diagnosis can be confirmed by a color flow duplex ultrasound study of the groin. Ultrasound-guided compression at 10-minute intervals for approximately 30 minutes will close approximately 90% of such pseudoaneurysms. Aneurysm size and duration, as well as arterial sheath size, do not appear to affect success. However, anticoagulation at the time of compression reduces the chance of pseudoaneurysm closure from 98% to 86%. If ultrasound-guided compression therapy does not succeed, surgical exploration with closure may eventually be required. Compressive bandages, sandbags, and C-compressive clamps generally do not work and may hide an expanding hematoma or pseudoaneurysm. Angiographic embolization is not currently recommended.

13. The answer is **D** (Rutherford, 4th ed., p. 1260).

Transaxillary arteriograms carry a higher (3–4%) complication rate than either transfemoral (1–2%) or translumbar (2–3%) arteriograms. The most common and the most potentially devastating risk of a transaxillary arteriogram is a progressive and sometimes permanent neurologic deficit of the hand due to an axillary sheath hematoma. Such a hematoma may be small but can tightly compress the axillary sheath contents (compartment-type syndrome). If hand tingling or weakness persists for 1 hour following a transaxillary arteriogram, the axillary sheath should be explored at the puncture site, with evacuation of any local hematoma. Delay of such an exploration can result in long-term neurologic disability of the hand.

14. The answer is **C** (Rutherford, 4th ed., pp. 1260–1261).

Acute lower-extremity arterial ischemia complicates approximately 10% of intra-aortic balloon pumps placed either percutaneously or surgically through the femoral artery. This complication is more common in patients who have underlying chronic arterial occlusive disease or aneurysms lined with atheroma and thrombus. Low cardiac output can contribute to worsening of the ischemia. Consequently, cardiac output must be maximized. If the lower extremity has only decreased pulses with maintenance of ankle Doppler signals and normal neurosensory examination, the extremity can usually be observed. However, loss of pulses and Doppler signal plus decreased motion and sensation indicate severe ischemia that must be corrected. If possible, the balloon pump should be removed from the femoral artery and moved to the contralateral femoral artery. If this is not possible, a femorofemoral cross-over graft occurs in approximately 5% of patients with intra-aortic balloon pumps.

15. The answer is **D** (Rutherford, 4th ed., p. 1260).

Local brachial artery thrombosis is a common complication of transbrachial arteriograms. Asymptomatic brachial artery occlusion may occur in as many as one third of patients. Although the occlusion may be asymptomatic initially, approximately 75% of such patients will eventually complain of forearm or hand fatigue and pain with vigorous exercise or in cold environments. Consequently, most experts would recommend immediate repair under local anesthesia. Such repairs are safe and restore a normal radial pulse in approximately 97% of patients. Delay beyond 24 hours should be avoided; the recurrent thrombosis rate jumps from 2% if the repair is performed in the first 24 hours to 12% if it is delayed beyond 24 hours. Most brachial artery thromboses are due to a local intimal injury; consequently, thrombolytic therapy without repair of the local arterial injury is not appropriate.

13

Visceral Ischemic Syndromes

1. Which of the following statements correctly characterize postprandial intestinal hyperemia?
   A. Intestinal hyperemia is maximal 30–90 minutes after eating.
   B. The duration of the postprandial intestinal hyperemic response is 4–6 hours.
   C. Both celiac and superior mesenteric artery flows increase markedly following a meal.
   D. Hyperemic response varies with the chemical composition of the ingested nutrients.
   E. Vasoactive intestinal peptide (VIP) is the most important humoral mediator of intestinal hyperemia.

2. The diagnosis of chronic intestinal ischemia can be reliably established by:
   A. Tests of intestinal absorptive ability.
   B. Angiography.
   C. Duplex scanning.
   D. History.
   E. None of the above, as a solitary investigation.

3. Nonocclusive mesenteric ischemia (NOMI) is:
   A. Common.
   B. Often associated with pre-existing shock.
   C. Most frequently seen following intestinal surgery.
   D. May be influenced by digitalis-mediated increases in visceral artery resistance.
   E. Confirmed by angiography demonstrating patent mesenteric arterial trunks with tapering visceral artery branch occlusions.

4. Which of the following statements concerning embolism and thrombosis of the superior mesenteric artery is/are true?
   A. Emboli to the superior mesenteric artery typically lodge just beyond the orifice of the artery, producing ischemia of the entire small bowel, whereas thrombosis typically occurs beyond the first few branches so that the ischemia that results spares the proximal jejunum.
   B. The mortality rate for treatment of embolic superior mesenteric artery occlusion is considerably higher (>80%) than that reported for treatment of acute superior mesenteric artery thrombosis (50–60%).
   C. Embolism may arise from cardiac or proximal arterial sources or as a complication of intra-arterial devices such as catheters, guidewires, etc. Thrombosis is usually caused by longstanding, progressive atherosclerotic stenosis of the proximal superior mesenteric artery.
   D. Patients with embolic superior mesenteric artery occlusion typically have chronic histories of abdominal pain and weight loss. Such symptoms are infrequently encountered in patients with thrombosis.
   E. Patients with superior mesenteric artery embolism typically have associated occlusive disease of other visceral artery branches. Such lesions are rare in patients with thrombosis.

5. Which of the following statements best describes the approach to surgical treatment of acutely ischemic intestine?
   A. If necrotic bowel is present, it should be resected and the patient should be evaluated by careful daily observation for the need for further treatment.
   B. Necrotic bowel should be resected, following which the cause of the intestinal ischemia should be determined by postoperative arteriography.
   C. The cause of the intestinal ischemia should be determined by operative findings. Necrotic bowel should be resected only if intestinal embolism is present, since the mortality rate associated with thrombosis is prohibitive.
   D. The cause of the intestinal ischemia should be determined by operative findings, and revascularization should be achieved by appropriate embolectomy or bypass procedure. Only bowel that is obviously necrotic following revascularization should be resected.
   E. Obviously necrotic bowel should be exteriorized, and patient condition stabilized by vigorous intensive care prior to diagnosing and treating the cause of the intestinal ischemia.

6. Which of the following methods has been objectively shown to be superior to clinical judgment for determining intestinal viability?
   A. Doppler ultrasound.
   B. Laser Doppler velocimetry.
   C. Infrared photoplethysmography.
   D. Surface oximetry.
   E. None of the above.

7. "Second look" procedures should be performed following initial operative treatment of acute intestinal ischemia:
   - **A.** Whenever bowel of uncertain viability has not been resected and patient condition does not rapidly improve.
   - **B.** Whenever bowel of uncertain viability has not been resected and objective parameters such as leukocyte count, temperature, pulse rate, and acid/base balance remain abnormal.
   - **C.** Whenever bowel or uncertain viability has not been resected regardless of patient condition.
   - **D.** In all cases.
   - **E.** In all cases except those in which revascularization has been performed.

8. Nonocclusive mesenteric ischemia (NOMI) is most often associated with:
   - **A.** Hemorrhagic hypovolemic shock.
   - **B.** Persistent shock-induced vasospasm.
   - **C.** Ergot poisoning.
   - **D.** Hyperreninemia.
   - **E.** None of the above.

9. All of the following disorders may cause nonocclusive mesenteric ischemia *except:*
   - **A.** Polyarteritis nodosa.
   - **B.** Digitalis toxicity.
   - **C.** Coarctation of the aorta.
   - **D.** Atrial fibrillation.
   - **E.** Sepsis.

10. Pharmacologic management of nonocclusive mesenteric ischemia may include any or all of the following measures *except:*
    - **A.** Captopril.
    - **B.** Sodium nitroprusside.
    - **C.** Digitalis.
    - **D.** Steroids.
    - **E.** Intra-arterial papaverine.

11. Splanchnic venous thrombosis has been associated with:
    - **A.** Protein C deficiency.
    - **B.** Protein S deficiency.
    - **C.** Antithrombin III deficiency.
    - **D.** Lupus anticoagulant.
    - **E.** All of the above.

12. The following problems are common presenting features of splanchnic venous thrombosis *except:*
    - **A.** Colon infarction.
    - **B.** Worsening ascites.
    - **C.** Variceal hemorrhage.
    - **D.** It may be asymptomatic.
    - **E.** Abdominal pain.

13. Which of the following statements about the evaluation of mesenteric venous thrombosis is/are *false?*
    - **A.** Arteriography, computerized axial tomography (CT) with contrast, or abdominal duplex scanning may confirm the diagnosis
    - **B.** The CT triad of hypodensity in the superior mesenteric vein, thickening of the small intestinal wall, and peritoneal fluid suggest laparotomy is indicated.
    - **C.** Standard therapy for venous intestinal infarction has been intestinal resection and anticoagulation.
    - **D.** For venous intestinal infarction, colonoscopy and upper GI endoscopy are diagnostic.
    - **E.** Development of ascites in patients with mesenteric venous thrombosis warrants surgery in those initially treated nonoperatively.

14. The following statements about mesenteric venous thrombosis is/are true:
    - **A.** Recurrent thrombosis is rare.
    - **B.** Anticoagulation does *not* reduce recurrent thrombosis.
    - **C.** Recurrent intestinal infarction after repeated venous thrombosis involves the area adjacent to prior infarction in 60% of patients.
    - **D.** Intra-abdominal infectious processes are *not* an important cause of portomesenteric venous thrombosis in children.
    - **E.** Mesenteric venous thrombosis has occurred as a complication of variceal sclerotherapy.

15. Which of the following statements regarding the natural history of *asymptomatic* visceral artery occlusion is/are true?
    - **A.** A small number (5–10%) of individuals with asymptomatic visceral artery occlusions will develop catastrophic acute intestinal ischemia.
    - **B.** Acute intestinal ischemia develops in individuals with asymptomatic visceral artery occlusions only when all three mesenteric vessels are involved.
    - **C.** Acute intestinal ischemia develops in individuals with asymptomatic visceral artery occlusions only when the superior mesenteric artery is occluded.
    - **D.** The natural history of asymptomatic intestinal artery occlusions is unknown.
    - **E.** Acute intestinal ischemia never develops in individuals with visceral artery occlusions without a preceding period of chronic symptoms (abdominal pain and weight loss).

16. Which of the following is *not* an indication for visceral arterial reconstruction?
    - **A.** Superior mesenteric artery occlusion in a patient with typical abdominal pain and weight loss.
    - **B.** Abdominal pain and weight loss in a patient with >60% stenosis of the superior mesenteric and celiac arteries and occlusion of the inferior mesenteric artery.
    - **C.** Celiac artery occlusion with normal superior mesenteric and inferior mesenteric arteries in a young man with an 18-month history of abdominal pain without weight loss.
    - **D.** Asymptomatic occlusions of both the superior mesenteric and celiac arteries in a patient scheduled for elective abdominal aortic aneurysm repair.
    - **E.** Normal celiac and superior mesenteric arteries in a patient scheduled for repair of a thoracoabdominal aortic aneurysm.

17. Which of the following may be associated with early postoperative occlusion of intestinal arterial revascularizations?
    - **A.** Abdominal pain, leukocytosis, fever, hemodynamic instability.
    - **B.** Abdominal pain, leukocytosis, without fever or hemodynamic instability.
    - **C.** Occult gastrointestinal blood loss without other signs or symptoms.
    - **D.** No signs, symptoms, or laboratory findings.
    - **E.** Any of the above.

18. Which of the following statements best describes current knowledge regarding graft material for intestinal arterial bypass?
    - **A.** Saphenous vein grafts are clearly superior to prosthetic materials for this application.
    - **B.** Prosthetic grafts are clearly superior to vein grafts for this application.
    - **C.** Most authors prefer vein grafts, reserving prosthetic grafts for patients with absent or inadequate veins.
    - **D.** Most authors prefer prosthetic grafts, reserving vein grafts for situations with necrotic or perforated bowel and the risk of graft sepsis.
    - **E.** Vein grafts and prosthetic grafts are equally acceptable.

QUESTIONS 19–21 CONCERN THE FOLLOWING PATIENT:

19. A 64-year-old man underwent emergency aortic reconstruction for a ruptured infrarenal aneurysm. During his second postoperative day he develops increasing abdominal pain and distention, an elevated temperature, and has had two nonbloody bowel movements. Your plan should include:
    - **A.** Monitor serum phosphorus, LDH, CPK, alkaline phosphatase, arterial pH, white cell count, and platelet count.
    - **B.** Flexible colonoscopy to rule out ischemic colitis.
    - **C.** Start oral Vancomycin to treat pseudomembranous colitis.
    - **D.** Change his antibiotics to cover both gram-negative bacteria and anaerobic bacteria if colonic ischemia is present.
    - **E.** Perform a sigmoid colectomy with an end colostomy and Hartman's pouch if mucosal ischemia is present.

20. Colonoscopy confirms the presence of mucosal ischemia. The patient has a benign abdomen and a normal white blood cell count. Which of the following is/are appropriate treatment at this point?
    - **A.** Monitor the white blood cell count, arterial pH, and platelet count.
    - **B.** Broad-spectrum antibiotics.
    - **C.** A barium enema to try to identify perforation or stricture.
    - **D.** Repeat colonoscopy within 12 to 24 hours.
    - **E.** A pulmonary artery catheter is essential to assess the adequacy of volume replacement.

21. Despite appropriate treatment, progressive clinical deterioration occurs. You elect to explore the patient and find a necrotic nonperforated descending colon. You perform a:
    - **A.** Transverse loop colostomy.
    - **B.** Left colectomy with colorectal anastomosis.
    - **C.** Left colectomy with an end colostomy and Hartman's pouch.
    - **D.** Total abdominal colectomy with ileostomy and Hartman's pouch.
    - **E.** Subtotal colectomy with ileoproctostomy.

22. Method(s) that may help prevent colonic ischemia following aortic reconstruction is/are:
    - **A.** Preoperative mechanical bowel preparation.
    - **B.** Immediate postoperative flexible sigmoidoscopy.
    - **C.** Routine reimplantation of the inferior mesenteric artery.
    - **D.** Maintenance of direct or indirect blood flow into at least one hypogastric artery.
    - **E.** Reimplantation of the inferior mesenteric artery using a Carrell patch if the stump pressure of the inferior mesenteric artery is less than 40 mm Hg.

13

Answers

1. The answers are **A, B, D** (Rutherford, 4th ed., pp. 1267–1270).

Intestinal hyperemia is a complex process involving humoral, metabolic, and probably neurofactors as well. While many intestinal peptides participate in post-prandial hyperemia, including Vasoactive Intestinal Peptide (VIP), cholecystokinin (CCK) is probably the most important. The hyperemic response varies with nutrient composition and appears strongest when a mixture of different nutrients (fat, carbohydrate, and protein) is ingested. Intestinal hyperemia is maximal 30–90 minutes after eating and lasts 4–6 hours. Whereas superior mesenteric artery flow increases dramatically after eating, flow increases in the celiac artery are much less or nonexistent.

2. The answer is **E** (Rutherford, 4th ed., pp. 1270–1274).

The diagnosis of chronic intestinal ischemia is made clinically in a patient with a suggestive history *and* appropriate angiographically proven celiac and superior mesenteric artery high-grade stenoses or occlusions. Tests of intestinal absorption and/or excretion have been inaccurate in the evaluation of chronic intestinal ischemia. Whereas lateral angiography and, in some centers, duplex scanning can reliably detect high-grade SMA and celiac artery stenoses, it is well recognized that such lesions may exist in asymptomatic patients; thus, their presence alone is not diagnostic of chronic intestinal ischemia. A combination of findings is required to verify the diagnosis.

3. The answers are **B, D, E** (Rutherford, 4th ed., p. 1276).

Nonocclusive mesenteric ischemia (NOMI) is an infrequently observed condition that can lead to intestinal infarction. It is virtually always associated with some form of systemic hypoperfusion state such as profound sepsis, severe congestive heart failure, and, more recently, low-output states following cardiac surgery. In the past, it has been anecdotally associated with the use of digitalis preparations. Experimental evidence suggests that baseline splanchnic arterial resistance is not altered by digitalis but that in digitalis-treated animals, mesenteric arterial resistance increases in response to splanchnic venous hypertension that may accompany profound cardiac shock. Although a number of chemical markers have been suggested as aiding in the diagnosis of NOMI, none have proven clinically useful. The diagnosis is best made by an appropriate level of physician suspicion in at-risk patients and confirmed by angiographic demonstration of patent mesenteric arterial trunks with tapering visceral artery branch occlusions.

4. The answer is **C** (Rutherford, 4th ed., pp. 1278–1280).

In the past, most emboli to the superior mesenteric artery arose from cardiac sources. Currently, arterial-arterial embolism is an increasingly important cause of superior mesenteric artery embolization. Similarly, arterial embolization may arise from diagnostic and/or therapeutic intra-arterial manipulation. Most sizable superior mesenteric artery emboli lodge at the site of a major change in arterial caliber, which in the superior mesenteric artery occurs beyond the first few branches. Thus, the ischemia associated with embolic occlusion usually spares the proximal jejunum, and this results in lower reported mortality figures compared with thrombosis. Superior mesenteric artery thrombosis usually results from progressive atherosclerotic stenosis. Such patients typically have occlusive lesions in multiple visceral vessels and histories of chronic abdominal pain and weight loss. The reported mortality for acute, symptomatic superior mesenteric artery thrombosis is close to 100%.

5. The answer is **D** (Rutherford, 4th ed., pp. 1280–1281).

Determination of the potential of ischemic bowel to recover following revascularization is very difficult. Logical management of acute intestinal ischemia requires accurate diagnosis of the cause of the ischemia, followed by revascularization by embolectomy or bypass, whichever is appropriate. Following revascularization, bowel that appeared hopelessly ischemic may return to normal appearance. Only bowel that remains ischemic after restoration of arterial flow should be resected. Delaying the revascularization in an attempt to stabilize the patient is futile. Resection alone is acceptable treatment only if there is no feasible means of revascularization, as occasionally occurs with multiple small emboli.

6. The answer is **E** (Rutherford, 4th ed., pp. 1281–1282).

Although each of the methods listed has been shown to have a high degree of reliability in differentiating viable and nonviable intestine, none is perfect, and none has been shown superior to clinical judgment alone. Only one prospective controlled study has been performed; in this study fluorescein injection was superior to clinical judgment, but this observation has not been duplicated by others. All currently available testing methods suffer from the same defect—namely, the occurrence of false negatives, the most dangerous incorrect result for patients.

7. The answer is **C** (Rutherford, 4th ed., pp. 1281–1282).

Clinical assessment of the viability of revascularized intestine is difficult. In cases with widespread involvement, resection of all abnormal bowel may result in an unacceptably short remaining intestine. Most authorities agree that when length is critical, only obviously necrotic intestine should be resected. Judgment regarding resection of questionable bowel is reserved for a "second look" procedure performed 24–48 hours after the initial operation. It is critically important that this procedure be performed *regardless* of patient condition, since revascularization and resection of the majority of the ischemic bowel may produce a deceptive improvement in patient condition. Second look procedures are not required when all the bowel remaining after the first procedure is clearly viable.

8. The answer is **B** (Rutherford, 4th ed., pp. 1284–1286).

Persistent vasoconstriction that fails to respond to local ischemia-related autoregulatory mechanisms represents the final common pathophysiologic pathway in the development of nonocclusive mesenteric ischemia (NOMI). Ergot poisoning and hemorrhagic shock are rare causes of NOMI, which is most frequently seen in *normovolemic* shock states associated with cardiac failure. The renin-angiotensin axis modulates the mesenteric vascular response to ischemia but does not appear to alter the incidence of the disease.

9. The answer is **D** (Rutherford, 4th ed., pp. 1284–1286).

Uncommon causes of nonocclusive mesenteric ischemia include polyarteritis nodosa (PAN), digitalis toxicity, repair of aortic coarctation, and systemic sepsis. Whereas PAN is more frequently complicated by diffuse aneurysm formation, the inflammatory phase of the disease may cause a necrotizing vasculitis with ischemia. Similarly, aortic-coarctation-related hypertension is occasionally necrotizing and may cause mesenteric ischemia. Sepsis and digitalis toxicity can produce persistent mesenteric vasoconstriction, with resultant bowel ischemia. Arterial fibrillation may lead to embolic intestinal infarction but does not cause nonocclusive ischemia in the absence of congestive heart failure.

10. The answer is **C** (Rutherford, 4th ed., pp. 1286–1287).

Optimization of cardiac output and mesenteric vasodilation form the basic management of this disease. These measures are usually accomplished with direct mesenteric infusion of papaverine and the use of systemic afterload reduction with an agent such as nitroprusside. Inhibitors of angiotensin like Captopril may also be useful because of the sensitivity of the mesenteric vasculature to the renin-angiotensin axis. Although digitalis may improve cardiac output, it also has a vasoconstrictive effect on the visceral vessels and has been implicated in the etiology of this disorder. It should not be used to treat mesenteric vascular insufficiency and should be discontinued if the problem is suspected in a patient already taking a cardiac glycoside. Steroids do not produce mesenteric vasodilation but are indicated to treat vasculitis, which can cause mesenteric ischemia.

11. The answer is **E** (Rutherford, 4th ed., pp. 1288–1293).

All of the hypercoagulable states listed have been reported as precipitating factors for splanchnic venous thrombosis. Certain malignancies have also been implicated. Portomesenteric venous thrombosis may complicate the course of those with cirrhosis or portal hypertension. Splanchnic venous thrombosis has been reported to occur spontaneously and to follow either sclerotherapy for esophageal varices or selective transhepatic portal angiography. Acute splanchnic venous occlusions are an uncommon cause of intestinal ischemia. Resection of infarcted intestine has been the standard approach to this problem, but those affected do not necessarily develop intestinal infarction and may occasionally be managed nonoperatively. One study reported that 0.38% of laparotomies done for an "acute abdomen" revealed mesenteric infarction, and only 17% of these infarctions were due to venous thrombosis. Prior understanding of the natural history and incidence of intestinal ischemia from venous thrombosis was biased because most cases were diagnosed at laparotomy or autopsy. Duplex ultrasound, computerized tomography (CT), and magnetic resonance imaging (MRI), as well as the aggressive use of arteriography for evaluation of patients with possible acute mesenteric ischemia, facilitate preoperative or antemortem diagnosis. A past history of portomesenteric or lower-extremity venous thrombosis in someone with abdominal pain, however, warrants inclusion of intestinal ischemia from venous thrombosis in the differential diagnosis. Most patients with this disorder had a history of prior venous thrombosis in one series. Splanchnic venous thrombosis has been associated with protein C or S deficiency, antithrombin III deficiency, presence of anticardiolipin antibody, and certain malignancies.

12. The answer is **A** (Rutherford, 4th ed., pp. 1289–1290).

Colon infarction is a rare complication of splanchnic venous thrombosis. When intestinal ischemia occurs secondary to splanchnic venous occlusion it usually affects the small intestine. Though splanchnic venous thrombosis may present with worsening ascites, variceal hemorrhage, or intestinal ischemia, occlusion of the portal or superior mesenteric veins can be asymptomatic.

13. The answer is **D** (Rutherford, 4th ed., pp. 1291–1292).

When the differential diagnosis suggests that mesenteric venous thrombosis is possible or likely, arteriography, CT with contrast, or abdominal duplex scanning may confirm the diagnosis. The CT triad of hypodensity in the superior mesenteric vein, thickening of the intestinal wall and valvulae conniventees in the small intestine, and a significant amount of peritoneal fluid suggests that laparotomy should be performed. The absence of ascites supports a decision to treat a patient with mesenteric venous thrombosis nonoperatively. In 1987, Clavien and colleagues suggested that development of ascites in such patients was an indication for surgery. In venous intestinal infarction, the mid small intestine is usually involved, thus eluding colonoscopy and upper GI endoscopy.

14. The answers are **C, E** (Rutherford, 4th ed., pp. 1295–1298).

Recurrent thrombosis can be expected in 29% of patients with mesenteric venous thrombosis. Anticoagulation reduces recurrence and overall mortality. Naitove and Weissman reported in 1965 that no deaths occurred in patients with primary mesenteric venous thrombosis who received anticoagulants postoperatively, whereas 50% of those who did not receive postoperative anticoagulation died. A literature review of mesenteric venous thrombosis reported that, of 173 patients who underwent bowel resection for mesenteric venous thrombosis, 22% had recurrent thrombosis. Of those treated surgically, recurrence was significantly lower in heparin-treated patients. Only 14% treated with heparin recurred, whereas 26% not treated with heparin recurred, a statistically significant difference. Of those with recurrence, 22% treated with anticoagulants died, whereas 59% of those not treated with heparin died. Recurrent infarction from repeated venous thrombosis involves the area adjacent to the anastomosis in 60% of patients. Intra-abdominal infection predisposes to portomesenteric infarction in children. Mesenteric venous thrombosis *has* been reported as a complication of variceal sclerotherapy (see question 11).

15. The answer is **D** (Rutherford, 4th ed., pp. 1301–1302).

Atherosclerotic obstruction of visceral arteries is frequently encountered, occurring in 6–10% of unselected autopsies and on 14–24% of aortograms. Both acute and chronic intestinal ischemia are rare syndromes, although clearly some individuals with visceral artery occlusions present with catastrophic acute intestinal ischemia without preceding symptoms of abdominal pain and weight loss. At present, the frequency with which this happens is unknown. The large number of patients with the arterial lesions and the infrequency with which the clinical syndrome is encountered both suggest that this is a rare event.

16. The answer is **C** (Rutherford, 4th ed., pp. 1301–1302, 1304).

Although symptoms of chronic intestinal ischemia are variable, abdominal pain and weight loss occur in nearly all patients. Patients with these typical symptoms and occlusions involving the superior mesenteric artery together with other visceral arteries should undergo operation. Occlusions of the celiac artery are well tolerated. Chronic abdominal pain without weight loss is most likely unrelated to intestinal ischemia. Asymptomatic occlusions of the visceral arteries should be repaired at the time of other indicated aortic surgery because of the well-documented occurrence of intestinal infarction if this is not done. Obviously, revascularization of the intestinal arteries is an essential part of thoracoabdominal aneurysm repair.

17. The answer is **E** (Rutherford, 4th ed., pp. 1308–1310).

Postoperative occlusion of visceral artery repairs may be difficult to diagnose. Completely typical postoperative findings may include abdominal pain, leukocytosis, fever, moderate hemodynamic instability, and some gastrointestinal blood loss. Alternately, occlusion of visceral bypass grafts may occur without any accompanying signs or symptoms. Symptoms may recur only when patients resume unrestricted oral intake, sometime postoperatively. For this reason, all visceral bypass patients should have postoperative arteriography to confirm the patency of repairs. If occlusion of the grafts is discovered in the early postoperative period, reoperation and revision are possible. If this is delayed until symptoms recur, scarring may have developed, preventing safe reoperation.

18. The answer is **D** (Rutherford, 4th ed., pp. 1304–1310).

Published experience with saphenous vein grafts for superior mesenteric and celiac artery revascularization reports inferior patency rates when compared to those achieved with prosthetic grafts. For this reason most authors prefer prosthetic grafts for elective operations and reserve vein grafts for those situations with an unacceptable risk of graft infection. The reasons for this strategy are related to the high flow rates present in visceral arteries and to the particular susceptibility of vein grafts to kinking and twisting because the mesentery is mobile.

19. The answers are **B, D** (Rutherford, 4th ed., pp. 1303–1309).

Colonic ischemia may occur in up to 60% of patients after aortic aneurysm rupture and repair. The diagnosis should be suspected if a combination of low-grade sepsis, diarrhea (often bloody), and abdominal distention develops. Diarrhea usually begins within 24 to 48 hours of operation in 75% of patients with ischemic colitis. Endoscopy is the most reliable diagnostic modality available. Visual signs of early mucosal ischemia include circumferential petechial hemorrhage and edema. Unexplained metabolic acidosis, leukocytosis, oliguria, and thrombocytopenia may be nonspecific markers of ischemic colitis and should raise suspicion for the diagnosis. Fluid resuscitation and broad-spectrum antibiotic administration should be initiated when the diagnosis is entertained. Mucosal ischemia can be followed conservatively with repeat colonoscopy and clinical observation over several days. If transmural ischemia or overt necrosis develops, then colectomy and colostomy are required. Vancomycin should be administered only if a definitive diagnosis of pseudomembranous colitis is established at colonoscopy.

20. The answers are **A, B, D** (Rutherford, 4th ed., pp. 1303–1309).

Patients with mucosal ischemia require vigorous monitoring, resuscitation, and support. If sepsis develops, the white blood cell count usually rises and the platelet count and arterial blood pH fall. Fluid requirements may be large; a pulmonary artery catheter can help guide volume replacement, but it is not absolutely essential in every case. Attempts should be made to decrease the colonic intraluminal bacterial load with intravenous antibiotics; oral antibiotics are not effective because of postoperative ileus. Barium contrast studies are contraindicated—if a perforation exists, barium peritonitis could ensue. Strictures form late in the course of ischemic colitis. Serial colonoscopy (to 40 cm if at all possible) is required to document possible progression of the disease process. Reversible lesions should improve within 7 to 10 days. Progressive clinical deterioration associated with advancing colonic ischemia requires operative exploration.

21. The answer is **C** (Rutherford, 4th ed., pp. 1313–1319).

The involved colon and all questionably viable colon need to be resected. Primary anastomosis following resection should not be attempted. Colostomy with Hartman's pouch or distal mucous fistula construction is required. During bowel resection, isolation of the retroperitoneum and the recently placed aortic prosthesis is necessary to prevent graft contamination.

22. The answers are **A, D, E** (Rutherford 4th ed., pp. 1313–1319).

Preoperative bowel preparation, reimplantation of the inferior mesenteric artery when the stump pressure is less than 40 mm Hg, and preoperative arteriography as a guide to reimplantation have all been described as useful methods to prevent postoperative ischemic colitis. In addition, blood flow to at least one hypogastric artery should be assured. If every patient underwent postoperative flexible sigmoidoscopy after aortic reconstruction, 6% of the patients would show signs of mucosal ischemia. Only 0.2% would have clinical signs of intestinal ischemia; 40–50% of these patients would die. Reimplantation of every patent inferior mesenteric artery is not necessary and only increases the rate of postoperative hemorrhagic complications.

14

Portal Hypertension

1. Which of the following statements is/are true regarding balloon-tube tamponade for acute variceal bleeding?
   A. It controls acute variceal bleeding in most patients if correctly used.
   B. Recurrent acute variceal bleeding is uncommon after removal of the tube.
   C. If recurrent upper gastrointestinal hemorrhage occurs in a patient with a tube in place, then the tube is either incorrectly positioned or the patient is invariably bleeding from a lesion other than esophageal varices.
   D. Severe aspiration pneumonia is a frequent complication of the use of the tube; thus comatose or stuporous patients should have their airways protected by endotracheal intubation.
   E. Correct inflation of the esophageal balloon is essential because this is the important functional component of the tube for controlling esophageal variceal bleeding.

2. Which of the following statements is/are true concerning gastric varices?
   A. They are rarely associated with esophageal varices prior to treatment of the esophageal varices.
   B. When present, they remain localized to the fundus of the stomach.
   C. When associated with segmental or left-sided portal hypertension, the cause is usually isolated splenic vein thrombosis.
   D. When treatment for recurrent gastric variceal bleeding is required, reported successful management options include pharmacologic therapy with propranolol, portacaval shunts, and devascularization and transection operations.
   E. When they appear after successful eradication of esophageal varices, they are not of clinical significance because bleeding is very rare.

3. Which of the following statements is/are true regarding emergency injection sclerotherapy for the treatment of acute esophageal variceal bleeding?
   A. If active variceal bleeding is noted at the time of emergency diagnostic endoscopy, sclerotherapy treatment should be delayed until the bleeding stops spontaneously or is controlled by pharmacologic therapy.
   B. A single-injection sclerotherapy treatment controls the variceal bleeding in about 70% of patients.
   C. When the patient has a second acute variceal bleed after emergency injection sclerotherapy treatment, sclerotherapy usually fails.
   D. Failure of sclerotherapy is defined as another acute variceal bleeding episode after two emergency sclerotherapy treatments during a single hospital admission.
   E. Patients in whom sclerotherapy fails should be subjected to an emergency portacaval shunt opertion.

4. Long-term survival of patients with bleeding esophageal varices treated with endoscopic methods is *equal or superior to* survival in those treated with:
   A. Selective splenorenal shunt.
   B. Nonselective portocaval shunt.
   C. Propranolol.
   D. Medical therapy (vasopressin or balloon tamponade as needed).
   E. All of the above.

5. In contrast to endoscopic sclerotherapy, endoscopic elastic band ligation is associated with:
   A. Significantly increased risk of nonbleeding complications.
   B. Signifantly decreased risk of nonbleeding complications.
   C. Higher incidence of splanchnic venous thrombosis.
   D. Higher rate of rebleeding.
   E. Improved survival.

6. The treatment for acutely bleeding esophageal varices that results in the best short-term (40-day) survival is:
   A. Endoscopic sclerotherapy.
   B. Endoscopic ligation.
   C. Medical therapy (vasopressin or balloon tamponade as needed).
   D. Emergency shunt insertion.
   E. None of the above.

7. The transjugular intrahepatic portosystemic shunt (TIPS) is hemodynamically similar to the following surgical shunts:
   A. End-to-side portocaval shunt.
   B. Side-to-side portocaval shunt.
   C. Distal splenorenal shunt.
   D. Mesocaval shunt.
   E. Proximal splenorenal shunt.

8. TIPS should *not* be attempted in patients who have:
   - **A.** Cavernous occlusion of the portal vein.
   - **B.** Right internal jugular vein occlusion.
   - **C.** Budd-Chiari syndrome.
   - **D.** Polycystic liver disease.
   - **E.** All of the above.

9. The potential advantages of TIPS over surgical shunts include all of the following *except:*
   - **A.** The procedure can be performed using local anesthesia.
   - **B.** Ascites clears gradully following TIPS.
   - **C.** There is less postshunt encephalopathy following TIPS.
   - **D.** The outflow of a TIPS is to the suprahepatic inferior vena cava (IVC).
   - **E.** Initial cost is less for TIPS.

10. All of the following are true about TIPS *except:*
    - **A.** The main limitation of TIPS is that it interferes with hepatic transplantation.
    - **B.** Primary patency of TIPS at one year is greater than 90%.
    - **C.** The portosystemic gradient following TIPS is typically reduced to about 10 mm Hg.
    - **D.** TIPS can still be performed when the hepatic veins are occluded.
    - **E.** TIPS may be repeated if late occlusion occurs.

11. Which of the following statements is/are *not* true about the epidemiology of portal hypertension?
    - **A.** In developing countries this condition's most common causes relate to viral or parasitic disorders of the liver.
    - **B.** Risk of the late development of hepatocellular carcinoma equally threatens individuals with alcoholic or postnecrotic cirrhosis.
    - **C.** Hepatic cirrhosis ranks ninth among all causes of death in the United States.
    - **D.** Chronic alcoholism is the cause of cirrhosis in most affected subjects in industrialized countries.
    - **E.** Development of ascites and/or jaundice is an ominous prognostic sign in previously stable cirrhotics.

12. Which of the following statements is/are true about the role of liver transplantation in patients with variceal hemorrhage?
    - **A.** Patients with variceal hemorrhage who undergo liver transplantation have a worse outcome than patients transplanted for other indications.
    - **B.** Chronic alcoholism is an absolute contraindication to liver transplantation.
    - **C.** A prior portasystemic shunt does not negatively impact survival following orthotopic liver transplantation.
    - **D.** The primary indication for liver transplantation is terminal, irreversible liver failure.
    - **E.** Graft rejection is a relatively uncommon complication of orthotopic liver transplantation.

13. A 48-year-old cirrhotic man, abstinent from alcohol for one year, develops massive variceal hemorrhage. An initial effort at endoscopic therapy fails, and variceal bleeding is controlled temporarily by balloon tamponade. He is jaundiced, has tense ascites, and manifests significant encephalopathy. Presuming each of the following treatment modalities is readily available, which is the *least* indicated procedure?
    - **A.** Orthotopic liver transplantation.
    - **B.** Repeat endoscopic therapy.
    - **C.** Portacaval shunt.
    - **D.** TIPS (angiographic portacaval shunt).
    - **E.** Esophageal transection using the EEA stapler.

14. Liver transplantation would be contraindicated in each of the following *except:*
    - **A.** A 24-year-old AIDS patient with hepatitis C-associated cirrhosis.
    - **B.** A 76-year-old man with cirrhosis due to alpha-1 antitrypsin deficiency who has an FEV_1 of 900 cc.
    - **C.** A 48-year-old woman with chronic active hepatitis B.
    - **D.** A 56-year-old man who has hemochromatosis, end-stage cirrhosis, and a 2-cm hepatoma in hepatic segment 4 found on perioperative imaging evaluation.
    - **E.** A 36-year-old woman with diffuse portal, splenic, and superior mesenteric venous thrombosis secondary to congenital antithrombin III deficiency.

15. All of the following statements about portacaval shunt are true *except:*
    - **A.** Prophylactic portacaval shunt to treat large or extensive esophageal varices that have never bled substantially reduces mortality.
    - **B.** Partial or complete portal vein thrombosis is a risk factor for portacaval shunt thrombosis.
    - **C.** Restricting the size of a portacaval anastomosis (partial portal decompression) may result in improved outcome.
    - **D.** An enlarged caudate lobe should not significantly complicate performance of a portacaval shunt.
    - **E.** Hypersplenism is predictably relieved by portacaval shunt.

16. Which of the following is/are *not* a contraindication to distal splenorenal shunt?
    - **A.** Intractable ascites.
    - **B.** Bleeding from gastric varices.
    - **C.** Active variceal hemorrhage requiring emergency portal decompression.
    - **D.** Hypersplenism.
    - **E.** A 4-mm left renal vein.

17. All of the following statements about nonalcoholic cirrhotic causes of portal hypertension are true *except:*

A. Optimal management for an 18-year-old male patient with Budd-Chiari syndrome and currently intact hepatocellular function is liver transplantation.

B. Chronic endoscopic therapy will suffice in most children with portal hypertension and bleeding varices.

C. A good long-term prognosis can be anticipated in patients with extrahepatic portal vein thrombosis.

D. Bleeding from gastric varices resulting from splenic vein thrombosis can be cured by splenectomy.

E. Patients with diffuse splanchnic venous thrombosis and variceal hemorrhage may require a devascularization procedure to control bleeding.

14

Answers

1. The answers are **A, C, D** (Rutherford, 4th ed., pp. 1328–1330).

Meticulous attention to detail is required for the correct use of balloon tube tamponade of bleeding esophageal varices. However, if the tube is correctly inserted by an expert, balloon tube tamponade will control acute variceal bleeding in most patients. If recurrent upper gastrointestinal hemorrhage occurs in the patient with a balloon tube in place, an expert should check that the tube is correctly placed. Persistent bleeding despite a correctly inserted tube invariably means that the patient is bleeding from an upper gastrointestinal lesion other than varices. Further immediate diagnostic endoscopy is therefore recommended. Although a balloon tube is highly successful in controlling acute variceal bleeding, approximately 60% of patients rebleed after removal of the tube. Therefore, a definitive procedure is required at the time of removal of the tube, usually injection sclerotherapy. If incorrectly handled, the tube is dangerous. Patients frequently develop severe aspiration pneumonia, which can be fatal. All stuporous or comatose patients should have their airways protected by an endotracheal tube prior to commencing balloon-tube tamponade. The most important component of a balloon tube is the gastric balloon. It is essential to pull this up tight against the esophagogastric junction to control esophageal variceal bleeding. Some authorities do not inflate the esophageal balloon at all.

2. The answers are **C, D** (Rutherford, 4th ed., pp. 1326–1328, 1332–1333).

There are three types of gastric varices. The first variety includes those associated with esophageal varices and are usually a direct continuation of the esophageal varices. They frequently disappear after successful eradication of esophageal varices by sclerotherapy but may persist. The second variety includes those that appear for the first time after successful eradication of varices by sclerotherapy or esophageal transaction. Although bleeding from gastric varices is generally unusual, they have been reported to be a problem by some groups. When hemorrhage does occur it is difficult to manage. If sclerotherapy fails, which it often does, then either a portal systemic shunt or a devascularization operation may be successful, as may pharmacologic therapy with propranolol for long-term management. The third variety of gastric varices includes isolated gastric varices that occur in association with segmental portal hypertension caused by splenic vein thrombosis. These varices tend to be localized in the fundus of the stomach and are not associated with esophageal varices. The condition is cured by gastric devascularization and splenectomy.

3. The answers are **B, D** (Rutherford, 4th ed., pp. 1328–1332).

Sclerotherapy is currently the accepted definitive treatment for acute variceal bleeding in most centers. Sclerotherapy should be performed at the time of the first emergency endoscopy whenever possible. A single-injection treatment will control acute variceal bleeding in about 70% of patients. Some 30% of patients require a further injection treatment, which results in final definitive control in 90–95% of patients. This means that 5–10% of patients fail to respond to one- or two-injection sclerotherapy treatments. Such patients should be identified early and some other form of emergency treatment instituted. Failure has been defined as another variceal bleeding episode occurring after two emergency injection treatments during a single hospital admission. When failure is diagnosed, the variceal hemorrhage should be recontrolled by balloon-tube tamponade. The patient should be resuscitated and then urgently given another form of therapy. There are several options for treatment of sclerotherapy failures, and a surgical shunt is only one. The two main surgical treatments are surgical shunt or a simple esophageal transection using stapling techniques. There is also evidence to suggest that either TIPS or esophageal variceal banding is a successful alternative to a major operative procedure for failures of emergency sclerotherapy.

4. The answer is **E** (Rutherford, 4th ed., pp. 1340–1341).

Long-term endoscopic treatment for bleeding esophageal varices has been compared with all of the methods listed in prospective randomized trials (see Tables 102–1 and 102–2). Whereas acute endoscopic treatment is aimed at control of active hemorrhage, long-term endoscopic therapy is aimed at eradication of esophageal varices in order to prevent recurrent bleeding. Both selective and nonselective shunt operations provide excellent long-term control of bleeding from esophageal varices. The price of bleeding control, in addition to initial mortality and morbidity associated with the operation, is a higher incidence of hepatic encephalopathy and eventual liver failure as a result of deprivation of portal blood flow to the liver. Reduction of portal blood flow to the liver eventually occurs regardless of the type of shunt employed and results in decreased hepatic functional capacity in shunt patients when compared to those treated with endoscopic methods. On the other hand, patients treated by endoscopic methods experience a greater risk of recurrent bleeding than those who have shunts. Five of six trials that compared shunts with endoscopic sclerotherapy showed no differences in overall survival between treatments. In one trial—which did demonstrate improved survival for endoscopically treated patients when compared to those treated initially with a selective shunt—approximately one third of the endoscopic group eventually required a shunt operation to control recurrent hemorrhage. Medical treatment, including administration of pharmacologic agents (i.e., vasopressin) and mechanical balloon tamponade, are effective in the actively bleeding patient for temporary control of hemorrhage. These treatments do not diminish the long-term risk of recurrent hemorrhage. Five of eight prospective randomized trials that compared endoscopic sclerotherapy with medical treatment showed a survival advantage for the patients treated with endoscopic sclerotherapy. Beta–adrenergic antagonist drugs such as propranolol are effective for preventing recurrent hemorrhage from esophageal varices in some patients. These drugs are not indicated for control of acute hemorrhage and may be associated with significant adverse side effects. Four prospective trials compared propranolol with endoscopic therapy for long-term prevention of recurrent hemorrhage in selected good-risk patients. Survival rates were similar in propranolol- and endoscopic sclerotherapy-treated patients in each study.

5. The answer is **B** (Rutherford, 4th ed., pp. 1342–1344).

Endoscopic ligation is a new form of endoscopic therapy performed with an elastic band ligating device similar to those used for treatment of internal hemorrhoids. Varices are individually ligated with small elastic "O" rings that cause strangulation and thrombosis of the vascular channel. Ischemic necrosis at the site of treatment occurs over the subsequent 24–48 hours, followed by ulceration and healing. Submucosal structures such as varices are obliterated and prevented from reforming because the submucosal layer is replaced by scar tissue. The endoscopic ligation technique was developed to provide a safe alternative to endoscopic sclerotherapy for treatment of bleeding esophageal varices. All evidence to date indicates that the risk of local treatment-related complications known to be associated with endoscopic sclerotherapy (e.g., esophageal stricture, chemical necrosis of the esophagus, and mediastinal and pleural effusions) is significantly reduced in patients treated with the mechanical ligation technique. Systemic complications such as adult respiratory distress syndrome, splanchnic venous thrombosis, and renal failure occur in small numbers of sclerotherapy-treated patients as a result of systemic dissemination of sclerosant. In contrast, systemic sequelae of endoscopic ligation have not been observed. The incidence of recurrent bleeding and overall survival in patients treated with endoscopic ligation has not been conclusively shown to be superior to that obtained in patients treated with endoscopic sclerotherapy.

6. The answer is **E** (Rutherford, 4th ed., pp. 1340–1341, 1342–1344).

The patient who presents with acutely bleeding esophageal varices is at high risk for dying from one of three major causes: exsanguination, liver failure, or complications of treatment employed to stop bleeding. Both endoscopic sclerotherapy and endoscopic ligation are effective for control of acute bleeding (85–95%), but neither treatment has been shown to affect short-term survival favorably when compared with standard medical therapy. Patients who have acutely bleeding varices treated with endoscopic techniques experience a lower incidence of recurrent hemorrhage than those treated medically, but this reduction in recurrent bleeding does not result in improved *short-term* survival. Emergency shunt insertion is effective for control of acute bleeding but in most centers is associated with prohibitive operative mortality and should be avoided unless other measures fail. Because the diagnosis of bleeding esophageal varices must be made endoscopically, many practitioners favor instituting endoscopic therapy at the time the diagnosis of bleeding esophageal varices is made. Short-term survival may not be altered by early endoscopic treatment, but those who do survive and undergo repeated endoscopic treatments to eradicate esophageal varices benefit.

7. The answers are **B, D, E** (Rutherford, 4th ed., pp. 1349–1352, 1354).

Like the mesocaval and *proximal* splenorenal shunts, blood flow through a TIPS is hemodynamically equivalent to a side-to-side portocaval shunt. Thus, patients with intractable ascites generally improve after this type of shunt.

8. The answer is **D** (Rutherford, 4th ed., pp. 1352–1354).

Although technically more challenging, TIPS can be successfully performed in some patients even when the portal or hepatic veins are occluded. The procedure may also be performed from a left internal jugular vein approach when the right vein is occluded. The only anatomic contraindication to TIPS is polycystic liver disease; because the stents are porous, the shunt depends on intact hepatic parenchyma as its lining. If a TIPS were performed in a patient with polycystic liver disease, blood could flow through the stent into the cystic spaces.

9. The answers are **A, D** (Rutherford, 4th ed., p. 1354).

The rate of portosystemic encephalopathy following TIPS is similar to that of surgical shunts and is higher than found with the distal splenorenal shunt. Over 20 patients have had successful hepatic transplants after TIPS procedures. Of the other choices listed, the only controversial one involves cost. Whereas the initial cost for TIPS is probably less than for operative shunts, this difference becomes smaller if repeat TIPS procedures are required. Moreover, the cost of stents is not inconsequential, averaging over $700 per stent.

10. The answer is **B** (Rutherford, 4th ed., p. 1354).

Although long-term experience is still being accumulated with patients who have undergone TIPS, it is clear that durability is a problem. Most series that have evaluated TIPS patency have found shunt stenosis and occlusion rates of 30–50% at one year. However, redilation of stents has been occasionally successful when stenosis occurs.

11. The answer is **B** (Rutherford, 4th ed., pp. 1323–1325).

Worldwide the leading cause of portal hypertension and variceal bleeding is either the cirrhosis that results from hepatitis B or C infection or the presinusoidal scarring following schistosomal infestation of the liver. Patients whose cirrhosis is derived from prior hepatitis are at substantially increased risk of developing hepatocellular carcinoma when compared to patients who have not had viral hepatitis (8–23-fold). Laennec's cirrhosis—the entity associated with chronic alcoholism—does not appear to be associated with an increased risk of hepatoma. The vast majority—more than 90%—of patients manifesting the complications of advanced cirrhosis and portal hypertension in industrialized countries have *alcoholic cirrhosis*. As many as 30 million adults in North America manifest signs and symptoms of chronic alcoholism. The development of ascites is associated with a one-year survival rate of only 10%, whereas cirrhotics with jaundice due to hepatocellular dysfunction have a median survival of only four months, according to the Boston Interhospital Liver Group. The mortality risk approaches 100% one year following the concurrent development of ascites, jaundice, cachexia, and spontaneous encephalopathy.

12. The answers are **C, D** (Rutherford, 4th ed., pp. 1365–1368).

Liver transplantation has emerged as a curative treatment for various manifestations of liver failure. Because of the substantial operative risk, expense, and scarcity of donor organs, the operation should be reserved for patients with terminal hepatocellular dysfunction. Whereas variceal hemorrhage is commonly associated with advanced liver disease, its presence alone does *not* necessarily warrant liver transplantation if other nontransplant therapies are available and potentially effective. However, orthotopic liver transplantation is at least as successful in patients with variceal hemorrhage as in those undergoing liver transplantation without concomitant bleeding. Similarly, whereas liver transplantation is *not* warranted in patients who are actively consuming alcohol, those who have a documented period of abstinence from alcohol consumption may have an excellent outcome from liver transplantation; recidivism rates appear to be acceptably low. Although subhepatic scarring associated with a prior portasystemic shunt may make liver transplantation more tedious and difficult, survival following successful operation is at least as good as that observed in patients who have not had a prior shunt. One third of successful orthotopic liver transplants may undergo chronic rejection, requiring consideration of a repeat transplantation.

13. The answer is **C** (Rutherford, 4th ed., pp. 1323–1325, 1365–1368).

Because the patient has end-stage liver failure and has been abstinent from alcohol for one year, he is a very good candidate for liver transplantation. His likelihood of survival is equivalent to that of subjects undergoing liver transplantation to treat a nonalcoholic cause of terminal liver failure. Although the initial effort at endoscopic therapy in this patient failed, a repeat effort under more controlled circumstances is warranted; at least short-term control of variceal hemorrhage can be anticipated in two thirds of patients so managed. Angiographic portacaval shunt (TIPS) is an excellent alternative in this patient as a "bridge" to transplantation because it decompresses the portal system without requiring a major operation or a general anesthetic. Esophageal transection is a relatively minimally invasive operative procedure that effectively controls esophageal varices bleeding, although hemorrhage from gastric variceal or portal hypertensive gastropathy is not manageable by this means. While highly effective at halting variceal bleeding, a portacaval shunt may result in significant scarring of the right upper quadrant and the hilum of the liver, therefore complicating subsequent liver transplantation. Additionally, the patient is Child-Pugh Class C and would have a substantial risk of early postoperative mortality following portacaval shunt. A prior portasystemic shunt does not worsen perioperative mortality in patients undergoing orthotopic liver transplantation, but transplant operations are more difficult, and blood loss greater, in such patients. In a potential liver transplant candidate requiring operative portal decompression, a shunt that avoids the right upper quadrant is best—mesocaval or splenorenal shunts being optimal.

14. The answer is **D** (Rutherford, 4th ed., pp. 1324–1325, 1356, 1365–1368).

Liver transplantation is generally reserved for patients with end-stage (Child-Pugh Class C) liver failure due to nonalcoholic liver disease (or, occasionally, for patients with alcoholic cirrhosis and a demonstrated period of alcohol abstinence). Advanced age, especially when complicated by extrahepatic medical comorbidity, is a contraindication to liver transplantation, as is the presence of the acquired immunodeficiency syndrome. Splanchnic venous thrombosis, as seen in certain hypercoagulable states, profoundly complicates liver transplantation. Although occasional patients with isolated portal vein thrombosis may be transplanted, diffuse splanchnic venous thrombosis prevents liver transplantation. Hepatitis B infection is a contraindication to liver transplantation; although the procedure technically can be performed, the likelihood of graft reinfection with hepatitis B virus is prohibitively high. The presence of hepatic malignancy isolated to the liver (especially a hepatocellular carcinoma of the fibrolamellar variety) has been treated successfully by orthotopic liver transplantation. Postnecrotic cirrhosis secondary to hepatitis C is now the most common condition requiring liver transplantation in adults in the United States.

15. The answer is **A** (Rutherford, 4th ed., pp. 1355–1365).

Portacaval shunt is highly effective in controlling variceal hemorrhage, with well over 95% of patients permanently protected from recurrent bleeding. The occasional patient who rebleeds from varices due to portacaval shunt thrombosis frequently is characterized by a history of partial or complete thrombosis of the portal vein at the time of the original shunt; although the portal vein can occasionally be thrombectomized, the likelihood of shunt occlusion is very high, and an alternative portal decompressive procedure should be considered. The major complications attendant upon standard portacaval shunt—portasystemic encephalopathy and accelerated liver failure—*may* be mitigated by partial portal decompression, usually by use of a small-stoma direct side-to-side portacaval anasmosis or interposition of an 8- or 10-mm PTFE portacaval H-graft. Hypersplenism is predictably and permanently relieved by total portasystemic shunts.

16. The answers are **B, D** (Rutherford, 4th ed., p. 1365).

The distal splenorenal shunt of Warren is based on two concepts: decompression of the gastrosplenic circulation into an adequate left renal vein and meticulous ligation of all potential collaterals from the hypertensive portomesenteric venous circulation toward the shunt. Because hepatic sinusoidal hypertension is not lowered after distal splenorenal shunt (and may even rise postoperatively), ascites production is not relieved by this procedure and may even be worsened by it; refractory ascites is thus a contraindication to the distal splenorenal shunt. Similarly, absence of an adequate systemic outflow vein, due to small size, remote anatomic location, or disease of the left renal vein, interdicts performance of the distal splenorenal shunt. Because a properly performed distal splenorenal shunt requires an extensive dissection of the entire splenic vein from its pancreatic bed, as well as meticulous collateral ligation, the procedure is lengthy and tedious and is not warranted when immediate control of active variceal hemorrhage is required. Hypersplenism is successfully resolved by the distal splenorenal shunt, as is bleeding from gastric varices.

17. The answer is **A** (Rutherford, 4th ed., pp. 1323–1325, 1355–1368).

In the Budd-Chiari syndrome, liver transplantation can be curative but should be reserved for patients with terminal liver failure. In the majority of Budd-Chiari patients who have a patent inferior vena cava, side-to-side portacaval shunt will suffice. Children with portal hypertension and bleeding varices generally have this condition because of extrahepatic portal vein thrombosis; their liver function and coagulation parameters are *normal*, and variceal bleeding can usually be controlled by chronic endoscopic therapy. For adults with extrahepatic portal vein thrombosis, splenorenal or mesocaval shunts can effectively control portal hypertension. Because shunt surgery requires a major splanchnic vein for inflow, diffuse splanchnic venous thrombosis cannot be managed by shunt surgery. Patients whose esophageal varices continue to bleed or who develop gastric variceal bleeding require some form of nonshunt devascularization procedure—splenectomy, EEA staple transection of the esophagus, and gastric devascularization. Patients with splenic vein thrombosis, usually resulting from pancreatitis, have "isolated" or "left-upper quadrant" portal hypertension. Portal pressure is normal, and if a portasystemic shunt is performed, it inevitably fails. However, these patients can be cured by splenectomy.

15

Renovascular Disorders

1. Which of the following factors is *most* suggestive of the presence of renovascular hypertension in an adult Caucasian patient?
   A. Age less than 30 years.
   B. Absence of a family history.
   C. Presence of an abdominal bruit.
   D. Diastolic pressure greater than 120 mm Hg.
   E. Systolic pressure of 160 mm Hg.

2. Which of the following screening tests is most accurate for identification of a patient with hemodynamically significant main renal artery stenosis?
   A. Peripheral plasma renins.
   B. Rapid sequence intravenous pyelography.
   C. Renal duplex sonography.
   D. Intravenous digital subtraction angiography.
   E. Blood pressure response to angiotensin-converting enzyme (ACE) inhibitors.

3. Successful control of blood pressure by drug therapy in a patient with renovascular hypertension provides a similarly effective stabilization of renal function in the affected kidney. **True** or **false?**

4. Which of the following statements is/are true regarding maintenance of the hypertensive state due to renal artery stenosis?
   A. Unilateral renal artery stenosis with a normal contralateral kidney in humans is primarily angiotensin II dependent, analogous to the two-kidney, one-clip Goldblatt rat model.
   B. The degree of hypertension is directly related to the level of systemic renin, which is a potent vasoconstrictor.
   C. A normal serum renin is rare in patients with unilateral renal stenosis.
   D. Bilateral renal artery stenosis in humans is mostly volume dependent, analogous to the one-kidney, one-clip Goldblatt rat model.
   E. In the one-kidney rat model, angiotensin II inhibitors, such as saralasin, produce a striking drop in blood pressure *only* when sodium restriction has been accomplished.

5. Plasma renin activity:
   A. Is uniformly elevated in patients with renovascular hypertension.
   B. Is best indexed against sodium excretion.
   C. Should be measured after salt depletion and administration of loop diuretics.
   D. Is increased by blocking angiotensin II (saralasin) or converting enzyme (ACE inhibitors) to a greater extent in patients with renovascular hypertension than in those with essential hypertension.
   E. Is low in malignant hypertension, which is almost always associated with essential hypertension.

6. With respect to the diagnosis of renovascular hypertension in unilateral renal artery disease, ACE inhibitors (captopril, enalapril):
   A. Decrease the glomerular filtration rate in the kidney *with renal artery stenosis* because *efferent* arteriolar tone is decreased.
   B. Decrease the glomerular filtration rate in the *normal* kidney because *afferent* arteriolar tone is decreased.
   C. Can enhance the diagnostic accuracy of isotopic renograms by accentuating differences in renal blood flow and GFR.
   D. Will improve renal function and produce a decrease in serum creatinine by vasodilatation.
   E. When given as a provocative test, provide sensitivity and specificity equivalent to the intravenous urogram

7. Currently, the most accurate screening method for diagnosis of a renal artery stenosis is:
   A. Radionuclide urography.
   B. Intravenous urography.
   C. Duplex ultrasound.
   D. Intravenous digital subtraction angiography.
   E. Peripheral plasma renins.

8. Angiographic features that suggest fibromuscular hyperplasia include all of the following *except:*
   A. Irregular stenosis that involves the proximal 2 cm of the renal artery.
   B. Beaded appearance.
   C. Weblike stenosis in the peripheral segment of the main renal artery.
   D. Aneurysms involving renal artery branches.
   E. Renal artery occlusion.

9. Balloon angioplasty is *least* successful in the treatment of:
   A. Focal atherosclerotic stenosis of the main renal artery.

B. Fibromuscular hyperplasia of the main renal artery.
C. Atherosclerotic lesions involving the renal artery ostium.
D. Anastomotic stenosis following renal transplantation.
E. Fibromuscular hyperplasia in a renal artery branch.

10. Which of the following statements is/are true concerning clinical clues of renovascular hypertension due to fibromuscular dysplasia (FMD) of the renal arteries?
   A. Episodic hypertension is common in patients with FMD.
   B. Hypertension is present in a pediatric-aged individual who has no other obvious signs of renal parenchymal disease.
   C. Systolic hypertension is greater than 160 mm Hg in patients under 45 years of age.
   D. Malignant hypertension more commonly accompanies hypertension due to FMD than essential hypertension.
   E. Hypertension caused by renal artery FMD usually responds well to antihypertensive drug therapy.

11. Which of the following provide evidence of a hemodynamically significant stenosis found on renal angiography?
   A. The presence of definable collateral vessels in the area of the renal artery stenosis.
   B. The finding of a severe stenosis on *intravenous* digital subtraction angiography.
   C. A pressure gradient across the renal artery stenosis measuring 10 mm Hg or greater.
   D. Demonstration of nonparenchymal renal artery branches functioning as collaterals by pharmacologic agents such as acetylcholine or epinephrine.
   E. All of the above.

12. Which of the following statements is/are true concerning the role of percutaneous transluminal angioplasty (PTA) in the management of renal artery stenoses?
   A. There are fewer complications after PTA for renal artery stenoses caused by fibromuscular dysplasia (FMD) than for stenoses caused by arteriosclerosis.
   B. Twenty-five percent of renal artery FMD lesions are not amenable to PTA.
   C. The best results for PTA of FMD lesions are for lesions caused by intimal fibrosis.
   D. PTA is more effective for renal artery stenoses in the pediatric-age patient than in the adult patient
   E. For all patients with renal artery stenoses who require therapy, a trial of PTA should be undertaken as the initial form of treatment

13. Which of the following statements is/are true concerning dilation of aortorenal saphenous vein grafts?
   A. The frequency of late aortorenal saphenous vein graft dilation is the same in pediatric-aged patients as it is in adult patients.
   B. Marked aneurysmal dilation eventually occurs in more than 80% of documented instances of vein graft dilation.
   C. Once aortorenal saphenous vein graft dilation is identified, complications frequently require reoperation.
   D. The most common complication of dilation of aortorenal saphenous vein graft is rupture.
   E. Treatment of dilated aortorenal saphenous vein grafts always requires graft replacement.
   F. None of the above.

14. Which of the following factors is/are most predictive of retrieval of renal function by revascularization in patients with ischemic nephropathy?
   A. Unilateral total occlusion of the renal artery with visualization proximal of a normal distal vessel on arteriography.
   B. Renal vein renin assays that show a 2:1 ratio between the involved and uninvolved side.
   C. Slow rate of deterioration in renal function during period before operation.
   D. Bilateral proximal occlusion with visualization of normal vessels distally by arteriography.
   E. Creatinine of 3.0 or less.

15. Approximately what percentage of patients with ischemic nephropathy who have successfully undergone correction of severe bilateral renal artery lesions will have retrieval of clinically important amounts of renal function?
   A. 25%.
   B. 45%.
   C. 65%.
   D. 85%.
   E. 100%.

16. Once deterioration of renal function reaches end-stage renal disease (dialysis dependence) in patients with ischemic nephropathy secondary to correctable renal artery lesions, one has less than a 20% chance of functional retrieval and removal from dialysis dependence. **True** or **false?**

17. Continuous perfusion of the kidney with a preservation solution during ex-vivo reconstructions is required to ensure protection against loss of function during the prolonged ischemia time. **True** or **false?**

18. Autotransplantation of the kidney to the ipsilateral pelvis is recommended following ex-vivo renal artery reconstructions to facilitate renal vein reimplantation. **True** or **false?**

19. The most important component of ex-vivo perfusion for protection of renal function during ex-vivo renal artery reconstruction is not components of the perfusate but maintenance of hypothermia **True** or **false?**

20. Renal artery aneurysms should be surgically repaired for which of the following indications?
    A. Renovascular hypertension.
    B. Heavily calcified aneurysm.
    C. Aneurysm greater than 2.5 cm in size.
    D. Chronic dissection.
    E. Rupture

21. A renal artery aneurysm in a pregnant patient:
    A. Is less likely to rupture than in a nonpregnant patient.
    B. Is more likely to rupture than in a nonpregnant patient.
    C. Should be repaired as a surgical emergency.
    D. Should be repaired electively regardless of size.
    E. Usually causes hypertension.

22. The best *screening* test for postbiopsy renal arteriovenous fistula is:
    A. Magnetic resonance imaging.
    B. Intravenous pyelography.
    C. Duplex Doppler ultrasound.
    D. Renal angiography.
    E. Intavenous digital angiography.

23. Transcatheter embolization of renal arteriovenous fistulas is likely to be successful in which of the following types?
    A. Postoperative fistula.
    B. Postbiopsy fistula.
    C. Congenital fistula.
    D. Neoplastic fistula.
    E. All of the above.

24. Acute thrombosis of the renal artery is always a surgical emergency; retrieval of renal function is uncommon unless operation can be undertaken within *two* hours. **True** or **false?**

25. Which of the following statements regarding renal artery trauma is/are true?
    A. Absence of hematuria effectively excludes the presence of renal artery trauma.
    B. Absence of a distal vessel or nephrogram visualized by arteriography does not predict that the kidney is irretrievable.
    C. Greater than 25% of patients with blunt abdominal trauma will have injuries to the renal vasculature.
    D. Correction of traumatic renal artery lesions uncommonly result in retrieval of preoperatively absent renal function.
    E. All of the above.

26. Acute spontaneous renal artery dissections most commonly are silent and occur in previously anatomically normal vessels. **True** or **false?**

15

Answers

1. The answer is **D** (Rutherford, 4th ed., pp. 1371–1373).

The incidence of renovascular hypertension is low in the general hypertensive population if all patients with even mild hypertension are included. Because the renovascular form tends to be relatively severe, its prevalence in the large subpopulation of mildly hypertensive patients (untreated diastolic blood pressure less than 105 mm Hg) is probably negligible. In contrast, it occurs frequently in the smaller group of severely hypertensive people. One shopping center screening study demonstrated that none of the 102 patients with diastolic blood pressure between 90 and 115 mm Hg had renovascular hypertension. In contrast, 9 of the 35 patients (26%) with diastolic blood pressure of 118 mm Hg or higher did have it. Further, if one breaks down these numbers according to race, the results are even more informative. Of those individuals with severe hypertension, none of the 13 black patients had renovascular hypertension, whereas the disorder occurred in 9 of the 22 white patients (41%). Similarly, another study showed a 31% incidence of renovascular hypertension in 85 patients initially evaluated for malignant hypertension.

2. The answer is **C** (Rutherford, 4th ed., pp.1373–1374).

Renal duplex sonography (RDS) has been proposed by several investigators as a useful screening test to identify candidates for arteriography. In an RDS validity analysis, 74 consecutive patients were evaluated who had 77 comparative RDS and standard angiographic studies of the arterial anatomy to 148 kidneys. RDS results from six kidneys (4%) were considered inadequate for interpretation. When single renal arteries were present (122 kidneys), RDS provided a 93% sensitivity, 98% specificity, 98% positive predictive value, 94% negative predictive value, and an overall accuracy of 96%. These results were adversely affected when kidneys with multiple (polar) renal arteries were examined. Thus, RDS can be a valuable screening test in the search for correctable renovascular disease causing global renal ischemia. Whereas blood pressure may fall particularly effectively when a patient with renovascular hypertension is given an ACE inhibitor, this medication is also efficacious in patients with essential hypertension. Combining administration of an ACE inhibitor with isotopic renograms may turn out to be a useful screening test (see questions 6 and 7 and Chapter 106). The other studies listed are either relatively insensitive or invasive when compared with duplex sonography.

3. The answer is **false** (Rutherford, 4th ed., pp. 1374–1375).

Data regarding the natural history of changes in renal functions during drug therapy are underscored by the changes that occurred in the 41 patients with atherosclerotic lesions in the medical arm of a randomized prospective study of medical versus surgical treatment of renovascular hypertension at Vanderbilt University reported in 1981 (see Table 105–6). In 19 of the patients, serum creatinine levels increased 25–120%. The glomerular filtration rates dropped 25–50% in 12 patients. Fourteen patients (37%) lost more than 10% of renal length. In four patients (12%), a significant stenosis progressed to total occlusion. Seventeen patients (41%) had deterioration of renal function or loss of renal size that led to operation. One patient required removal of a previously reconstructable kidney. Interestingly, of the 17 patients in whom renal function deteriorated, 15 had acceptable control of blood pressure during the period of nonoperative observation.

4. The answers are **A, D, E** (Rutherford, 4th ed., pp. 1377–1380).

Hypertension from renovascular disease may be maintained by overfilling of the arterial system (volume hypertension), by arteriolar constriction without increased volume (vasoconstrictor hypertension), or by an inappropriate interaction of these two factors. In all three settings, there is an excess volume *relative to* the capacity of the arterial tree. The renin–angiotensin–aldosterone system exerts major control over these variables through both angiotensin II–induced vasoconstriction and aldosterone-induced volume expansion. In the setting of unilateral arterial stenosis with a normal, contralateral kidney, there is decreased renal blood flow to the diseased kidney, and glomerular filtration rate (GFR) decreases. This leads to renin release and angiotensin II formation. The renin secretion from the stenotic kidney increases markedly, which is manifested by an increased peripheral renin activity level when indexed against concurrent 24-hour sodium excretion. Because the contralateral kidney senses increased pressure, it will suppress its renin secretion to zero. With the elevation of blood pressure, there is a resultant natruresis from the normal kidney. Accordingly, sodium and water retention, which is due both to the hemodynamic alterations in the stenotic kidney and to aldosterone secretion, that would serve to feed back and shut off renin secretion is limited. Thus, abnormal renin secretion is sustained, and the patient is hypertensive mostly because of unilateral hypersecretion of renin, resulting in angiotensin II–induced vasoconstriction. In contrast, a renal artery lesion in the presence of *contralateral* renal disease or *bilateral* renal artery disease is analogous to the one-kidney, one-clip Goldblatt rat model. Because the disease is bilateral, the opposite kidney is *not* able to compensate for the increased sodium retention with natruresis. Thus, volume expansion serves to return the renin secretion to normal (manifested by a normal peripheral plasmin renin activity level), decreasing vasoconstriction induced by angiotensin II generation. However, there is increased total body sodium and water, resulting in volume-dependent hypertension. Thus, the degree of hypertension with bilateral disease is unrelated to the level of systemic renin. Moreover, renin itself is not a vasoconstrictor but serves to transform angiotensinogen to angiotensin I. Although a *low* serum renin is unusual in renal vascular disease, a *normal* serum renin may be found both with unilateral and bilateral renal artery disease, depending on the volume status of the patient. In the one-kidney, one-clip rat model of hypertension, renin secretion is suppressed to normal quite rapidly by volume expansion caused by sodium water retention. However, when animals are *sodium restricted,* there is a striking drop in blood pressure by administration of the angiotensin II inhibitor saralasin. In contrast, these same animals fail to show a response to acute angiotensin II inhibition following sodium repletion.

5. The answers are **B, D** (Rutherford, 4th ed., pp. 1380–1385).

As noted in the previous discussion, plasmin renin activity is not uniformly elevated in patients with renovascular hypertension, depending on volume status. Although it is rarely low, it may be within the range of normal. This inconsistency may be explained by two factors. First, it is now recognized that the peripheral plasma renin activity level must be indexed against some marker of the state of sodium balance. In 1992, Laragh and co-workers suggested indexing renin activity with the concurrent daily rate of sodium excretion. In normal subjects, plasma renin activity falls as the sodium excretion increases. Second, it is clear that essentially all diuretic and antihypertensive drugs influence the renin angiotensin system. Thus, for accurate assessment of actual renin secretion utilizing the peripheral plasma renin activity level indexed against sodium excretion, patients must not receive any antihypertensive or diuretic drug therapy for at least three weeks. Moreover, patients should be on normal salt intake rather than salt depletion to obtain accurate levels. A useful approach to identify renin hypersecretion is to measure plasma renin activity in response to angiotensin II blockade. It has been shown that saralasin, an angiotensin II inhibitor, induces increases in plasma renin activity to a greater extent in patients with renovascular hypertension than in patients with essential hypertension. In patients with malignant hypertension, which is commonly due to atherosclerotic renovascular disease, peripheral plasma renin levels are often high.

6. The answers are **A, C** (Rutherford, 4th ed., pp. 1380–1385).

Administration of angiotensin II–converting enzyme inhibitors, such as captopril and enalapril, can be very helpful to establish the diagnosis of renovascular hypertension. After giving captopril to patients with renovascular disease, in the kidney with the renal artery stenosis and marked reduction of glomerular filtration rate (GFR), the GFR drops even further as *efferent* arteriolar tone is reduced. (In effect, the normalization of the pressure head across the glomerulus decreases filtration pressure.) In contrast, in the normal contralateral kidney, the role of angiotensin II as an *afferent* constrictor is removed, and the renal blood flow and thereby glomerular filtration go up. The net difference between the two kidneys then is apparent utilizing a scanning agent that measures GFR or renal blood flow. In patients with bilateral renal artery disease, administration of ACE inhibitors will cause deterioration of renal function with increases in creatinine because of the effect on efferent arterioles. As a provocative test, captopril has been shown to provide a sensitivity of 100% and a specificity of 95%. This is in sharp contrast to intravenous urography, which gives a sensitivity of 75% and a specificity of 86% for renovascular disease.

7. The answer is **C** (Rutherford, 4th ed., pp. 1390–1399).

Although it was used for many years as the primary screening procedure in hypertensive patients, intravenous urography has been shown to have very poor specificity and sensitivity, and its use has been largely abandoned for this purpose. Similarly, the initial enthusiasm for intravenous digital angiography as an imaging modality for the aorta and renal arteries has been replaced by skepticism, and this procedure is now only rarely used. Conventional radionuclide urography is also insufficiently accurate for routine screening, although there is considerable evidence to support the accuracy of this imaging technique when it is used in conjunction with angiotensin-converting enzyme (ACE) inhibitors (see Chap. 106). Duplex ultrasound is now the best noninvasive way to image the renal arteries. This method provides information about both the anatomy of the renal artery and the extent of flow restriction (see questions 2 and 6).

8. The answer is **A** (Rutherford, 4th ed., pp. 1394–1399).

Fibromuscular hyperplasia is generally grouped into three major types: intimal, medial, and adventitial (see Chap. 108). The medial variety has a typical beaded appearance, which spares the proximal segment of renal artery and commonly extends into one or more segmental branches. The intimal variety appears as a weblike, short focal stenosis of the distal main renal artery or a segmental branch vessel. Patients with fibromuscular hyperplasia commonly have associated aneuryms, particularly at the bifurcation of the main renal artery. Lesions involving the most proximal segment of the renal artery, especially those involving the ostium, are usually atherosclerotic, although in younger age groups this segment of vessel can be involved in patients with neurofibromatosis and Takayasu's disease. Although it is relatively unusual, renal artery fibromuscular hyperplasia can progress to occlusion, occasionally in the setting of acute dissection.

9. The answer is **C** (Rutherford, 4th ed., pp. 1399–1401).

The *best* results of balloon angioplasty of renal arteries have consistently been reported in the treatment of stenoses caused by fibromuscular hyperplasia (FMH: also denoted as fibromuscular dysplasia [FMD]). Originally, the use of balloon angioplasty was limited to the main renal artery, but with the development of small, low-profile balloons and better coaxial techniques, the application of angioplasty for branch lesions has increased, and the results of dilating these smaller vessels is comparable to the results reported for angioplasty of fibromuscular disease in the larger, main renal vessel. The results of angioplasty for focal atherosclerotic disease have been almost as good as for FMH as long as the ostial segment of the vessel is free of disease. The use of balloon angioplasty for transplant anastomotic stenosis has been controversial. Some centers have reported excellent success and long-term patency, whereas other reports have been much more pessimistic. It is probable that these discrepant results reflect differences in the nature of the lesion that develops at different centers based on different surgical techniques. Clearly, when the lesion responsible for the stenosis is intimal hyperplasia at the anastomosis, angioplasty can be highly successful. Conversely, when the lesion is a desmoplastic reaction in the adventitia around the anastomosis, PTA is far less effective. Atherosclerotic lesions involving the ostium of the renal artery have had the worst results from balloon angioplasty because the wall of the aorta around the ostium is affected, and this segment of aorta is not easily dilated with a balloon catheter. Recent experience has shown that the results may be improved using expandable metallic stents. However, long-term benefit has not yet been demonstrated.

10. The answer is **B** (Rutherford, 4th ed., pp. 1404–1406).

Clinical clues that suggest renovascular hypertension due to fibromuscular dysplasia (FMD) include occurrence of hypertension in pediatric-aged patients unaccompanied by obvious renal disease or the sudden onset of diastolic hypertension greater than 115 mm Hg in women under 45 years of age. Elevated systolic hypertension is common to virtually all forms of hypertension. Malignant hypertension does not occur more frequently in patients with fibromuscular dysplasia. Renovascular hypertension is, in general, more resistant to conventional drug therapy than essential hypertension.

11. The answers are **A, C, D** (Rutherford, 4th ed., pp. 1404–1406).

Indications for operation in the management of fibrodysplastic renovascular hypertension include the demonstration of the presence of a hemodynamically significant stenosis and evidence of its functional importance. In most institutions, renal angiography has proved to be the most useful test in assessing the relevance of a renal artery stenosis in these patients. Evidence of a hemodynamically significant renal artery stenosis includes the demonstration of collateral vessels that evolve as a pressure gradient across the renal artery approaches 10 mm Hg. In addition, demonstration of nonparenchymal renal artery branches functioning as collateral vessels by pharmacoangiographic techniques using agents such as epinephrine and acetylcholine can be useful in defining the significance of renal artery stenosis. *Intravenous* digital subtraction angiography is not recommended in patients suspected of having fibrodysplastic renovascular hypertension because it inadequately demonstrates significant detail concerning the severity and extent of renal artery disease, especially stenoses involving segmental branches.

12. The answer is **B** (Rutherford, 4th ed., pp. 1405–1406).

Percutaneous renal angioplasty can be effective treatment for patients with renal artery stenoses caused by fibromuscular dysplasia (FMD). However, complications are not rare, averaging 11% (2.5–38.5%), and are sometimes quite serious. Complications accompanying PTA of FMD lesions are not as common as those associated with PTA of atherosclerotic renal arterial stenoses. Adult patients with fibrodysplastic renovascular hypertension benefit from PTA in approximately 85% of cases. Failures in most reported series do not include patients whose lesions were not technically able to be dilated. Unfortunately, as many as 25% of the stenoses in patients with renal artery fibrodysplasia are not amendable to PTA. The best results for PTA of FMD renal artery stenoses are obtained in adult patients with unilateral medial fibrodysplasia. Intimal fibroplasia, in particular when associated with congenital defects, is more resistant to dilation. Transluminal angioplasty is contraindicated in patients who have renal artery stenoses secondary to FMD when these stenoses occur in the presence of macroaneurysms, involve multiple segmental branches, or are associated with dissections.

13. The answer is **F** (Rutherford, 4th ed., p. 1414).

Dilation of saphenous vein aortorenal grafts occurs in 20–44% of aortorenal saphenous vein grafts performed in pediatric-aged patients. Vein graft dilation usually appears as a nonprogressive, uniform increase in graft diameter. Marked aneurysmal dilation is distinctly uncommon and occurs in approximately 2% of aortorenal vein grafts in adults and 20% of vein grafts in pediatric-aged patients. Rupture of dilated aortorenal vein grafts has not been reported. The most common complication is luminal thrombus formation and distal embolization. When such dilated vein grafts require repair, they may either be plicated or replaced.

14. The answer is **D** (Rutherford, 4th ed., pp. 1419–1426).

Reduction in measures of global excretory renal function requires that global renal dysfunction be present. The most reversible cause of global dysfunction is correctable global ischemia. By definition, therefore, occlusive disease affecting *both* kidneys or the vessel to a *solitary* kidney is the desired anatomic variety of disease. When this is the case, retrieval of function occurs in over one half of patients. Another factor predictive of benefit is *rapid* deterioration of function.

15. The answer is **C** (Rutherford, 4th ed., pp. 1420–1425).

A 1991 review of the results of correction of lesions by Dean and his associates in 53 patients with ischemic nephropathy has shown that approximately two thirds of patients with severe bilateral lesions or a severe lesion to a solitary kidney will have significant retrieval of renal function following renal revascularization. In contrast, only approximately one third of patients who underwent correction of a unilateral lesion were similarly benefited (see Tables 109–1 and 109–2).

16. The answer is **false** (Rutherford, 4th ed., pp. 1420–1425).

According to their 1991 publication, the experience of Dean and his associates suggests that a patient with severe bilateral correctable lesions and dialysis-dependent renal failure has greater than a 75% chance of removal from dialysis by bilateral revascularization. Favorable results in patients with only a unilateral correctable lesion is very unusual (see Table 109–3).

17. The answer is **false** (Rutherford, 4th ed., pp. 1433–1434).

Methods of temporary renal perfusion vary among centers in which ex-vivo renal artery reconstructions are performed. Complex perfusion pump systems have been developed by several centers to allow continuous perfusion during the period of total renal ischemia. Although continuous perfusion may have comparative superiority for prolonged renal preservation during storage periods, simple intermittent flushing with the chilled preservative solutions provides equal protection during the shorter periods of two to three hours required for ex-vivo dissection and complex renal artery reconstruction. In this method of intermittent flushing, a liter of the Collin's solution to be used for flushing is refrigerated overnight. Immediately before its use, the additional components are added, and the liter of chilled (5–10° C) solution is hung on an intravenous stand so as to provide at least 2 m of gravitational perfusion pressure. Five hundred ml of solution is flushed through the kidney as soon as it is removed from the renal fossa. At the completion of each anastomosis, an additional 150–200 ml of solution is flushed through the kidney, a procedure that also allows examination of the suture line for leaks.

18. The answer is **false** (Rutherford, 4th ed., pp. 1434–1438).

Autotransplantation of the kidney to the iliac fossa has become the accepted method for reattachment of the ex-vivo reconstructed renal artery. This technique was initially borrowed from the renal transplant surgeon without consideration of the significant differences in the two patient populations. Since many ex-vivo procedures are performed in relatively young patients, durability of operation should be measured in terms of decades. For this reason, attachment of the kidney to the iliac arterial system within or below sites commonly susceptible to significant atherosclerotic occlusive disease can subject the autotransplanted kidney to atherosclerotic occlusive lesions that may reduce the durability of the renovascular operation. In addition, subsequent management of peripheral vascular disease may be complicated by the presence of an autotransplanted kidney. Furthermore, after the kidney has been replaced into the original renal fossa, the attachment of renal artery graft to the aorta at a more proximal site should approximate standard aortorenal bypasses with a high probability of success. To replace the kidney into its original location, Gerota's capsule is removed from the kidney during mobilization. At the point of renal vein transection, a large vascular clamp is placed to occlude partially the vena cava at the site of renal vein origin. An ellipse of vena cava containing the renal vein origin is then excised, and the kidney is removed for ex-vivo perfusion and reconstruction. When the microvascular renal artery/graft anastomoses are completed, the kidney is replaced in its original bed and the ellipse of vena cava is reattached. This technique decreases the likelihood of renal vein anastomotic stenosis due to technical misadventures. After this, the renal artery graft is attached to the aorta in standard fashion.

19. The answer is **true** (Rutherford, 4th ed., p. 1434).

Maintenance of profound renal parenchymal hypothermia during the period of total ischemia is of greatest importance in preserving renal function. Studies in canines have shown that warm ischemia times in excess of 30 minutes are associated with increasing permanent loss of function. Thus, ex-vivo perfusion of the kidney is performed with a chilled preservative solution. Although lowering the renal core temperature dramatically slows energy-dependent metabolism of the cortical cells, it also inactivates the cellular membrane sodium-potassium pump with subsequent cellular swelling occurring as a result of entrance of salt and water into the cell.

20. The answers are **A, E** (Rutherford, 4th ed., pp. 1442–1444).

There are four reasons to operate on renal artery aneurysms. The first is renal hypertension, as shown by many studies. The second is acute dissection, which is a surgical emergency. The chronic "healed" dissection is a more difficult problem. The risk of future dissection or rupture is probably small, and operation should not be performed unless the patient has severe hypertension. The third indication is rupture, also an emergency. The fourth indication is the risk of rupture. This indication is controversial because the risk cannot be estimated with certainty. The decision to resect may result in loss of a functioning kidney if reconstruction is unsuccessful. Small aneurysms, less than 2.5 cm, can be safely observed. Aneurysms larger than 4 cm should be resected. Mid-sized aneurysms, 2.5–4 cm, should be regarded with some suspicion, but should not be resected unless additional indications are present. The old dictum that heavily calcified aneurysms should be resected has not been confirmed. Uniform calcification of the aneurysm wall is not associated with increased risk of rupture. Partial or incomplete calcification, however, may predispose to rupture.

21. The answer is **B** (Rutherford, 4th ed., pp. 1442–1444).

Pregnancy increases the risk of rupture of renal artery aneurysms. In 1987, Cohen and Shamash reviewed 18 cases of rupture during pregnancy, suggesting that renal artery aneurysms are more likely to rupture during pregnancy. In 1990, Pliskin et al. reported a giant aneurysm with associated fistulas diagnosed postpartum. This probably resulted from rupture of an aneurysm into the renal vein during the pregnancy. Removal of smaller renal artery aneurysms in women who may become pregnant may be indicated. The published experience is too limited to allow recommending a precise size limit, but it would seem reasonable to remove any aneurysm over 2.5 cm. What about the woman who is already pregnant? Such a large operation may be unwise during pregnancy; but the risk of rupture should be communicated to the patient. Operation for ruptured aneurysm is clearly a surgical emergency.

22. The answer is **C** (Rutherford, 4th ed., pp. 1445–1447).

Duplex Doppler ultrasound is the best *screening* test for postbiopsy renal arteriovenous fistula. In 1989, Middleton et al. used the color Doppler instrument to diagnose eight such fistulas following renal transplantation and biopsy. Five of the eight fistulas closed under observation with sonography; angiography was not necessary. Intravenous pyelography may show a mass displacing a portion of the caliceal system, but the test is not very sensitive. Computed tomography may be used to show the lesion, but sensitivity is not particularly good, and the study is expensive. Magnetic resonance imaging is no better than computed tomography and is even more expensive. Magnetic resonance angiography eventually may prove to be useful, but it is currently an experimental modality for this application. Intravenous digital angiography is more invasive than duplex examination and gives less detail than standard renal angiography. Renal angiography is the definitive diagnostic study, although it is too invasive and expensive for a *screening* test. It should be performed if either operative surgery or catheter embolization is contemplated.

23. The answers are **B, D** (Rutherford, 4th ed., pp. 1147–1450).

A number of techniques of transcatheter embolization have been used by interventional radiologists. Materials embolized include blood clot, lead shot, Gelfoam, and Gianturco coils. The best results have been obtained in postbiopsy fistulas, which are typically small, single, and located peripherally. Neoplastic fistulas have also been embolized successfully; operation is an undesirable alternative for an unresectable tumor. On the other hand, postoperative fistulas are typically large fistulas between the remnants of the renal artery and vein. They are large, central, and unlikely to be successfully embolized, whereas operation is straightforward and poses no risk of loss of a kidney. Congenital fistulas are typically multiple, and although embolization may well be attempted in order to salvage the kidney, it is less likely to be successful.

24. The answer is **false** (Rutherford, 4th ed., pp. 1452–1455).

Acute thrombosis of a renal artery is usually silent and is a manifestation of progression of the underlying atherosclerotic lesion. In most instances, collateral perfusion to the kidney has developed to such an extent that the event is totally silent and goes unrecognized. Occasionally, however, the lesion is recognized acutely because of its adverse effect on excretory function of a solitary kidney or in the only kidney with previously significant residual function. Although all patients with acute renal artery thrombosis have a history of hypertension, the acute presentation produces acceleration of the hypertension and development of oliguric acute renal failure. Operation should be undertaken only after the patient is properly evaluated. Postponement of operation for evaluation and management of co-morbidities have no impact on the probability or degree of renal function retrieval. When collaterals have *not* developed, such as occurs in acute renal artery thrombosis from trauma, expeditious revascularization is essential. In this setting, most authors recommend against attempted renal artery repair once the "warm ischemia" time exceeds several hours.

25. The answer is **D** (Rutherford, 4th ed., p. 1452).

Renal artery trauma is an uncommon clinical problem, occurring in less than 10% of penetrating and 1% of blunt abdominal and back injuries. Common signs and symptoms of renal trauma include flank pain and tenderness and microscopic or gross hematuria; however, approximately 20% of patients with significant renal artery injury have no hematuria. Loss of the nephrogram and nonvisualizations of the distal vessel beyond the injury are strong predictors that lost renal function is *not* retrievable. Unfortunately, in most series less than 25% of revascularized kidneys will have significant retrieval of renal function.

26. The answer is **false** (Rutherford, 4th ed., pp. 1454–1455).

Acute spontaneous renal artery dissections usually occur as a complication of underlying atherosclerotic or fibromuscular dysplastic renovascular disease. In one review, upper abdominal or flank pain with radiation to the epigastrium was the most common presenting complaint (92%); hematuria was present in 33% of patients; all patients had severe hypertension; and 40% had acceleration of pre-existing hypertension.

16

Extracranial Cerebrovascular Disease

1. Carotid territory transient ischemic attacks (TIAs) are:
   A. An absolute indication for carotid endarterectomy.
   B. Have been shown to produce no structural damage to brain tissue.
   C. Episodes of monocular or hemispheric dysfunction that clear completely and without residual symptoms within 24 hours.
   D. Episodes of monocular visual loss, sensory or motor dysfunction, dizzy spells, or vertigo.
   E. All of the above.

2. The risk of stroke following carotid territory transient ischemic attacks associated with a hemodynamically significant stenosis:
   A. Is greatest within six months of the ischemic event.
   B. Is greater in women than in men.
   C. Is greater when the symptom is amaurosis fugax rather than hemispheric dysfunction.
   D. Is about 80% in five years.
   E. Is about 30% in five years.

3. Asymptomatic, hemodynamically significant carotid stenosis:
   A. Will cause subsequent stroke in over half of individuals with this disorder.
   B. Is no longer a potential cause of stroke once it has proceeded to *asymptomatic* occlusion.
   C. Is of no clinical significance until the patient begins to experience transient ischemic symptoms.
   D. Has been shown to produce fewer combined events of transient cerebral ischemia and stroke when treated by carotid endarterectomy.
   E. Should always be repaired before another surgical procedure requiring general anesthesia.

4. A *dominant* hemisphere middle cerebral artery infarction may result in which of the following deficits?
   A. Broca's aphasia (motor or nonfluent aphasia).
   B. Wernicke's aphasia (sensory or fluent aphasia).
   C. Gerstmann's syndrome.
   D. Neglect and findings of agnosagnosia, agraphesthesia, astereognosis, and impaired double simultaneous stimulation.
   E. Akinetic mutism.

5. Which of the following statements is/are true of cardiologic testing in stroke patients?
   A. All patients with a new stroke should have an electrocardiogram (ECG).
   B. All patients with a new first stroke require echocardiography.
   C. Transthoracic echocardiography and transesophageal echocardiography are equally sensitive for finding an embolic cardiac source in stroke patients.
   D. Holter monitoring is recommended in all stroke patients under the age of 50 who have no obvious cause for the stroke.
   E. Stroke patients with angina require clinical evaluation for coronary artery disease independent of the patient's age.

6. Which of the following studies should be performed routinely in patients with new onset of stroke?
   A. Electroencephalography (EEG).
   B. Lumbar puncture.
   C. Magnetic resonance angiography (MRA).
   D. Complete blood count (CBC).
   E. Transcranial Doppler imaging.

7. Patients with a stroke in the posterior cerebral artery (PCA) distribution may have:
   A. Transient monocular blindness.
   B. Cortical blindness (Anton's syndrome).
   C. Metamorphopsia.
   D. Palinopsia.
   E. Peduncular hallucinosis.

8. Anomalies in the anatomy of the aortic arch and its branches include:
   A. Common ostial origin of the left common carotid and left subclavian arteries.
   B. Common ostial origin of the innominate and left common carotid artery.
   C. Separate origin of the right vertebral artery directly from the ascending aortic arch.
   D. Aberrant right subclavian artery originating from the proximal descending thoracic aorta.
   E. Aberrant course of the left subclavian artery behind the first rib and beneath its inferior surface.

9. The circle of Willis:
   A. Is complete in its "textbook" description in about 50% of individuals.
   B. Consists of (1) the A1 segments of the anterior cerebral arteries, (2) the anterior communicating artery, (3) posterior communicating arteries, (4) posterior cerebral arteries.
   C. Most commonly has anomalies involving the anterior communicating artery (hypoplasia, absence, or duplication).
   D. Is interrupted by hypoplasia or absence of one or both posterior communicating arteries in about 25–30% of cases.
   E. May have connections of "fetal origin" such as an enlarged posterior communicating artery with hypoplasia of the initial (P1) segment of the posterior cerebral artery.

10. Complications of cerebrovascular angiography:
    A. Are more often neurologic than associated with the puncture site or administration of contrast material.
    B. Produce death or stroke or require operations in less than 0.2% of cases.
    C. Are decreased by administration of systemic heparin.
    D. Are reduced by systemic sedation to decrease patient movement and oxygen demands by the brain.
    E. Include transient ischemic attacks in 0.9% of cases.

11. Indirect tests such as periorbital Doppler examination and ocular pneumoplethysmography can detect which of the following?
    A. Bifurcation stenosis with 25–50% diameter reduction.
    B. Bifurcation stenosis greater than 60% diameter reduction.
    C. Tight stenosis versus occlusion.
    D. Siphon stenosis greater than 60%.
    E. All of the above.

12. Carotid duplex scan can:
    A. Detect bifurcation stenosis with 25–50% diameter reduction.
    B. Detect bifurcation stenosis greater than 60% diameter reduction.
    C. Distinguish tight stenosis from occlusion.
    D. Detect siphon stenosis greater than 60%.
    E. All of the above.

13. Vertebral artery disease can be evaluated using:
    A. Ocular pneumoplethysmography.
    B. Duplex scan.
    C. Transcranial Doppler.
    D. All of the above.
    E. None of the above.

14. In the presence of a tight stenosis of an internal carotid artery, the extent of collateral development can be assessed using:
    A. Ocular pneumoplethysmography.
    B. Carotid duplex scan.
    C. Transcranial Doppler.
    D. All of the above.
    E. None of the above.

15. In the first few hours after ischemic stroke onset, a brain CT scan:
    A. Is often normal in appearance.
    B. Is required to exclude intracerebral hemorrhage.
    C. Is inferior to MRI scanning of the brain.
    D. Usually demonstrates lacunar infarctions well.
    E. All of the above.

16. MRI scanning of nonhemorrhagic infarcts after several days:
    A. May be normal in appearance.
    B. May have high intensity on T1-weighted images.
    C. May have high intensity on T2-weighted images.
    D. May be low intensity on T2-weighted images.
    E. None of the above.

17. MRI scanning of hemorrhagic infarcts *more than several days after an event:*
    A. Is less capable than CT scanning in demonstrating a hemorrhagic component.
    B. Is more capable than CT scanning in demonstrating a hemorrhagic component.
    C. May show areas of bright signal on T2-weighted images.
    D. May show areas of low signal on T2-weighted images.
    E. Is no different than MRI scanning in the first 24 hours after an event.

18. Magnetic resonance angiography (MRA) has the following characteristics:
    A. Ability to image aneurysm clips.
    B. Freedom from artifacts.
    C. Accurately determines the exact degree of vessel stenosis.
    D. Requires substantial postacquisition processing for accurate vessel depiction.
    E. Can be obtained using standard MRI software.

19. Immediate anticoagulation in acute cardioembolic stroke:
    - **A.** Is indicated in nonvalvular paroxysmal atrial fibrillation.
    - **B.** Should aim for a prothrombin time-control ratio of approximately 2.
    - **C.** Is indicated in the primary prevention of noncardiogenic ischemic cerebrovascular attacks.
    - **D.** Is indicated in patients with a massive clinical stroke but a normal CT brain (which was performed within six hours of the stroke onset).
    - **E.** All of the above.

20. With regard to treatment of arterial hypertension in acute ischemic stroke:
    - **A.** Previously normotensive and hypertensive patients should be treated similarly.
    - **B.** Blood flow to the area of cerebral infarction is improved because autoregulation is preserved in the ischemic penumbra.
    - **C.** Initial therapy of a drowsy hypertensive patient with midline shift on CT of the brain should include prompt lowering of the BP.
    - **D.** Labetalol is useful because there is frequently an excessive sympathetic tone.
    - **E.** Captopril is useful because renin levels are frequently elevated.

21. Regarding fluid administration in acute ischemic stroke:
    - **A.** In general, fluids should be restricted so as to avoid raised intracranial pressure, which would impair cerebral blood flow.
    - **B.** A combination of a hypotonic solution, such as 5% dextrose, and an isotonic solution, such as normal saline, is desirable.
    - **C.** *All* patients with ischemic stroke should receive 1 g/kg of 50% dextrose so as to avoid missing those patients whose hemiplegia may be due to hypoglycemia.
    - **D.** Continuous hypertonic glucose solutions are useful to decrease cerebral edema.
    - **E.** None of the above.

22. The NASCET trial demonstrated that patients with carotid artery stenoses of 70% or greater:
    - **A.** And transient ischemic attacks had fewer strokes following carotid endarterectomy than those treated with medical management alone.
    - **B.** And history of prior mild stroke had fewer subsequent strokes following carotid endarterectomy than those receiving medical management alone.
    - **C.** With prior symptoms of either transient ischemic attack or prior mild stroke had fewer subsequent deaths following carotid endarterectomy than those managed medically alone.
    - **D.** Have outcomes similar to those of patients with cartoid artery stenosis of 50–70%.
    - **E.** All of the above.

23. The indication for carotid endarterectomy that is most controversial is:
    - **A.** A patient with transient ischemic attacks and a documented 70% carotid stenosis.
    - **B.** A patient with a prior mild stroke and a stenosis of 75% without ulceration.
    - **C.** Amaurosis fugax in a patient with a 70% carotid stenosis with an "A" ulcer.
    - **D.** "Global" cerebral ischemia with a *unilateral* 75% carotid stenosis.
    - **E.** Asymptomatic 90% stenosis.

24. All of the following statements concerning shunting of the carotid artery at the time of carotid endarterectomy are true *except*:
    - **A.** Air emboli can occur with a shunt.
    - **B.** Shunts will reverse EEG abnormalities that occur with temporary carotid clamping.
    - **C.** Routine shunting will reduce perioperative stroke rate.
    - **D.** Most patients in selective shunt series actually do not require shunting.
    - **E.** Measurement of cartoid back pressure is a widely accepted method to determine the need for a shunt.

25. The following statements about vertebrobasilar insufficiency are true *except:*
    - **A.** The presence of orthostatic hypotension with a 20-mm-Hg systolic pressure drop upon standing excludes a patient from further work-up.
    - **B.** A head CT scan is mandatory to rule out tumors and assess the integrity of the brain.
    - **C.** In labyrinth disease, the sudden inertial changes when the patient's head turns briskly result in immediate symptoms and often marked nystagmus, whereas in vertebral artery compression, it takes a few seconds before the patient fears for his balance.
    - **D.** A 24-hour ECG (Holter monitoring) should be obtained in *all* patients evaluated for vertebrobasilar insufficiency.
    - **E.** MRI is superior to CT scan for demonstrating brain stem infarctions.

26. With respect to indications for vertebral artery (VA) reconstructions:
    - **A.** In patients with orthostatic hypotension, symptoms may not respond to medical treatment, and only the reconstruction of a diseased or occluded VA will render the patient asymptomatic.

B. When VAs are reconstructed in patients for diffuse cerebrovascular disease with unreconstructable carotid arteries, the presence of large undiseased middle cerebral arteries increases success rates.
C. The morbidity from combined-concomitant carotid and VA repair is greater than from isolated carotid or VA reconstruction.
D. In VA reconstructions (both isolated and concomitant with a carotid operation), only severely stenosed (>75% luminal narrowing) and clearly dominant or single VAs are operated upon.
E. In patients with an embolic source in a vertebral or subclavian artery, a normal artery on the opposite side supplies blood to the basilar artery and obviates repair of the diseased side.

27. Regarding arteriographic evaluation of the vertebral arteries, the following statements are true *except:*
A. The most common congenital anomaly is the left VA arising from the aortic arch proximal to the left subclavian artery.
B. The most common atherosclerotic lesion of the VA is severe stenosis of its origin.
C. The second segment of the vertebral artery (V_2), which extends from C_6 to C_2, is the segment of the VA most commonly compressed by osteophytes.
D. V_2 is the second most common site for atherosclerotic involvement of the VA.
E. V_3, which extends from the top of C_2 to the atlanto-occipital membrane at the base of the skull, is the segment most frequently affected by dissection due to fibromuscular dysplasia and/or trauma.

28. Standard surgical techniques for treatment of vertebrobasilar insufficiency include:
A. Transposition of the VA into the common carotid artery.
B. Cervical sympathectomy as a concomitant procedure.
C. Bypasses to the V_4 segment.
D. Bypasses to the V_2 segment.
E. Bypasses to the V_1 segment.

29. Symptoms of kinking of the internal carotid artery:
A Include hemiparesis, monocular blindness, dizziness, ataxia, and dysarthria.
B. May occur with rotational changes of the head and neck.
C. May be absent despite acute angulation of the kinked segment.
D. Should be ascribed to coexistent atherosclerotic bifurcational disease rather than to tortuous or kinked arterial segments.
E. Are relieved by aspirin.

30. Which of the following is the best test to determine functional significance of disease in a patient with symptoms of carotid insufficiency due to a kink or coil of the carotid artery?
A. Electroencephalography (EEG).
B. Technetium-pertechnetate cerebral perfusion scan.
C. Extracranial and intracranial angiography.
D. Carotid duplex scan.
E. Oculoplethysmography (OPG).

31. You are asked to consult on a patient with a tortuous internal carotid artery. Which of the following preoperative and operative decisions is/are true?
A. A standard endarterectomy will usually eliminate the kinking.
B. Kinks can be eliminated with reimplantation of the internal carotid artery more proximally on the common carotid artery.
C. Even if asymptomatic, an S-shaped or spiral-looped internal carotid artery is an indication for surgical repair.
D. Most commonly, the distal extracranial internal carotid artery is the tortuous segment.
E. Completion angiography is recommended after endarterectomy in patients with tortuous carotid arteries.

32. Which of the following statements regarding fibromuscular dysplasia (FMD) of the internal carotid arteries (ICAs) is/are true?
A. It is the third most common site of predilection for FMD.
B. The most common type at this site is medial fibrodysplasia.
C. Unlike the renal arteries, there is no gender predilection for FMD of the ICA.
D. If FMD is found in one ICA, there is a better than 50:50 chance a similar lesion will be found in the opposite ICA.
E. FMD lesions involve the cervical ICA in the following order of segmental localization: upper third > middle third > lower third.

33. Which of the following statements regarding lesions associated with FMD of the cervical carotid artery is/are true?
A. Because of the much younger age of patients with FMD of the ICA, concomitant carotid atherosclerosis is characteristically absent.
B. Vertebral artery involvement with FMD may occur as an isolated finding and is present in over 5% of cases with carotid FMD.
C. Intracranial internal carotid aneurysms are found in association with cervical FMD in 2–5% of cases, approximately as frequently as they are with symptomatic carotid bifurcation atherosclerosis.
D. Renal artery involvement is found in nearly two thirds of patients with carotid FMD.
E. Based on careful histopathology, dissection of the ICA can be attributed to an underlying FMD lesion in close to one third of cases without a history of trauma.

34. Which of the following statements regarding the clinical course and management of carotid FMD is/are true?

A. Because more than half of the patients in reported surgical series are symptomatic, and stroke with permanent neurologic deficit occurred in well over 10% in most series, carotid dilation is justified in asymptomatic good-risk patients with a tight carotid stenosis.
B. If present, renal FMD should routinely be corrected *before* carotid FMD.
C. In a patient with an asymptomatic but high-grade (85–90%) carotid artery stenosis due to FMD, an associated ipsilateral 12-mm diameter intracranial aneurysm takes priority in treatment.
D. For bilateral asymptomatic 80% FMD carotid stenoses, both should be dilated but as staged procedures, employing a 5–7-day interval.
E. Balloon dilation has no place in the treatment of carotid FMD because of the small but definite risk of causing stroke.

35. The one most frequent cause of extracranial carotid artery aneurysms is:

A. Infection.
B. Fibromuscular dysplasia.
C. Blunt trauma.
D. Penetrating trauma.
E. Atherosclerosis.

36. The one most common mode of presentation of extracranial carotid aneurysms is:

A. Central nervous system deficit.
B. Peripheral (cranial) nerve dysfunction.
C. Hemorrhage.
D. Painful cervical mass.
E. Asymptomatic cervical mass.

37. Distal extracranial internal carotid aneurysms are best managed by:

A. Carotid ligation.
B. Aneurysmorrhaphy
C. Endoluminally placed coils, balloons, etc.
D. Resection and interposition grafting.
E. Resection and end-to-end anastomosis.

38. Which of the following statements is/are true regarding characteristics of atherosclerotic aneurysms of the extracranial carotid arteries?

A. They are associated with a relatively low incidence of other peripheral aneurysms.
B. The male to female ratio is higher than for abdominal aortic aneurysms.
C. There is evidence for a generalized arterial abnormality as the underlying etiology.
D. Hypertension is infrequently present and is not considered to be an important etiologic factor.
E. The natural history is very favorable, characterized by slow enlargement and lack of symptoms in most cases.

39. Extracranial–intracranial bypass may be indicated for which of the following situations?

A. Occlusion of the internal carotid artery associated with one or two transient ischemic attacks (TIAs).
B. TIAs due to severe middle cerebral artery stenosis.
C. Minor stroke due to severe stenosis of the intrapetrous (intracranial) segment of the internal carotid artery.
D. Recurrent, progressively severe TIAs due to carotid artery occlusion that are refractory to anticoagulation.
E. Carotid bulb ulceration.

40. Cerebral hemodynamic insufficiency can be demonstrated by:

A. Transcranial Doppler measurements of middle cerebral artery velocity responses to changes in arterial PCO_2.
B. Transcranial Doppler measurements of middle cerebral artery velocity responses to acetazolamide infusion.
C. Xenon/computerized tomography measurements of cerebral blood flow before and after acetazolamide infusion.
D. All of the above.
E. None of the above.

41. Which of the following vessels may be used to construct an extracranial–intracranial anastomosis?

A. Superficial temporal artery.
B. Occipital artery.
C. Saphenous vein graft from the external carotid artery.
D. All of the above.
E. None of the above.

42. The diagnostic studies *most* helpful in evaluating a large carotid artery paraganglioma include which of the following?

A. Color-flow duplex sonography.
B. Carotid angiography.
C. CT scan of the neck.
D. MRI of the neck.
E. *Intravenous* digital angiography.

43. Ten days after resection of an intraoral carcinoma, partial mandibulectomy, and a radical neck dissection, a patient develops a postoperative salivary fistula followed two days later by a "sentinel bleed" from the neck wound. Which of the following statements is the best course of action?

A. Reopen the neck wound and resect the infected segment of the common carotid artery, insert an interposition vein graft, and drain and close the wound.

B. Prepare the patient for immediate definitive surgical intervention to include extra-anatomic rerouting of the carotid circulation through clean uninvolved tissue followed by closure of the salivary fistula and establishment of adequate drainage of the infected neck wound.
C. Place the patient on nursing alert with instructions to apply pressure to the neck wound should further bleeding occur.
D. Reopen the neck wound, ligate the common carotid artery, debride the area, and drain it.
E. Reopen the neck wound, ligate the common carotid artery, and perform extracranial-intracranial bypass.

44. Which of the following statements regarding temporal arteritis (giant cell arteritis) is/are true?

A. Temporal arteritis is also called Horton's arteritis.
B. This disease is unresponsive to corticosteroid therapy.
C. The majority of symptoms associated with temporal arteritis result from gradual occlusion of branches of the carotid and vertebral arteries.
D. Temporal arteritis is histopathologically related to Takayasu's disease.
E. All of the above.

45. Which of the following statements is/are true regarding cranial nerve dysfunction associated with carotid endarterectomy?

A. Cranial nerve injuries occur in less than 2% of patients and generally are unpreventable.
B. Most injuries result in temporary dysfunction of the vagus and hypoglossal nerves.
C. The glossopharyngeal nerve fails to enter the surgical field even during high dissection of the internal carotid artery and, therefore, cannot be injured.
D. Vagus nerve dysfunction may be asymptomatic, so the integrity of the vocal cords should be confirmed by direct inspection before proceeding with elective contralateral carotid endarterectomy.
E. None of the above.

46. After carotid endarterectomy under general anesthesia with primary closure of the arteriotomy, a patient awakens uneventfully and remains neurologically asymptomatic for two hours before the abrupt onset of a profound contralateral hemiplegia. Under these circumstances, the following statements are true:

A. If a shunt had been used during the primary operation, this complication would not have occurred.
B. Thrombosis of the internal carotid artery must be assumed to be the most likely explanation for the delayed neurologic event.
C. Surgical intervention is not warranted unless it can be performed within 30 minutes of the onset of neurologic symptoms.
D. Internal carotid shunting and patch angioplasty probably are indicated during a reoperation.
E. Severity of neurologic symptoms should not be a factor in the decision to return to the operating room.

47. Which of the following statements most accurately describe(s) recurrent stenosis occurring within two years after previous carotid endarterectomy?

A. It probably is related to myointimal hyperplasia rather than recurrent atherosclerosis.
B. It is likely to become symptomatic and should be corrected by a reoperation as soon as it is discovered.
C. Its development and/or clinical course *may* be ameliorated by patch angioplasty during the primary operation.
D. It is more common in men than in women.
E. All of the above.

48. The following statement(s) is/are true regarding the results of carotid endarterectomy for *acute stroke:*

A. Carotid endarterectomy is contraindicated in *all* patients presenting with an acute stroke.
B. Clinical criteria may be used to select patients for operation.
C. It is best to delay operation for six weeks or longer after an acute stroke, considering the high risk of operation during an acute stroke and the low incidence of recurrent stroke during the six-week observation interval.
D. Operation in the presence of an acute stroke in properly selected patients can be performed with similar morbidity and mortality as in patients presenting remotely after a stroke.
E. Sudden worsening of a patient recovering from an acute stroke is a contraindication for surgery.

49. The following have been shown to influence the results of *external* carotid endarterectomy *except:*

A. Bilateral carotid occlusion.
B. Preoperative fixed neurologic deficit.
C. Symptomatic internal carotid artery occlusion.
D. Disease in the vertebral arteries.
E. Specific hemispheric or retinal symptoms.

50. The following statement(s) is/are true regarding prospective randomized studies of carotid artery disease in patients with *symptomatic* carotid artery stenosis:

A. Patients with stenosis >75% had similar outcomes whether treated medically or surgically.
B. Patients with carotid artery stenoses between 50 and 75% had significantly increased risk of stroke from carotid endarterectomy.
C. Patients with stenosis >75% in the ipsilateral carotid artery had fewer strokes when treated by aspirin than by endarterectomy.
D. Patients with stenosis <30% in the ipsilateral carotid artery were found to have a benign course, with no improvement offered by surgical intervention.
E. None of the above.

51. The following statement(s) is/are true regarding patients with *asymptomatic* carotid stenosis:
    A. The NASCET trial established that patients with high-grade asymptomatic carotid stenosis do better with carotid endarterectomy than with conservative medical management.
    B. The Canadian Aspirin Trial showed that patients with asymptomatic carotid stenosis do better with aspirin than without therapy.
    C. The risk of stroke of a carotid stenosis >80% in the asymptomatic patient is 10% per year of observation.
    D. An acceptable morbidity and mortality for asymptomatic patients offered carotid endarterectomy is 5%.
    E. None of the above.

52. Ticlopidine:
    A. Is an anticoagulant that inhibits thrombin formation.
    B. Is an inhibitor of adenosine diphosphate pathway of platelet aggregation.
    C. Is an adenylate cyclase inhibitor that also inhibits thromboxane and prostacyclin production.
    D. Is an antiplatelet agent that has not been shown to be better than aspirin in the treatment of symptomatic patients with carotid artery disease.
    E. Inhibits most of the known stimuli to platelet *adhesion*.
    F. Has a significant incidence of neutropenia, which is on the order of 10–20%.

16

Answers

1. The answer is **C** (Rutherford, 4th ed., pp. 1457–1458, 1464–1471, 1474–1476).

By definition, TIAs are limited to episodes of monocular or hemispheric dysfunction. These can produce symptoms of transient monocular visual loss such as visual blurring or altitudinal defect. They can also cause motor or sensory dysfunction involving the face, arm, and/or lower extremity. Often there are mixed sensory and motor symptoms. When the events are purely sensory or purely motor, the differential diagnosis includes lacunar syndrome. In the past TIAs were assumed to cause no anatomic abnormalities in the brain. However, recent studies have demonstrated that TIAs are often associated with structural damage, as documented by magnetic resonance imaging. Nonfocal symptoms such as light-headedness, dizziness, and vertigo are very nonspecific and do not reflect neurologic dysfunction caused by a carotid artery lesion. Finally, TIAs alone are not an absolute indication for operation. TIAs in association with a specific arterial lesion, particularly a stenosis compromising the lumen by 70% or greater, represent proven indications for operation.

2. The answers are **A, E** (Rutherford, 4th ed., pp. 1457–1458).

The risk of stroke in patients with carotid territory TIAs becomes less as the time interval between the event and evaluation occurs. In general, the six-month interval after the last transient ischemic event represents the period of highest risk. Few data exist concerning the risk of TIAs in women compared with men. However, the data that are available suggest that women with TIAs experience fewer strokes than men. Amaurosis fugax represents a less dire prognostic event than a hemispheric TIA. Finally, TIAs herald strokes in roughly one third of patients.

3. The answer is **D** (Rutherford, 4th ed., pp. 1458–1459, 1666–1667).

Asymptomatic carotid stenosis remains the focus of intense investigation with regard to prognosis and best methods of management. The prospective randomized trial conducted by the Veterans Administration conclusively demonstrated that the *combined* events of transient cerebral ischemia and stroke were statistically significantly reduced by carotid endarterectomy compared to medical management. Of note, most patients who suffer strokes with documented carotid artery stenosis fail to have premonitory TIAs. Unfortunately, the study was not designed to look at the event of stroke alone, which has been the basis for criticism. Patients with an asymptomatic carotid artery occlusion remain at risk for subsequent stroke in the distribution of that artery at the rate of 5% per year. In the past, it was recommended that high-grade asymptomatic carotid stenoses be repaired prior to other nonvascular or vascular operations, prophylactically to prevent stroke. However, the incidence of postoperative strokes—even after open heart procedures—is quite low. It is therefore difficult to justify *routine* prophylactic carotid endarterectomy in this setting, and the carotid lesion should be treated on its own merits.

4. The answers are **A, B, C** (Rutherford, 4th ed., pp. 1474–1476).

A main stem middle cerebral artery (MCA) occlusion may present with hemiplegia, hemisensory loss, and hemianopsia, and a tonic gaze deviation toward the side of the lesion can be seen. MCA occlusion presents with a decreased level of consciousness in about 25% of patients. If only the *upper* division of the MCA is involved, the infarct involves the cortical surface of the frontal and anterior parietal lobes. The lower two thirds of the face and the arm are primarily affected, with relative sparing of the leg. In the *dominant* hemisphere, the aphasia is predominantly a motor (Broca's) aphasia. In the *nondominant* hemisphere, the neglect and anosagnosia are less prominent than in the more proximal arterial occlusions. Emboli traveling to the *lower* division of the MCA tree may produce very little weakness and sensory loss. The patient has a visual field deficit. In the dominant hemisphere, the patient has a fluent (Wernicke's) aphasia. An isolated nondominant parietal lobe lesion results in abnormalities in stereognosis (the ability to recognize objects by sense of touch alone), double simultaneous stimulation, and graphesthesia (the ability to recognize figures written on the skin). A dominant hemisphere parietal occipital lesion may result in a Gerstmann's syndrome, consisting of finger agnosia (inability to recognize one's own fingers), acalculia (inability to calculate), right–left disorientation, and agraphia (inability to write). Akinetic mutism is associated with bilateral anterior cerebral artery infarctions, not with MCA infarctions.

5. The answers are **A, D, E** (Rutherford, 4th ed., p. 1478).

An ECG is important in all patients with cerebrovascular disease. New-onset ECG abnormalities are frequently seen in the setting of acute stroke. Only in patients in whom there is reason to suspect cardiac embolism or valvular disease is an echocardiogram warranted. An echocardiogram should be performed on all patients under the age of 50 years presenting with a stroke syndrome of uncertain cause or when they have known coronary artery disease, prior recent myocardial infarction, cardiomyopathy, known valvular disease, or chest x-ray indicating cardiomegaly. In patients in whom an embolic source is suspected, a transesophegeal echocardiogram should be performed even if the transthoracic echocardiogram is normal. Transthoracic echocardiography is not as sensitive in identifying left atrial masses or other potential sources of emboli. Echocardiography is not justified in the older patient in whom the cause of stroke is known who has no evidence of cardiac disease. In patients in whom arrhythmia is suspected, an ambulatory ECG (Holter monitor) is useful. Holter monitoring is unlikely to find previously unsuspected atrial fibrillation. However, other arrhythmias are found often enough to warrant Holter monitoring in acute stroke patients who have otherwise unexplained strokes. It must be remembered that an arrhythmia alone without associated embolization usually causes global ischemia with diffuse rather than focal cerebral symptoms. The association of cerebrovascular disease and cardiovascular disease is well established. Approximately 40% of stroke patients with no symptoms of coronary artery disease will have severe stenosis in at least one coronary artery. Coronary artery evaluation, including exercise electrocardiograms and resting and exercise radionuclide cardiac studies, should be undertaken on an individual basis. Dipyridamole-thallium myocardial imaging can be useful in diagnosing asymptomatic ischemic heart disease in stroke patients unable to exercise. Stroke patients who have an abnormal ECG or clinically significant angina pectoris should be considered for coronary angiography independent of chronological age.

6. The answer is **D** (Rutherford, 4th ed., pp. 1477–1479).

In current clinical practice, outside the operating room and in the absence of stroke-related seizures, EEG has a very limited role in the clinical evaluation of the patient with acute cerebrovascular disease. Brain mapping and other forms of computerized analysis of EEG hold a promise of being valuable tools in clinical evaluation of these patients, but right now they remain research tools. The role of routine cerebrospinal fluid (CSF) examination in cerebrovascular disease is controversial. Certainly, it must be tested if subarachnoid hemorrhage, vasculitis, embolic infective endocarditis, or infection is suspected. In patients under the age of 40 years who do not have a clear atherosclerotic or embolic cause of stroke, a lumbar puncture should be done routinely as part of the stroke work-up. CSF examination is especially useful in stroke patients presenting with unexplained fever, elevated white blood cell count, stiff neck, prior unexplained headache, or a history of syphilis or lupus. In the absence of a traumatic spinal tap, the presence of blood in the CSF is the sine qua non of intracranial bleeding. However, although in certain circumstances a CSF examination may be helpful, it is not a required routine study in all stroke patients. MRA is a noninvasive method of imaging both the extracranial and intracranial vasculature. The study is expensive and requires a lot of patient cooperation. The spatial resolution is not adequate for reliably detecting ulcerated plaques. It tends to overestimate carotid stenosis. With improvements in both software and hardware, this technique may play a larger role in routine evaluation of stroke patients. However, in current clinical practice, the angiogram remains the "gold standard" in evaluating the vascular tree in stroke patients. A CBC is useful in screening for anemia or polycythemia. In cerebrovascular disease, a highly elevated hematocrit may be hazardous because sludging may occur and may contribute to impaired cerebral blood flow. An elevated white count may be the first indication of an underlying infection. Obtaining a CBC is low risk, low cost, and potentially very helpful. It should be ordered as a routine test in *all* new stroke patients. When done properly, transcranial Doppler studies can detect severe intracranial stenosis involving major arteries at the base of the brain. It is useful for monitoring patients with subarachnoid hemorrhages. In ischemic stroke, it has limited clinically utility at present.

7. The answers are **B, C, D** (Rutherford, 4th ed., pp. 1474–1476).

Transient monocular blindness is usually due to ischemia in the distribution of the ophthalmic artery, a branch of the internal carotid artery. It is not associated with posterior cerebral artery ischemia. With bilateral PCA infarction, the patient may have bilateral homonymous hemianopsia with or without macular sparing (cortical blindness). A patient with cortical blindness (Anton's syndrome) may not admit to being blind and will confabulate when asked to name objects in the room. The patient may also have metamorphopsia (visual distortion of objects) or palinopsia (persistence of an image after it has left the visual field). Peduncular hallucinosis consists of nonhorrendous, often pleasurable, colorful hallucinations. It can be associated with occlusion at the distal end of the basilar artery, causing rostral brainstem ischemia. Whereas occlusion of the distal basilar artery may be associated with PCA stroke, PCA ischemia without basilar occlusion will not cause peduncular hallucinosis.

8. The correct answers are **B, D** (Rutherford, 4th ed., pp. 1481–1483).

In approximately 95% of all patients, the aortic arch gives rise to three major branches: the innominate artery (right brachiocephalic trunk), the left common carotid artery, and the left subclavian artery. One of the most common variants is a common osteal origin of the innominate and left common carotid arteries, which occurs in approximately 10% of patients. However, a true brachiocephalic trunk of more than a few millimeters in length that then divides into the innominate and left common carotid is relatively rare. The left carotid and left subclavian arteries do *not* arise from a common osteum. Likewise, the right vertebral does *not* take origin from the ascending aortic arch. However, separate origin of the left vertebral artery directly from the aorta proximal to the left subclavian artery is a relatively common anatomic variant, occurring in approximately 5% of patients. The right subclavian artery normally originates from the innominate artery and arches laterally and posteriorly, passing posterior to the anterior scalene muscle. The most common aortic arch anomaly compatible with long-term survival is an aberrant right subclavian artery that originates from the proximal descending thoracic aorta and passes posterior to the esophagus. Unless this anomaly causes dysphasia in the neonatal period, it may escape detection until the patient is examined angiographically later in life. Anomalies such as double aortic arch, interrupted arch, right arch, and cervical arch are often associated with complex congenital heart disease or symptoms caused by pressure on the trachea or esophagus and, thus, require surgical correction in the neonatal or pediatric-age group. The left subclavian artery originates directly from the aorta and is usually its third branch. It extends vertically within the mediastinum, then arches laterally en route to the neck to pass posterior to the anterior scalene muscle. Subclavian arteries exit the neck by passing over the superior surface of the first rib, posterior to the clavicle, in close relationship to the lower portion of the brachial plexus.

9. The correct answers are **B, D, E** (Rutherford, 4th ed., pp. 1488–1489).

The circle of Willis is a unique vascular ring that encircles the diencephalon, including the sella turcica and pituitary. It consists of the A1 segments of the anterior cerebral arteries and the anterior communicating arteries at the anterior portion of the ring, which connect the internal carotid systems to each other. The short posterior communicating arteries originate from the internal carotid arteries at or near the bifurcation into anterior and middle cerebral arteries. The posterior communicating arteries run posteriorly to connect with corresponding proximal segments of the posterior cerebral arteries, thus connecting the internal carotid system and the anterior circulation with the vertebral basilar system, the posterior circulation. Only *20%* of patients actually have the "textbook" symmetrical circle of Willis; hypoplasia of one or more components occurs in most individuals. Hypoplasia or absence of one or both *posterior* communicating arteries occurs in approximately 25–30% of individuals, thus effectively isolating the anterior and posterior circulation to a greater or lesser degree. Anomalies of the anterior communicating artery, including hypoplasia, absence, or duplication, occur in approximately 10% of individuals. Hypoplasia of the initial (P1) segment of the posterior cerebral artery with primary or sole flow to the posterior cerebral artery via an enlarged posterior communicating artery from the internal carotid occurs in approximately 15–20% of cases and is termed a "fetal origin." Persistence of additional fetal communications between the carotid and vertebral-basilar systems include the trigeminal, otic, hypoglossal, and proatlantal intersegmental arteries, but it occurs rarely.

10. The correct answers are **B, E** (Rutherford, 4th ed. pp. 1496–1497).

Most complications associated with cerebrovascular angiography are due to problems at the puncture site or to administration of radiographic contrast material and are discussed elsewhere in the textbook (Section II). Fortunately, true neurologic complications are uncommon during cerebral angiography. The incidence of major complications (death, stroke, access site problems requiring surgical intervention) has been found to be approximately 0.16% in a recent large study. Transient neurologic deficits (TIAs) were reported to occur with a frequency of approximately 0.9% in another study. The use of systemic heparin anticoagulation during aortic arch and selective common carotid angiography has been shown to be *ineffective* in reducing the incidence of complications. There is a unanimity of opinion regarding avoidance of significant sedation in most cerebrovascular angiographic procedures in order to prevent masking neurologic complications as a result of the procedure.

11. The answers are **B, D** (Rutherford, 4th ed., pp. 1508–1511).

Indirect tests such as periorbital Doppler and ocular pneumoplethysmography rely on detecting physiologic changes distal to the carotid bifurcation. The periorbital Doppler test depends upon changes in the collateral pathways of the face, whereas ocular pneumoplethysmography detects a decrease in ophthalmic artery pressure. A 50–60% stenosis is required to produce enough of a drop in the distal internal carotid artery pressure to be detected by either of these methods. Both techniques depend on an abnormality measured at the level of the ophthalmic artery. For this reason a tight stenosis of the internal carotid at the bifurcation or of the siphon can be detected. One of the drawbacks of the indirect tests is that one cannot distinguish a tight stenosis from an internal carotid artery occlusion. In some cases of occlusion there is a very great decrease in ophthalmic artery pressure. However, typically there is not much difference between tight stenosis and occlusion with respect to the ophthalmic artery pressure due to compensation from collateral branches.

12. The answers are **A, B, C** (Rutherford, 4th ed., pp. 1511–1514).

The carotid duplex scan is highly accurate in assigning carotid bifurcation disease to categories of stenosis ranging from a normal artery to a total occlusion. Image interpretation combined with Doppler wave form analysis permits separation of early degrees of stenosis as well as identification of tight lesions. With suitable experience with patients having advanced pathology, it is usually possible to distinguish a tight stenosis from a total occlusion, although an occasional "string sign" with extremely sluggish flow may be misdiagnosed. Whereas the scan is quite accurate in identifying low grades of stenosis in the area of the bifurcation, it cannot detect similar lesions in the region of the siphon. Severe lesions at the siphon (greater than 80% diameter reduction) may be detected indirectly by abnormalities of the internal carotid wave forms, but less severe lesions do not alter the wave form sufficiently to be reliably detected.

13. The answers are **B, C** (Rutherford, 4th ed., pp. 1508–1514).

The examination of the lower portion of the vertebral arteries has become a routine part of a cerebrovascular duplex scan. In many cases it is possible to detect a tight stenosis by the high-velocity jet detected at the origin of the vertebral artery. In some cases it may not be possible to study the origin of the vessel; however, indirect evidence of occlusive lesions can be detected by low-velocity flows away from the takeoff of the vessel. Of course, detection of reversed flow identifies a vascular "steal." A complete transcranial Doppler examination includes evaluation of the posterior circulation. The basilar artery together with distal portions of both vertebrals are examined. Severe asymmetry of flow velocities in the two vertebrals points to occlusive disease, and reverse flow documents a steal. Ocular pneumoplethysmography provides no information about the vertebral arteries.

14. The answers are **A, C** (Rutherford, 4th ed., pp. 1509–1514).

A large gradient (>10 mm Hg) between the two ophthalmic artery pressures is highly suggestive of poor collateralization, and examination with compression of the ipsilateral common carotid artery provides an indirect measure of the back pressure. Experience has shown that these indirect values correspond closely to stump pressure measurements made during operation. Transcranial Doppler examination of velocities in the anterior and posterior communicating branches helps provide a qualitative impression of collateralization. Normally there is relatively little flow through these collateral pathways. No information is provided to indicate extent of collateralization by the routine carotid duplex scan.

15. The answers are **A, B** (Rutherford, 4th ed., pp. 1517–1523, 1529).

In the first several hours after onset of ischemic stroke, a CT scan is often normal in appearance. After hours or days, areas of low density can be seen, and there may be a progressive mass effect with distortion of underlying ventricles and overlying sulci. Lacunar infarcts are often quite small; on anatomical sections, they may be only a few millimeters in cross-sectional diameter, so that they could remain below the resolution of many scanners. In a patient presenting with an abrupt strokelike clinical syndrome, a CT scan is advisable in the initial hours in order to exclude mass lesions that may simulate an ischemic event, including primary intracerebral hemorrhages and subdural hematomas. CT scan is still considered the imaging procedure of choice in the acute period. In contrast to MRI studies, uncooperative patients can be imaged quickly, and there is easier access to patients who may require intravenous lines or ventilatory support. In some cases, when the patient is more stable, a follow-up MRI scan may be advantageous for evaluation in order to provide additional detail.

16. The answers are **A, C** (Rutherford, 4th ed., pp. 1523–1530).

MRI scans typically show areas of infarction after several days; however, small lacunar infarcts may still be missed, as with CT scanning. On T1-weighted images, *nonhemorrhagic* infarcts have *low* intensity; high intensity is seen only if petechial hemorrhage is associated with the infarct or if frank hemorrhage develops later. Typically, high-intensity patches are seen on T2-weighted images.

17. The answers are **B, C, D** (Rutherford, 4th ed., pp. 1523–1530).

The appearance of hemorrhage on MRI scanning depends on when the scan is obtained. In the first day the lesion may be isointense on T1-weighted images and of low signal on T2-weighted images. Typically, several days later a very bright area is seen on T1-weighted images due to the appearance of methemoglobin; the signal may be either bright or low in intensity on T2-weighted images. Later on, due to the presence of hemosiderin, areas of low signal are often seen in sites of old hemorrhage on T2-weighted images.

18. The answer is **D** (Rutherford, 4th ed., pp. 1531–1535).

Magnetic resonance angiography (MRA) requires both special computer software and a cooperative patient because movement, coughing, and swallowing can seriously degrade image quality owing to characteristic artifacts. Patients with ferromagnetic aneurysm clips should not be imaged on an MRI scanner. Although patients with certain kinds of metallic clips can be safely imaged, the magnetic field surrounding the clips is distorted, which degrades image quality in the adjacent brain tissue. Magnetic resonance angiograms often overestimate the degree of stenosis due to a variety of effects, including intravoxel dephasing due to turbulent flow and saturation effects. Although it is often important to look at thin-section source images, vascular anatomy can be better appreciated by utilizing a variety of procedures, including maximum-intensity projection techniques and special editing procedures that allow for visualization of selected segments of the vessel. A major problem in the interpretation of MRA is that vessels have a tendency to overlap, thereby obscuring views of underlying or overlying structures. Resolution of vessel overlap can be accomplished by looking at multiple rotated planes of projection or by the independent processing of selected volumes of tissue.

19. The answer is **A** (Rutherford, 4th ed., pp. 1547–1551).

Recent trials have shown that warfarin is of benefit in patients with nonvalvular atrial fibrillation who have at least one of the following risk factors: history of hypertension, recent congestive cardiac failure, previous thromboembolic event, left ventricular dysfunction, or left atrial enlargement. Low-dose warfarin (prothrombin time: control ratio of 1.2:1.5) has been shown to be as effective as higher doses. The value of warfarin in the primary prevention of noncardiogenic ischemic cerebrovascular attacks is questionable and generally not routinely recommended given the potential adverse side effects. Caution is warranted when considering anticoagulation in a patient with a profound stroke because the individual may be more likely to have an expedited CT brain scan, which may not identify infarcts that are fated to undergo hemorrhagic conversion. Furthermore, patients with large aseptic cardioembolic brain infarcts who are anticoagulated are more likely to have symptomatic hemorrhagic conversion of their infarct. Therefore, normotensive patients with a small- to moderate-size stroke should be anticoagulated at 24 hours, and those with large infarcts at 5–7 days, provided there is no evidence of hemorrhagic conversion of the infarct on brain imaging.

20. The answer is **D** (Rutherford, 4th ed., pp. 1544–1545).

Hypertensive persons who suffer strokes, in contrast to normotensive persons, maintain a constant cerebral blood flow over a higher range of mean blood pressure (BP), as indicated by a shift to the right of their autoregulatory curve. Therefore, BP should be lowered less in patients known to be hypertensive before their strokes or in those whose clinical status deteriorates with control of hypertension. The area of brain affected by a stroke, including the ischemic penumbra, is devoid of autoregulation with blood flow proportional to blood pressure. Therefore, treatment of hypertension may impair blood flow to the ischemic penumbra and extend the size of the cerebral infarct. Hypertension poststroke, in the presence of elevated intracranial pressure, may reflect a physiologic response by an ischemic brainstem to maintain blood flow to this vital area. In this instance, lowering BP, without treatment of raised intracranial pressure, is likely to cause neurologic deterioration. Hypertension poststroke is frequently associated with elevated cathecolamines and high sympathetic nervous system activity; thus, when hypertension is treated, the combined alpha- and beta-adrenoreceptor-antagonist labetalol or the beta blocker propranolol are useful agents. Although renin may be produced by the brain, it has not been specifically implicated in post-stoke hypertension.

21. The answer is **D** (Rutherford, 4th ed., pp. 1541–1543, 1545–1547).

Recent evidence suggests that fluid restriction may be harmful in acute ischemic stroke. It may decrease the intravascular volume, cause hypotension, and produce increased blood viscosity, which may aggravate the ischemic injury. In general, the fluid of choice in stroke is one that is isotonic, such as normal saline. Hyperglycemia in acute stroke is associated with an adverse prognosis. Intravenous fluids containing glucose are thus probably best avoided, and certainly hypertonic glucose solutions are usually disadvantageous unless hypoglycemia is documented. This can be done quickly using the "finger-stick" method. A patient with a focal neurologic deficit due to hypoglycemia should be rapidly given 1 g/kg of 50% glucose intravenously, followed by a 5–10% dextrose infusion.

22. The answers are **A, B, C** (Rutherford, 4th ed., pp. 1555–1556).

In the NASCET trial, the subset of patients with stenoses ranging from 70 to 99% and symptoms of either transient ischemia or prior mild stroke had significantly fewer strokes and late deaths after carotid endarterectomy and best medical management compared with the control group, who received best medical management alone. The subset of patients with stenoses <70% continues to be the basis of an ongoing trial (see Table 119–1).

23. The answer is **D** (Rutherford, 4th ed., pp. 1554–1555).

The greatest controversy exists as to whether "global" ischemic symptoms are truly related to extracranial arterial occlusive disease. Patients with multiple extracranial arterial occlusive lesions and global symptoms probably have reasonable justification for unilateral operation in order to improve total blood flow. However, *unilateral* lesions should be considered in the same category as an asymptomatic lesion.

24. The answer is **C** (Rutherford, 4th ed., pp. 1559–1563).

Most patients who undergo temporary carotid clamping and observation of their neurologic status, either awake or with general anesthesia, with documentation by EEG, tolerate temporary clamping without neurologic dysfunction. Approximately 10–15% of patients who demonstrate temporary dysfunction can be reversed using an intraluminal shunt. Shunts carry a risk, which includes the inadvertent embolization of either air or particulate material unless special care is taken to avoid this complication. No study has demonstrated that the routine use of shunting results in a better outcome than series in which selective shunting is used and in certain reports in which no shunt has been used. Although the exact value that compels insertion of a shunt is controversial, measurement of carotid back pressure has proven to be a reliable method to determine the need for a shunt.

25. The answer is **A** (Rutherford, 4th ed., pp. 1574–1575).

Common systemic causes of vertebrobasilar insufficiency are orthostatic hypotension, overzealous antihypertensive therapy, arrhythmias, and malfunction of pacemakers, anemia, brain tumor, and subclavian steal. A 20-mm-Hg systolic pressure drop upon standing is generally arbitrarily chosen as a criterion for diagnosis of orthostatic hypotension. However, the presence of orthostatic hypotension does *not* necessarily exclude a patient from further work-up. A CT scan is mandatory to rule out tumors and to assess the integrity of the brain. Unsuspected hemorrhagic infarction may be found, but brainstem infarctions are often missed because they tend to be smaller in size and the resolution of the CT scan in this area is poor. Therefore, MRI is superior to CT scan to demonstrate these lesions. Inner ear problems frequently produce symptoms consistent with vertebrobasilar insufficiency. Patients often complain of symptoms upon turning their heads, which can also occur when osteophytes compress the vertebral artery in its second portion. In labyrinth disease, the sudden inertial changes when the patient's head turns briskly result in immediate symptoms and often marked nystagmus; however, in vertebral compression, it takes a few seconds before the patient fears for his balance. Some patients with vertebrobasilar insufficiency due to arrhythmias will recognize the association of palpitations with the appearance of their symptoms, the latter being secondary to decreased cardiac output resulting from the arrhythmia. A 24-hour ambulatory ECG (Holter monitoring) should be obtained in all patients evaluated for vertebrobasilar insufficiency before operation is performed.

26. The answers are **A, C, D** (Rutherford, 4th ed., pp. 1574–1575).

Patients with symptoms of vertebrobasilar insufficiency and systemic hypotension may or may not have concomitant vertebral artery stenosis or occlusion. In some patients the cause of decreased mean arterial pressure can be corrected by readjustment of antihypertensive medication, by antiarrhythmic drugs, or by insertion of a pacemaker. In patients with orthostatic hypotension, the problem may not respond to the medical treatment, and only reconstruction of a diseased or occluded vertebral artery will render the patient asymptomatic despite persistent auscultation of blood pressure due to poor sympathetic venous tone control. Another indication for vertebral artery reconstruction occurs when one or both carotid arteries are occluded and the patient has diffuse cerebral hypoperfusion without possible carotid artery reconstruction. In this group, the presence of large posterior communicating arteries (not middle cerebral arteries) increases the likelihood of success. The third group of indications for vertebral artery repair involves patients with severe carotid lesions who also have severe disease of the origin of the dominant or single vertebral artery on the same side as the planned carotid operation. Treatment of these patients is controversial. Some investigators recommend concomitant repair through a single incision. However, patients undergoing concomitant internal carotid vertebral artery repair experience greater morbidity compared to those undergoing isolated carotid or vertebral artery reconstructions. Similar to lesions in the carotid artery, vertebral artery reconstructions should be corrected only when the lumen is severely stenosed (>75% lumenal narrowing) in a clearly dominant or single vertebral artery. In patients with embolic sources in one vertebral artery or the subclavian artery, the source of the embolus is corrected regardless of the status of the opposite vertebral artery.

27. The answer is **D** (Rutherford, 4th ed., pp. 1575–1577).

The most common anatomic variant of the vertebral artery is an origin arising from the aortic arch just proximal to the left subclavian artery. Less commonly, the right vertebral artery takes origin from the innominate or right common carotid artery. The most common atherosclerotic lesion of the vertebral is severe stenosis of its origin. Thus, this lesion may be missed in standard arch views because of supraimposition of the subclavian over the first segment of the vertebral artery. Oblique projections may be helpful in this instance, along with recognition of poststenotic dilatation of the first centimeter or two of the vertebral artery. While redundancy and kinks are common, only the most severe are associated with hemodynamic significance. Selective subclavian injections are required to evaluate the second segment of the vertebral artery, which extends from C_6 to the top of the transverse process of C_2. The most common pathology of the V_2 segment is extrinsic compression by osteophytes. In patients with symptoms prompted by neck rotation, the V_2 segment must be evaluated with angiograms taken with the neck in right or left rotation. The vertebral artery may be perfectly normal in one projection and occluded in the other by extrinsic compression. This segment is rarely affected by atherosclerosis. The V_3 segment, which extends from the top of the transverse process of C_2 to the atlanto-occipital membrane at the base of the skull, is the section most frequently affected by dissection due to fibromuscular dysplasia and/or trauma. Importantly, when the vertebral artery is occluded proximally, it usually reconstitutes at the V_3 segment via the occipital connection, a collateral linking the occipital artery with the vertebral artery at this level. Because of this collateral, the distal vertebral and basilar arteries usually remain patent despite proximal VA occlusion.

28. The answers are **A, E** (Rutherford, 4th ed., pp. 1577–1588).

Most reconstructions of the VA attempt to relieve either an orificial stenosis (V_1 segment) or disease/occlusion of its intraspinal course (V_2 segment). A number of techniques are available. Transposition of the VA into the common carotid artery is a particularly popular method of repair. The V_4 segment is surgically inaccessible, and access to the V_2 segment is difficult because of its intraspinous course. Subclavian to vertebral bypass was popular in the 1970s. It is still useful when a contralateral carotid occlusion increases the risk of complete clamping the only carotid supply during a transposition operation. Inadequate length of the VA for transposition also generally requires a bypass procedure. Subclavian VA endarterectomy is another useful procedure, particularly for limited orificial VA stenosis. Cervical sympathectomy is not a part of VA surgery. Horner's syndrome is a complication to be avoided, although most patients tolerate these symptoms relatively well.

29. The answers are **A, B, C** (Rutherford, 4th ed., pp. 1588–1591).

Most patients with tortuous carotid arteries are asymptomatic because there is compensatory flow through the contralateral normal carotid artery, the vertebral arteries, and the circle of Willis. However, in the presence of a severe unilateral kink, a patient may present with hemiparesis, monoparesis, amaurosis fugax, monocular blindness, aphasia, or stroke. Bilateral kinks are often associated with symptoms of global ischemia such as syncope, vertigo, or other signs of posterior circulatory insufficiency. The most common causative mechanism for symptoms is axial twisting when the patient turns his head to the ipsilateral side of the kink. When atherosclerotic disease coexists it may not be possible to determine whether the symptoms are caused by the kink or the plaque. The efficacy of aspirin to prevent symptoms due to tortuous carotid segments is unknown.

30. The answer is **C** (Rutherford, 4th ed., p. 1591).

An electroencephalogram (EEG) is of little value in the evaluation of tortuous carotid segments. Changes during head rotation have been observed, but they are not pathognomonic. Likewise, cerebral perfusion scans have demonstrated cerebral ischemia associated with carotid kinking, but the significance of the findings are usually insufficient to predict surgical benefit. Carotid duplex scanning can identify and map the course of a tortuous vessel, but its use in diagnosing the *functional* significance of a kink is unclear as yet. Positional OPG is able to unmask reductions in carotid blood flow, but it may include a high incidence of false positive examinations. Angiography remains the definitive diagnostic test. Evaluation is completed with views during flexion, extension, and bilateral rotation. In addition, atherosclerotic plaques and ulcers can readily be identified.

31. The answers are **B, E** (Rutherford, 4th ed., pp. 1590–1593).

The proximal half, rather than the distal half, of the extracranial internal carotid artery is the tortuous segment. Tortuosity alone is not an indication for reconstruction; symptoms or an associated critical stenosis must be present. Endarterectomy of a tortuous internal carotid artery will often aggravate the tortuosity and produce kinking because the internal stenting plaque is removed. A segmental resection of the internal carotid artery with a primary end-to-end anastomosis is technically difficult. A patch angioplasty of the internal carotid artery will correct mild tortuosity. An eversion endarterectomy of the internal carotid artery with reimplantation of the ostium proximally on the common carotid artery is effective treatment for markedly tortuous vessels. Segmental resection and reanastomosis of the common carotid artery can also be performed to eliminate an internal carotid artery kink. Completion angiography is recommended to ensure complete resolution of the kink.

32. The answers are **B, D** (Rutherford, 4th ed., pp. 1594–1595).

The ICA is the *second* most common site of predilection for FMD; the renal artery is *first* and the external iliac artery is *third*. Medial fibrodysplasia, with its characteristic "string of beads" appearance on arteriogram, occurs in 80–90% of internal carotid artery FMD. At this site, like the renal arteries, there is a strong preponderance of females, close to 90%. In reported series, from 38 to 89% have *bilateral* carotid FMD, on average over half. The middle third of the cervical ICA is the segment most commonly involved with FMD, followed by upper third involvement. The lower third of the ICA, where atherosclerosis is common, is least frequently affected by FMD.

33. The answer is **B** (Rutherford, 4th ed., pp. 1594–1596).

Patients with carotid FMD are characteristically older than those with renal FMD, well in the age range for carotid atherosclerosis, which is present in close to 20% of symptomatic cases. Thus atherosclerosis must be taken into consideration as an alternative cause of cerebrovascular symptoms. A range of 7–19% of concomitant vertebral artery involvement by FMD has been reported. However, this lesion is of little clinical consequence. Intracranial aneurysms are found in 10–50% of patients with cervical FMD and may pose management dilemmas, namely, the advisability of dilating a stenotic carotid FMD lesion proximal to an intracranial aneurysm. Renal artery involvement occurs in roughly 25–50% of patients with carotid FMD, not in two thirds of such patients. A small percentage of spontaneous carotid dissections has been attributed to an arterial dysplasia (not typical FMD lesions), but this has not been well established by histopathologic studies. Dissection has yet to be reported in prospective follow-up of typical carotid FMD (e.g., "string of beads") lesions, so that this threat certainly should *not* be used to justify *prophylactic* intervention for FMD lesions.

34. The answer is **C** (Rutherford, 4th ed., pp. 1594–1599).

Surgical series are heavily weighted with symptomatic cases; the risk of developing significant cerebrovascular symptoms by patients with asymptomatic FMD lesions is probably not much more than 10%, if that. This is not high enough to justify prophylactic intervention in most such patients. Each FMD lesion should not be corrected routinely but on the basis of symptoms or future threat to health. Normally, renal FMD should be treated by PTA or surgery only if it is causing hypertension or loss of renal function. Controlling hypertension prior to carotid surgery is appropriate management, but if the carotid lesion is symptomatic, normotension can usually be achieved with antihypertensive medications. Normally, the lesion presenting the greatest threat is treated first. An intracranial aneurysm of this size (12 mm) presents a danger of rupture greater than an asymptomatic FMD stenosis, and prior to relief of the stenosis would likely increase pulsatile pressure within the aneurysm and increase the risk of rupture. Moreover, data from the VA asymptomatic carotid stenosis trial must be extrapolated to FMD lesions in order to justify treatment of asymptomatic lesions. It is debatable whether asymptomatic FMD lesions should be surgically dilated, although a case can be made for treating one side where there are bilateral tight stenoses. In addition, the cumulative risk of staged carotid surgery is increased with intervals less than 10–14 days. While it is true that *percutaneous* balloon dilation of FMD carotid lesions is justifiably frowned upon because of risk of embolism or injury to the dysplastic vessels, *intraoperative* balloon dilation does not carry the same risks (because of back flushing and direct observation). Intraoperative balloon dilation is a useful adjunct for high (upper one third) lesions.

35. The answer is **E** (Rutherford, 4th ed. pp.1600–1608).

Aneurysms of the extracranial carotid artery are distinctly uncommon lesions. In the past, as reflected in the older literature, infection, especially syphilis, was cited as the usual etiology. In addition, infection originating in the pharynx, causing inflammation in the contiguous carotid arterial wall, was also a frequent etiology. These are now rare causes, although mycotic aneurysms still occur; the most frequent infectious cause now is infection involving a prosthetic patch used for carotid endarterectomy. Staphylococcus species have been the most common organisms recovered from these cases. The incidence of this type of carotid aneurysm is three to four times higher when a prosthetic patch is used than when the carotid arteriotomy is closed primarily. This is one reason many surgeons prefer to use an autogenous patch if a patch is used at all. Trauma has become increasingly common as a cause of extracranial carotid aneurysms. Most, of course, are pseudoaneurysms. Both blunt and penetrating injuries have been associated with these lesions, the former attributed to hyperextension, which causes stretching, twisting, or impalement of the distal extracranial internal carotid arteries against the transverse process of the cervical vertebrae. These pseudoaneurysms are typically located near the base of the skull. Dissection, also often the result of blunt trauma, is not considered an aneurysmal process. Overall, atherosclerosis is now the most frequently reported cause of extracranial carotid aneurysms. There are only a handful of reports from single institutions that contain more than 20 carotid aneurysms, so these data are somewhat soft; however, atherosclerosis accounted for 25–70% of cases in these reports. These aneurysms occur in elderly patients, are usually fusiform, and tend to occur at the common carotid bifurcation. When they occur more distally in the internal carotid artery, they can be saccular. They are usually unilateral but are associated in about 15% of cases with an aneurysm elsewhere in the body. The external carotid artery is rarely involved. Other less common causes may need to be considered, especially in young people who present with no antecedent history of infection or trauma. Among these are cystic medical necrosis and Marfan's syndrome. But in an elderly patient with a pulsatile neck mass and no previous neck surgery, atherosclerosis is the usual etiology.

36. The answer is **D** (Rutherford, 4th ed., pp. 1606–1607).

Obviously, the etiology of a carotid aneurysms will have a major impact on its mode of presentation. Since most extracranial carotid aneurysms are atherosclerotic and involve the carotid bifurcation, many are visible, and most are readily palpable unless they are very small. Aneurysms involving the distal extracranial internal carotid artery usually point inward and are visible or palpable in the pharynx. Most, but not all, are pulsatile, and the differential diagnosis, therefore, must include carotid body tumors, cervical lymph nodes, and congenital cysts. Overall, pain is the most common symptom. It was the most prominent symptom in 40% of patients in one recent review. The pain may be felt in the region of the mass, behind the ear, or in the auditory canal, or it may be manifest as headache. CNS deficits appropriate to the side of the aneurysm are also fairly common, including hemispheric and retinal transient ischemic attacks or frank stroke. Most are thought to be due to downstream embolization of fragments of mural thrombus. Thrombus of the internal carotid artery is less common. Compression of cranial nerves by the aneurysm can cause dysphagia, hoarseness, facial pain, and occasionally even Horner's syndrome. Hemorrhage from aneurysm rupture is now rare and occurs almost exclusively with infected pseudoaneurysms. In this situation a draining sinus or cellulitis is present in or around the cervical incision, and there may be episodes of minor bleeding before major hemorrhage occurs. Rupture can also occur internally into the pharynx. Perhaps as many as one third of extracranial carotid aneurysms are asymptomatic and are discovered on routine physical examination or by duplex ultrasound.

37. The answer is **D** (Rutherford, 4th ed., pp. 1607–1609).

For aneurysms near the carotid bifurcation, resection and restoration of arterial continuity is the preferred method of treatment. Replacement grafts are required most commonly, with autogenous grafts being preferred, although prosthetics seem to function adequately if no infection is present. Distal lesions, however, present a far greater challenge, largely because of problems with exposure and adjacent structures. Exposure of the distal extracranial internal carotid artery can be facilitated by division of the posterior belly of the digastric muscle, resection of the styloid process, detachment of the sternocleidomastoid muscle from its mastoid attachment, and anterior subluxation of the mandible. The use of a nasotracheal rather than an endotracheal tube for anesthesia also provides for an additional centimeter or so of room at the apex of the exposure. A balloon catheter (shunt) can also be used for distal arterial control. These methods, singly or in combination, allow for direct reconstruction of many distal extracranial carotid aneurysms. Resection and interposition grafting is the procedure of choice whenever possible. Small saccular aneurysms can sometimes be treated by aneurysmorrhaphy, but these may require no surgical treatment at all if they are asymptomatic. A few have been successfully treated by transcatheter placement of coils and detachable balloons. At this level in the neck it is usually not possible to resect the aneurysm and perform and end-to-end anastomosis because of lack of sufficient arterial length. Internal carotid arterial ligation should be used only if the aneurysm is large, produces significant symptoms, and cannot be treated by other means. When this becomes necessary, the incidence of stroke is high (20–40%), especially if the carotid back pressure is less than 60–70 mm Hg. If this is the case, serious consideration should be given to the performance of an extracranial to intracranial bypass.

38. The answer is **A** (Rutherford, 4th ed., pp. 1600–1608).

In most series, the incidence of other peripheral aneurysms in association with extracranial aneurysms is low, about 14–15%. This is a markedly lower incidence than the incidence of other aneurysms in patients with, for example, femoral or popliteal aneurysms in whom other aneurysms occur in 50–60%. The histologic appearance of the usual fusiform aneurysm in the carotid bifurication is that of internal elastic lamina disruption and thinning of the media. Flow disturbances in the carotid bifurcation have been well documented and may play a role in this process, but this is probably not a factor in those atherosclerotic aneurysms of the more distal extracranial internal carotid artery. It is in this location where saccular aneurysms most frequently occur. Hypertension may also be a contributing factor in the etiology in a general way due to its influence on the development of atherosclerosis, but not all of these patients have significant hypertension. The male to female ratio for extracranial atherosclerotic carotid aneurysm is about 2–3:1, lower than that for either abdominal aortic or other peripheral aneurysms. In this regard, the ratio is closer to the male to female ratio for atherosclerotic occlusive lesions. All of these characteristics make it unlikely that a single etiologic process such as a generalized arterial abnormality underlies these aneurysms. The natural history of these aneurysms is certainly not well understood. Most patients are symptomatic, and it is the symptoms that lead to the diagnosis. The fact that these lesions are so uncommon, even in asymptomatic patients undergoing cerebral angiography or carotid duplex scanning, suggests that there are probably not a large number of such lesions that go undetected. There are no good contemporary data regarding long-term follow-up of untreated patients; however, in the University of Michigan series there was a 50% stroke rate during a mean follow-up interval of 6.3 years in patients who did not undergo operation. Historically, older data are even worse, but include aneurysms of all etiologies.

39. The answer is **D** (Rutherford, 4th ed., pp. 1610–1612).

The International Extracranial–Intracranial (EC–IC) Bypass study concluded that this surgical procedure is not effective in preventing strokes in patients presenting with a few TIAs or a minor stroke due to internal carotid artery occlusion, middle cerebral artery stenosis, or inaccessible internal carotid artery stenosis. The EC–IC study did not include patients with carotid artery occlusion who had persistent TIAs that were refractory to anticoagulation. Such patients can be considered the "medical failure" group. If physiologic assessment of the cerebral hemodynamic status suggests inadequate collateral circulation distal to an occluded carotid artery (hemodynamic insufficiency), EC–IC bypass may be considered in order to relieve the patient of recurrent TIAs and potentially to reduce the risk of future stroke.

40. The answer is **D** (Rutherford, 4th ed., pp. 1612–1614).

All three of these techniques have been used to assess cerebrovascular reserve and to identify patients with cerebral hemodynamic insufficiency. These tests, which are analogous to a "brain stress test," determine the ability of the cerebral vasculature to dilate in response to a vasodilating stimulus. In areas of severe focal blood flow insufficiency, a cerebral steal can be seen after the administration of the vasodilating stimulus. Several groups have used these tests to predict stroke risks. It has been found that patients with severe occlusive disease and markedly impaired cerebrovascular reactivity have a much higher stroke risk than patients with normal cerebrovascular reactivity. The results of these tests may be used to select candidates for EC–IC bypass.

41. The answer is **D** (Rutherford, 4th ed., pp. 1615–1621).

The standard EC–IC bypass (and the procedure studied by the EC–IC study) consists of anastomosis of the superficial temporal artery (which is dissected from the scalp) to a superficial branch of the middle cerebral artery. In cases where the superficial temporal artery is extremely small, the occipital artery can be used for anastomosis to the middle cerebral artery. The occipital artery has also been used for anastomosis to vessels in the posterior circulation. In cases in which immediate high bypass flow is required, a large-diameter anastomosis may be constructed with a saphenous vein graft from the external carotid artery to a large proximal branch of the middle cerebral artery. When an excessively large saphenous vein poses a technical difficulty, the radial artery may be used as a conduit.

42. The answers are **A, B, D** (Rutherford, 4th ed., pp. 1622–1624).

Color-flow duplex sonography is helpful when the paraganglioma is small. It can easily delineate a hypervascular mass nestled in the carotid bifurcation and is now the most widely used diagnostic test. Carotid arteriography is essential in identifying the blood supply of large tumors so that preoperative embolization may be employed as a preliminary step before surgical excision. MRI is more helpful than CT scanning to determine the extent of tumor involvement of the distal carotid artery and the structures at the base of the skull. Intravenous digital angiography provides images with inadequate detail upon which to base operative decisions.

43. The answer is **B** (Rutherford, 4th ed., p. 1628).

The occurrence of a "sentinel bleed" under the circumstances described heralds a potentially disastrous hemorrhage if prompt surgical intervention is not undertaken at once. The best course of action is to reroute the carotid circulation through clean, uninvolved tissue. Following closure of these wounds, adequate drainage should be accomplished by re-exploring the neck wound and placement of drain. In-line placement of vein interposition grafts into an infected field results in an unacceptably high rate of anastomatic disruption. A "sentinel bleed" must not be ignored or exsanguinating hemorrhage may follow. Ligations of the carotid artery may result in stroke if collateral circulation is inadequate. Ligation of the common carotid artery **(E)** would preclude performance of extracranial-intracranial bypass; this strategy would be reasonable only if the infection were strictly limited to the internal carotid artery and ligation of the internal carotid (not common carotid artery) was performed.

44. The answers are **A, C, D**. (Rutherford, 4th ed., pp. 1628–1632).

Temporal arteritis is also called Horton's arteritis and *does* respond to the administration of corticosteroids. The gradual occlusion of the branches of the carotid and vertebral arteries is the cause of most symptoms in this disease. Both temporal arteritis and Takayasu's disease are characterized by infiltration of giant cells into the artery.

45. The answers are **B, D** (Rutherford, 4th ed., pp. 1641–1643).

Cranial nerve injuries associated with carotid endarterectomy often are asymptomatic, but several objective clinical studies have indicated that they occur in as many as 10–15% of patients. Most of these injuries involve the hypoglossal nerve or the recurrent laryngeal fibers within the anterior aspect of the vagus nerve, and they are manifest by temporary dysfunction of the tongue or the ipsilateral vocal cord, which often resolves spontaneously within a matter of weeks. Such injuries are presumed to result from blunt trauma from excessive retraction, hemostatic forceps, or vascular clamps. In many cases they may be avoided by adequate mobilization of the hypoglossal nerve together with direct visualization and avoidance of the vagus and superior laryngeal nerves. Injury to the glossopharyngeal nerve is exceedingly unlikely during standard carotid endarterectomy, but it can have severe nutritional consequences requiring supplemental tube feedings after high exposure of the internal carotid artery near the styloid process and the base of the skull. Since a unilateral vocal cord palsy may be clinically occult, it is prudent to perform a laryngoscopic examination of the cords before proceeding with elective contralateral carotid endarterectomy in order to preclude the possibility of simultaneous, bilateral recurrent laryngeal nerve injuries.

46. The answers are **B, D** (Rutherford, 4th ed., pp. 1643–1648).

Although factors related to intraoperative cerebral ischemia (e.g., clamp ischemia and/or atheromatous embolization) may deserve consideration whenever a patient awakens from general anesthesia with an established neurologic deficit following carotid endarterectomy, they probably are irrelevant in the setting of a delayed deficit discovered after a documented "lucent period." In this situation, it is safest to assume that platelet aggregation has occurred throughout the endarterectomy site and has precipitated a thrombus propagating into the internal carotid artery. The literature concerning this complication is not extensive, but there appears to be a consensus in collected series that expeditious thrombectomy enhances neurologic recovery in over half of those patients who experience postoperative occlusions. The severity of the postoperative symptoms and the circumstances encountered during the original operation inevitably influence the decision whether a patient who awakens with a neurologic deficit should undergo immediate reoperation, carotid angiography, or close observation. Furthermore, although a reoperation should be performed as promptly as possible, several reports have indicated that neurologic improvement is still feasible if it is done within two hours (and possibly within four hours) after thrombosis has occurred. In the absence of any evidence to the contrary, it seems prudent to use both carotid shunting and patch angioplasty during a reoperation in order to restore and maintain cerebral blood flow.

47. The answers are **A, C** (Rutherford, 4th ed., pp. 1649–1654).

Provided the primary operation was technically adequate, early recurrent stenosis occurring within three years after carotid endarterectomy is much more likely to be caused by myointimal hyperplasia than by recurrent atherosclerosis. Since hyperplastic lesions generally have a smooth, nonulcerated surface that discourages embolization, they rarely produce neurologic symptoms and often are discovered on the basis of routine postoperative surveillance with noninvasive imaging. For this reason, as well as the fact that at least some hyperplastic recurrences tend to regress under observation, there is considerable sentiment throughout the literature that elective reoperations are unnecessary unless recurrent stenosis becomes either symptomatic or preocclusive in its severity. Although the matter is still open to debate, a number of reports have suggested that patch closure of the original carotid arteriotomy reduces the subsequent incidence of recurrent stenosis, especially in women. This may eventually prove to be an important distinction, since myointimal hyperplasia otherwise appears to occur more frequently in women than in men (see Tables 126–6 and 126–7).

48. The answer is **B** (Rutherford, 4th ed., pp. 1663–1664).

Carotid endarterectomy is contraindicated in most patients presenting with an acute stroke. Nevertheless, a few selected patients who present with an acute stroke who have a demonstrable significant carotid artery stenosis and who on CT scan do not have a hemorrhagic infarct may be appropriately selected for surgery once they have reached a plateau in their clinical recovery. This may require days or weeks, depending on the particular patient. Acute neurologic worsening occurring in a patient recovering from the initial event is termed "stroke in evolution" and suggests an unstable carotid lesion, which in most instances should be surgically corrected. Loss of consciousness, dense neurologic deficit, and hemodynamic instability are contraindications to operation in the acute phase of a stroke. Delaying intervention for six weeks or longer has been proposed by some investigators but carries a risk as high as 21% for recurrent stroke during the 4–6-week observation period. Several studies have shown that if the CT scan is negative following an acute stroke, perioperative neurologic morbidity and mortality are not increased. On the other hand, most agree that the perioperative morbidity and mortality of carotid endarterectomy in the presence of an acute stroke are increased, compared to patients operated electively long after the acute event.

49. The answer is **D** (Rutherford, 4th ed., p. 1664).

External carotid artery revascularization has been found to be effective in the management of patients with significant collateralization between the external and the internal system in the presence of an internal carotid artery occlusion. Operation is aimed at removing a stenotic lesion in the origin of the external carotid, if present, and eliminating potential embolization from the cul de sac created by the occluded internal carotid artery. The combination of bilateral carotid occlusion and preoperative fixed neurologic deficit predicts the highest perioperative morbidity. Additional factors that increase morbidity and mortality include a severely diseased contralateral carotid artery and symptomatic patients with internal carotid artery occlusion. Best results are obtained when surgery is performed to relieve specific hemispheric or retinal symptoms. Disease in the vertebral arteries has no impact on the outcome of external carotid artery revascularization.

50. The answer is **D** (Rutherford, 4th ed., pp. 1667–1668).

The European Carotid Surgery Trialists Collaborative group, which reported their findings in 1991, divided patients into mild, moderate, and severe stenosis groups and randomized these patients to either surgical or medical therapy. Among the patients with severe stenosis, only 3.7% of surgically treated patients had disabling stroke compared to 8.4% in those treated medically. Patients in the mild carotid stenosis category (0–29%) had a very small three-year stroke risk of ipsilateral ischemic stroke when treated medically, so that the risks of surgery were not outweighed by its benefits. In the North American Carotid Endarterectomy Trial (NASCET), patients with >70% stenosis in the ipsilateral carotid artery and symptoms of TIA or stroke within three months were found to benefit substantially from carotid endarterectomy. Patients in the 30–69% category continue to be studied, and the results of this portion of the trial are not yet available. Thus, patients with lesser stenosis can be treated conservatively, whereas patients with high-grade stenosis should be treated surgically. Patients in the moderate stenosis category can be treated with either modality, depending on the patients' own wishes and general health.

51. The answer is **E** (Rutherford, 4th ed., pp. 1666–1668).

The NASCET trial, published in 1991, randomized *symptomatic* patients with carotid artery disease to either medical or surgical therapy. It showed conclusively that *symptomatic* patients with >70% stenosis did better after carotid endarterectomy than with medical management. To date, results of only the VA *asymptomatic* carotid artery stenosis trial have provided meaningful findings. Interpretation of the data has been controversial, but roughly 20% of medically treated patients had ipsilateral neurologic events (stroke, death from stroke, transient ischemic attacks) compared with 10% of surgically treated patients. The only other available prospective randomized trial in asymptomatic patients is the CASANOVA study, and due to multiple flaws in this trial, the results are questionable. There has been no study comparing aspirin to placebo in *asymptomatic* patients that has shown a benefit of aspirin therapy in these patients. The decision to recommend carotid endarterectomy in an asymptomatic patient should be based on an acceptable morbidity and mortality demonstrated by the surgeon (<3%), the patient's risk factors, plaque composition, and the patient's life expectancy.

52. The answer is **B** (Rutherford, 4th ed., pp. 1665–1666).

Ticlopidine is a potent platelet antiaggregant that functions primarily as an inhibitor of adenosine diphosphate pathway of platelet aggregation. It inhibits most of the known stimuli to platelet *aggregation* and in contrast to aspirin does not block the production of thromboxane or prostacyclin by platelets or endothelial cells, respectively. It alters the function of the platelet for its lifespan. The Ticlopidine-Aspirin Stroke study showed that the three-year event rate for nonfatal stroke or death from any cause was less for ticlopidine treatment than for aspirin treatment. Overall, there was a 12% risk reduction by ticlopidine for nonfatal stroke or death from any cause and a 21% risk reduction of nonfatal or fatal stroke at three years. The most common side effect of ticlopidine was diarrhea, which occurred in 21% of patients. There was an important, although small, incidence of neutropenia, which was reversible upon discontinuation of the drug.

17

Venous Disorders

1. Which of the following statements regarding venous flow in normal legs is/are true?

   A. In the standing position, hydrostatic pressure in the legs is markedly increased, whereas that in the right atrium remains unchanged (at a few mm Hg). The pressure gradient thus created is primarily responsible for the return of blood from the legs to the heart.
   B. Owing to the weight of the column of blood above the venous valves, valves in the legs remain closed during quiet standing and open only during calf muscle contraction.
   C. In the standing position, calf muscle contraction reduces venous pressure at the ankle by decreasing peripheral venous volume and by shortening the length of the hydrostatic column.
   D. Exercise (walking) reduces hydrostatic pressure equally in the arteries and veins of the leg.
   E. In the supine position, the rate of venous outflow from the legs fluctuates in response to changes in intra-abdominal pressure.

2. Which of the following statements regarding acute thrombotic venous obstruction is/are true?

   A. Peripheral venous pressure is always elevated.
   B. The hemodynamic effects are independent of the location and extent of the thrombotic process.
   C. It is often accompanied by venous valvular incompetence.
   D. Edema results from an elevation in mean capillary pressure.
   E. Has little effect on the phasic changes in venous outflow that accompany respiration.

3. Which of the following statements regarding ambulatory venous pressure in patients with chronic venous insufficiency is/are true?

   A. It returns rapidly to resting levels after cessation of exercise.
   B. It correlates poorly with the volume of blood remaining in the calf veins after exercise.
   C. It correlates poorly with the incidence of venous stasis ulcers.
   D. It may be "normalized" by ligation of the saphenous vein.
   E. It may exceed resting venous pressure when there is significant outflow obstruction.

4. The diagnosis of *superficial* thrombophlebitis of the forearm is *best* made by:

   A. Duplex scanning.
   B. Doppler velocity probe.
   C. Physical examination.
   D. Phlebography.
   E. Photoplethysmography.

5. Which of the following statements regarding *superficial* thrombophlebitis of the lower extremity is/are true?

   A. It is usually a limited process that will resolve spontaneously.
   B. Extension into the deep venous system can occur.
   C. It is usually associated with a demonstrable bacterial infection.
   D. The presence of varicose veins predisposes one to superficial thrombophlebitis.
   E. It often leads to a venous stasis ulcer.

6. *Superficial* thrombophlebitis is treated by:

   A. Hot wet compresses, bed rest, elevation.
   B. Elastic stockings.
   C. Excision.
   D. Antibiotics.
   E. All of the above.

7. Which of the following statements regarding the clinical diagnosis of acute *deep* venous thrombosis (DVT) is/are true?

   A. Unilateral limb swelling is one of the more reliable clinical signs.
   B. A positive Homan's sign in a bedridden patient is highly sensitive and specific for occult DVT.
   C. Palpation of a tender "cord" is indicative of DVT.
   D. The diagnosis of phlegmasia cerulea dolens can ordinarily be made on physical examination.
   E. Objective tests for DVT are unnecessary if another cause for the patient's symptoms and signs has been identified clinically.

8. Which of the following statements regarding physiologic tests for DVT (impedance plethysmography, Doppler ultrasonography) is/are true?

   A. They are reported to be about 90% sensitive and specific for detecting and ruling out extensive DVT in the above-knee veins of symptomatic patients.

B. They are insensitive to clots in the infrapopliteal veins.
C. They detect most nonocclusive clots in duplicated veins.
D. They accurately locate and define the extent of venous thrombi.
E. When they are negative in symptomatic outpatients, pulmonary embolism rarely occurs during follow-up.

9. Which of the following statements regarding the diagnosis of DVT with duplex scanning or color-flow imaging is/are true?

A. Failure to visualize a clot rules out DVT.
B. In all locations, failure of a vein to collapse with probe compression is a reliable sign of DVT.
C. Color-flow mapping, although not necessary, is a valuable adjunct to duplex scanning and facilitates the examination.
D. Examination of infrapopliteal veins is impractical and highly inaccurate and contributes little to the examination.
E. Advantages include the ability to identify nonocclusive clots, clots in duplicated veins, and masses causing extrinsic venous compression.
F. A negative duplex or color-flow scan of the legs rules out pulmonary embolism.

10. Which statement(s) regarding contrast venography for the diagnosis of acute lower-extremity deep venous thrombosis is/are true?

A. Multiple pathologic correlation studies have shown that venography is at least 95% sensitive for detection of acute thrombi.
B. Contrast venography is the imaging modality of choice initially to evaluate patients with symptoms suggestive of DVT.
C. Multiple studies have demonstrated that different experienced observers will concur regarding the presence or absence of DVT on at least 95% of venograms.
D. Interobserver variability is significantly *less* for venograms negative for DVT than for venograms that are positive.
E. Venograms carry negligible risk for potentially serious complications or patient discomfort.

11. Which of the following statements is/are true regarding the safety of contrast venography?

A. Although major contrast reactions (e.g., laryngospasm or cardiopulmonary arrest) are relatively rare, preventative measures have not been shown to be effective in reducing the risk in patients with a history of prior reactions.
B. Prospective randomized clinical trials have *not* proven that ionic contrast material has a higher rate of contrast-induced nephropathy than nonionic contrast material.
C. Other than causing local discomfort, extravasation of contrast medium into the subcutaneous tissues is of no clinical consequence.
D. Documented post-venography DVT occurs in approximately 20% of patients and is not related to the concentration of contrast medium.
E. None of the above.

12. Which of the technical modifications listed below is /are appropriate?

A. Closed system venography using an Esmark® bandage and a proximal blood pressure cuff inflated to a suprasystolic pressure improves definition of venous malformations.
B. Descending venography is primarily useful for identification of incompetent perforating veins.
C. In patients with malfunction of a hemodialysis arteriovenous fistula, inflation of a blood pressure cuff to suprasystolic levels prior to injection of contrast medium will afford improved opacification of the central (e.g., subclavian) veins.
D. In upper-extremity venography, use of a Wright's maneuver (head turned to the opposite side, arm abducted and externally rotated) is helpful for distinguishing subclavian vein thrombosis from inflow artifact.
E. All of the above.

13. Which of the following statements is/are true regarding measurement of ambulatory venous pressure (AVP)?

A. AVP reflects the hydrostatic pressure in the superficial system during ambulation.
B. The highest AVP levels are found in patients with valvular incompetence in the perforator and deep venous systems, including the popliteal vein.
C. AVP reflects *only* the pressure present in the deep venous system.
D. AVP should be measured in a deep vein of the calf.
E. Increasing AVP correlates with the incidence of leg ulceration.

14. Which of the following statements is/are true in regard to the assessment of lower-extremity venous function with air plethysmography (APG)?

A. It measures changes in the lower-extremity venous pressure in the superficial system.
B. It is an excellent screening tool for venous reflux; however, it does not allow *quantitation* of the degree of reflux.
C. The residual volume fraction calculated with APG correlates directly with direct measurements of the ambulatory venous pressure.
D. The venous filling index expressed in mL/sec is a reliable indicator of venous outflow obstruction.
E. APG gives quantitative information about the presence of venous reflux.

15. The most reliable way to elicit valve closure during the evaluation of venous reflux with duplex ultrasonography is:
   - **A.** With the patient in the supine position, using manual compression proximal to the insonation site.
   - **B.** With the patient in the standing position, using manual compression distal to the insonation site.
   - **C.** With the patient in the supine position, using a rapid deflation device proximal to the insonation site.
   - **D.** With the patient in the standing position, using a rapid deflation device distal to the insonation site.
   - **E.** All methods are equally reliable.

16. Which of the following statements is/are *most* accurate regarding the evaluation of incompetent calf perforating veins (ICPV)?
   - **A.** The evaluation of calf perforator incompetence is based on the identification of venous flow from the superficial to the deep venous system.
   - **B.** Ascending venography has been shown to be far superior to Doppler evaluation and duplex scanning in the diagnosis of ICPVs.
   - **C.** Ascending phlebography has a high rate of false negative findings in determining the presence or absence of ICPVs.
   - **D.** Clinical examination is the most accurate method in the diagnosis of the presence of ICPVs.
   - **E.** The evaluation of ICPVs is of little clinical significance; therefore, no methods have been developed for their evaluation.

17. Which of the following statements is/are true regarding the diagnosis of pulmonary embolism (PE)?
   - **A.** Westermark's sign had been observed in 35% of patients eventually studied by pulmonary angiography.
   - **B.** Classic ECG findings of atrial fibrillation/flutter indicate pulmonary embolism in 25% of patients with two or more lobar arteries obstructed.
   - **C.** Arterial blood gas results usually show widened A-a gradients with hypoxia and hypocarbia. However, up to 10% of patients with PE can have a normal PaO_2.
   - **D.** The V/Q scan is definitive in less than 30% of patients with suspected PE.
   - **E.** None of the above.

18. Important technical details of venous thrombectomy for unilateral iliofemoral venous thrombosis include all of the following *except*:
   - **A.** Balloon occlusion of the inferior vena cava to prevent pulmonary embolism during the thrombectomy, which is accessed from the contralateral femoral vein.
   - **B.** Completion iliofemoral phlebography to ensure adequate clearing of thrombus.
   - **C.** Creation of a ≤4 mm A-V fistula, usually in end-side fashion with the proximal saphenous vein to the proximal superficial femoral artery, improves patency.
   - **D.** Maintenance of perioperative anticoagulation along with the application of external pneumatic compression devices assist in maintaining patency.
   - **E.** An autotransfusion device is useful.

19. The reasons lytic therapy for DVT does not result in successful clearing of thrombus include which of the following?
   - **A.** Thrombolytic therapy is usually reserved for patients with the most extensive deep venous thrombosis, therefore leading to selection bias.
   - **B.** Patients with iliofemoral DVT treated with *systemic* lytic therapy fail to have the majority of the plasminogen activator reach the thrombus; therefore, activation of fibrin-bound plasminogen is suboptimal and lysis is inadequate.
   - **C.** Frequently patients have the lytic infusion terminated prematurely, leaving residual thrombus.
   - **D.** If streptokinase is used, antistreptococcal antibodies may minimize its lytic effect.
   - **E.** All of the above.

20. Given a patient with documented deep vein thrombosis and a contraindication to anticoagulation, under which of the following circumstances would insertion of a Greenfield vena caval filter be *contraindicated?*
   - **A.** Presence of systemic sepsis with bacteremia.
   - **B.** Second trimester pregnancy in a 20-year-old woman.
   - **C.** Vena caval thrombosis extending to the level of the renal veins.
   - **D.** None of the above.
   - **E.** All of the above.

21. Among the variety of percutaneous vena caval filters available, the early follow-up experience suggests that they are similar in their results with the *exception* of the incidence of:
   - **A.** Recurrent embolism.
   - **B.** Vena caval thrombosis.
   - **C.** Migration.
   - **D.** Vena caval penetration.
   - **E.** Local hemorrhage.

22. Significant advantage(s) of the titanium Greenfield filter over the original stainless steel Greenfield filter is/are:
   - **A.** Cost.
   - **B.** Time for insertion.
   - **C.** Elimination of filter misplacement.
   - **D.** All of the above.
   - **E.** None of the above.

23. Primary varicose veins are currently thought to be a consequence of:
   A. Arteriovenous fistulas, local trauma, weakness of the vein wall.
   B. Arteriovenous fistulas, weakness of the vein wall, valvular incompetence.
   C. Arteriovenous fistulas, local trauma, valvular incompetence.
   D. Local trauma, weakness of the vein wall, valvular incompetence.
   E. None of the above.

24. Isolated superficial venous insufficiency is *not* a cause of the chronic venous stasis syndrome. **True** or **false?**

25. Varicosities of the greater saphenous vein below the knee are always caused by valvular incompetence at the saphenofemoral junction. **True** or **false?**

26. Injury to the femoral artery at the time of high ligation and stripping of the greater saphenous system is best prevented by:
   A. Carefully noting the color and structure of the vessels.
   B. Passing the stripper from top to bottom (groin to ankle).
   C. Waiting until the leg is wrapped before removing the stripper.
   D. Passing the stripper from bottom to top (ankle to groin).
   E. Identifying the saphenofemoral junction.

27. Injection sclerotherapy is *most* useful for treatment of:
   A. Reticular veins.
   B. Varicose clusters.
   C. Palliation of varicose veins in the aged.
   D. Intradermal venectasias.
   E. All of the above.

28. Sources of venous hypertension that contribute to development of varicose veins and telangiectasias include:
   A. Gravitational reflux.
   B. Compartmental hypertension.
   C. Incompetent reticular networks.
   D. All of the above.
   E. None of the above.

29. Regarding injection sclerotherapy of varicose veins, intravenous thrombosis is:
   A. A desirable result.
   B. An undesirable result.
   C. A possibly fatal complication.
   D. An inconsequential event.
   E. An inevitable result.

30. From available data regarding the natural history of chronic venous insufficiency (CVI):
   A. Venous recanalization following DVT occurs many years after the initial event and is generally unrelated to the development of symptoms of CVI.
   B. Venous ulceration is never seen with isolated superficial venous valvular incompetence.
   C. Venous recanalization following deep venous insufficiency generally occurs early (within one year), whereas valvular incompetence occurs later.
   D. The appearance and localization of valvular insufficiency after DVT in an individual patient is predictable based on the extent and location of initial thrombus.
   E. All of the above.

31. Evidence for local ischemia within the microcirculation in CVI includes:
   A. Elevated magnetic resonance spectroscopy-determined levels of radio-labeled high-energy phosphates from gastrocnemius muscle in patients with CVI.
   B. Consistently low $TcPO_2$ levels in the gaiter area in patients with CVI.
   C. Lower resting skin blood flow demonstrated by laser Doppler techniques in CVI limbs compared to normals.
   D. None of the above.
   E. All of the above.

32. Pharmacologic agents that have been demonstrated to have some benefit in promoting healing of venous stasis ulcers include:
   A. Hydroxyrutosides
   B. Stanozolol
   C. Dimethyl sulfoxide
   D. Calcium dobesilate
   E. None of the above.

33. The "white cell trapping" theory of venous ulceration is supported by:
   A. Decreased femoral vein white cell counts after 30 minutes of dependency in limbs with CVI compared to controls.
   B. Lipodermatosclerotic skin biopsies demonstrating significantly more white blood cells per mm^3 than biopsies from controls.
   C. Capillary microthrombosis observed in perimalleolar skin in patients with CVI examined by capillary microscopy.
   D. All of the above.
   E. None of the above.

34. Which of the following pathologic conditions causing chronic venous reflux is/are most amenable to valvuloplasty (Kistner's internal technique).

A. Post-thrombotic reflux.
B. "Primary" valvular reflux.
C. Combined reflux/obstruction.
D. Perforator incompetence.
E. Primary varicose veins.

35. In evaluating post-thrombotic patients for valve reconstruction surgery for venous reflux, which of the following investigations is useful in delineating coexisting *hemodynamic* obstruction?

A. Ascending venography.
B. Descending venography.
C. Arm/foot venous pressure differential.
D. Color duplex examination.
E. All of the above.

36. Which of the following valve reconstructive procedures is the most durable?

A. Segment transfer procedure.
B. Internal valvuloplasty.
C. External valvuloplasty.
D. Axillary vein transfer.
E. The above are equally durable.

37. A high incidence of which of the following complications has been reported after direct valve reconstruction procedures?

A. Pulmonary embolism.
B. Thrombosis of repair after internal valvuloplasty.
C. Edema of the arm from which the axillary vein valve was harvested.
D. Wound breakdown.
E. None of the above.

38. Which of the following statements is/are true concerning venous claudication?

A. The pain is described as "burning sensation" in the calf with normal ambulation.
B. Venous claudication is caused by increased intramuscular pressure.
C. Diagnostic criteria for venous claudication include venous hypertension only with exercise.
D. Iliac vein obstruction is the etiology.
E. Pain is mediated by Bassini pain receptors.

39. Which of the following statements is/are true concerning diagnostic criteria for the patient undergoing venous bypass for chronic obstruction?

A. Venous pressure studies and phlebography are mandatory preoperative evaluations.
B. Phlebographic demonstration of venous obstruction with large, profuse collaterals is a contraindication for bypass surgery.
C. A femoral pressure gradient between limbs at supine rest that exceeds 2 mm Hg indicates a significant iliofemoral obstruction in the limb with elevated pressure.
D. An arm/foot venous pressure differential at rest of >4 mm Hg and a foot venous pressure elevation with reactive hyperemia of >6 mm Hg are indicative of hemodynamically significant venous obstruction.
E. Hemodynamic function is uniformly abnormal when phlebographic obstruction is documented.

40. Which of the following statements is/are true of operative techniques unique to bypass grafts in the venous system?

A. Bypass conduits interposed in the venous system should be longer than the excised vein segment.
B. Bypass conduits must be autogenous.
C. Adjunctive arteriovenous fistulas can improve long-term patency of both autogenous and prosthetic venous bypass conduits.
D. Adjunctive arteriovenous fistulas must be surgically closed after six months.
E. All of the above.

17

Answers

1. The answers are **C, E** (Rutherford, 4th ed., pp. 1673–1681).

Under most circumstances, hydrostatic pressure (–ρgh) at any point in the vascular system is perfectly balanced by the gravitational potential energy (ρgh) at that same point (see Chap. 3). Since these two components of Bernoulli's equation cancel, hydrostatic pressure has no influence on the return of blood to the heart. The pressure responsible for returning blood to the heart in a quietly standing individual is simply the "dynamic pressure" derived from contraction of the left ventricle and is approximately the same regardless of the position of the subject. Therefore, blood continues to flow cephalad in the standing position, and the venous valves remain open. Calf muscle contraction compresses intra- and intermuscular veins, forcing blood to flow cephalad. After the muscles relax, reflux is prevented by closure of competent venous valves. In accordance with the venous pressure–volume compliance curve, venous pressure falls as the venous blood volume decreases. Thus, the effective length of the hydrostatic column is reduced. Although calf muscle contraction reduces venous hydrostatic pressure, it has no effect on the hydrostatic pressure in arteries. Because venous pressure is reduced during walking while arterial hydrostatic pressure does not change, the pressure gradient across the capillary bed is increased. This mechanism, therefore, contributes to the augmentation of blood flow observed during exercise. In the supine position, pressure in the abdominal veins is quite low and fluctuates with intra-abdominal pressure. During inspiration, the diaphragm descends, temporarily increasing intra-abdominal pressure. Because peripheral venous pressure remains unchanged, the pressure gradient across the legs is decreased and venous outflow is reduced. With expiration, the diaphragm ascends, intra-abdominal pressure falls, and blood backed up in the leg veins now flows cephalad. These respiratory effects are characteristic of normal venous blood flow.

2. The answer is **D** (Rutherford, 4th ed., pp. 1682–1684).

Peripheral venous pressure is directly proportional to venous outflow resistance. Although peripheral venous pressure is usually increased in limbs with acute deep venous thrombosis, the increase may be imperceptible (or absent) when the thrombus is nonocclusive, is located in an intramuscular vein, is confined to one of the three major below-knee veins, or is isolated to one of a pair of duplicated superficial femoral or popliteal veins. On the other hand, a thrombus that occludes major veins (such as the common femoral or popliteal) and their associated inflow and outflow collaterals will elevate venous resistance significantly and will cause a marked increase in peripheral venous pressure. When the thrombotic process is very extensive, involving all the major deep veins and most of the superficial and deep collaterals, venous pressure may rise to levels that impair tissue perfusion (phlegmasia cerulea dolens). Thus, the location and extent of the thrombus is critically important in regard to its hemodynamic effects. Because capillary blood pressure must exceed that in the peripheral veins and venules, venous obstruction raises capillary pressure, upsets the Starling equilibrium, and forces fluid out of the capillaries into the interstitial space. Edema fluid continues to accumulate until tissue pressure rises to levels that re-establish the Starling equilibrium. Venous valvular incompetence ordinarily plays little role in the pathophysiology of *acute* deep venous thrombosis. Valvular incompetence becomes significant only with the resolution of the thrombus. Fluctuations in intra-abdominal pressure have less effect on the pressure gradient across the leg when the peripheral venous pressure is elevated. For this reason, blood flow in a major vein below a thrombotic obstruction usually varies little with respiration and may become "continuous."

3. The answers are **A, E** (Rutherford, 4th ed., pp. 1686–1691).

The term "ambulatory venous pressure" refers to the pressure measured in a dependent vein (usually a vein on the dorsum of the foot) after calf muscle exercise. In normal limbs with functioning valves, venous pressure in the foot is decreased to 20 mm Hg or less by exercise and then returns slowly over a period of 20 seconds or more as the calf veins are refilled by inflow from the capillaries. In limbs with incompetent venous valves, reflux of blood down the limb reduces the efficiency of the calf muscle pump and allows the veins to refill rapidly after cessation of exercise. Because the calf veins are incompletely evacuated, ambulatory venous pressure remains high and correlates well with the residual venous volume. The incidence of venous stasis ulceration increases with the level of ambulatory venous pressure, reaching 80% when pressures exceed 80 mm Hg (see Table 129–3). Thus, ambulatory venous pressure is often considered the physiologic "gold standard" for the severity of chronic venous insufficiency. Although ligation of the saphenous vein prevents reflux in the superficial system and may normalize ambulatory venous pressure in patients with simple varicose veins, this procedure has little effect on ambulatory venous pressure in limbs with chronic venous insufficiency since it does not prevent deep venous reflux. When venous outflow is obstructed, venous pressure may actually be increased by calf muscle contraction. This is the mechanism responsible for "venous claudication."

4. The answer is **C** (Rutherford, 4th ed., pp. 1696–1697).

Superficial thrombophlebitis usually presents as a tender, firm knot or cord just under the skin in one of the veins.

Probably it is most often seen during or following an intravenous infusion, especially if certain medications are administered through this route. Superficial thrombophlebitis occurs most often in the forearm of the upper extremity because this is the most frequent site of intravenous infusion. The diagnosis can usually be made by history and examination. In contrast, superficial thrombophlebitis may be difficult to diagnose in the thigh of an obese patient or in the subclavian vein. In these instances, duplex scanning or even phlebography may be required. The Doppler velocity probe, when used by a skilled technologist, may be able to establish the diagnosis in these instances. Photoplethysmography would be of little value, since it is designed to detect deep venous reflux.

5. The answers are **A, B, D** (Rutherford, 4th ed., pp. 1696–1697).

Superficial thrombophlebitis is usually a self-limiting disorder that resolves spontaneously. Although in most cases it regresses regardless of therapy, in others it can progress in severity and/or location and last for six weeks or more. Furthermore, there is increasing evidence that it extends into the deep system more than previously thought. Although upper-extremity septic thrombophlebitis is not uncommon, especially in the critically ill patient, in most cases of thrombophlebitis involving the lower extremity, bacteria cannot be cultured. Patients with varicose veins do have a predisposition for thrombophlebitis. In fact, it often occurs in varicose veins caused by deep vein thrombosis. Superficial thrombophlebitis, therefore, may be associated with a chronic venous ulcer, but is not thought to be an important factor in the development of the ulcer.

6. The answer is **E** (Rutherford, 4th ed., pp. 1696–1697).

Superficial thrombophlebitis, especially if limited, may resolve while the patient wears elastic stockings and continues normal activity. If more extensive thrombophlebitis is present, hot wet compresses, bed rest, and elevation afford relief, although the recovery period is protracted. Antibiotics have been recommended to treat atypical bacterial forms, which have been implicated as etiologic agents. However, most patients do not respond to antibiotics alone. Excision of the vein, while radical, has been associated with rapid recovery. Excision should be performed for septic thrombophlebitis, and the wound should be left open. If the thrombophlebitis in the saphenous vein extends to the groin, the vein should be ligated near the saphenofemoral junction to prevent deep vein thrombosis and pulmonary embolism. Whereas anticoagulation is not generally recommended, recognition of concurrent deep vein thrombosis may require anticoagulation.

7. The answers are **A, D** (Rutherford, 4th ed., pp. 1698–1700).

The clinical diagnosis of acute DVT is notoriously inaccurate—not much better than flipping a coin. Although there are many other causes of unilateral leg swelling, this sign should alert the clinician to the possible presence of a venous thrombosis. Indeed, it may be the only physical manifestation of DVT in some patients. Homan's sign is neither sensitive nor specific and is not recommended as a method for diagnosing DVT in bedridden patients. Thrombosed deep veins are seldom palpable. Tender "cords," however, are often felt in patients with *superficial* venous thrombosis, some of whom may also have DVT. Because DVT can coexist with any of the multiple conditions that mimic DVT, objective testing for venous thrombosis should be considered even when an alternative diagnosis appears likely. Phlegmasia cerulea dolens is an exception to the rule that DVT cannot be diagnosed on physical examination alone. In this life- and limb-threatening condition, the massive swelling of the leg, severe pain, deep cyanosis, bullae, and decreased pulses are practically diagnostic.

8. The answers are **A, B, E** (Rutherford, 4th ed., pp. 1701–1717).

There is ample evidence that experienced technologists are able to diagnose acute symptomatic DVT accurately in above-knee veins with impedance plethysmography (IPG) and Doppler ultrasonography. These methods, however, are unreliable for identifying clots below the knee, nonocclusive thrombi in major veins, and thrombi confined to one of a pair of duplicated veins. For these reasons, they are not suitable for surveillance studies of high-risk asymptomatic patients, in whom clots are often nonocclusive and are frequently isolated to the infrapopliteal veins. Although it may be possible to determine the approximate location and extent of large thrombi with the Doppler, the IPG is sensitive only to the presence of obstruction and provides little or no anatomic information. Despite these limitations, physiologic tests have the advantage of being portable, easily and quickly performed, and inexpensive. When they are clearly positive in a patient in whom extrinsic compression can be ruled out, no other diagnostic test is necessary. Moreover, many investigators have shown that pulmonary embolism occurs during follow-up in fewer than 1% of untreated symptomatic outpatients with negative physiologic test results.

9. The answers are **C, E** (Rutherford, 4th ed., pp. 1717–1722).

Duplex and color-flow scanning are recognized as the most accurate noninvasive tests for DVT. When these studies are performed by skilled technologists, additional tests are seldom required. Although visualization of a clot on the B-mode image is the most specific sign of DVT, many thrombi are hypoechogenic and are not clearly seen. To avoid overlooking clots, venous compressibility and venous flow patterns should be assessed. In most locations, failure of the vein to collapse with probe pressure is a reliable sign of DVT; however, some veins (such as the superficial femoral in the adductor hiatus, the profunda femoris, and the subclavian) are resistant to compression. Assessment of Doppler flow patterns in these and other areas will avoid many false positive and false negative errors. Color facilitates the examination by rapidly identifying veins and by visualizing flow over extended regions. It often obviates the need to assess compressibility and Doppler flow patterns. Symptomatic calf vein thrombosis can be diagnosed with reasonable accuracy with conventional duplex scanning, but the studies may be difficult because of the small size and large number of veins at risk. For this reason, some laboratories restrict their examination to the above-knee veins. Color-flow mapping greatly simplifies scanning of infrapopliteal veins by facilitating their identification, by making it easier to trace the veins throughout their courses, and by immediately revealing the absence of flow in occluded venous segments. Because DVT is frequently confined to below-knee veins, examination of this area is required in all symptomatic and high-risk asymptomatic patients when no thrombi are found in the proximal veins. Other major advantages of duplex and color-flow scanning include the ability to identify nonocclusive (free-floating) clots, thrombi in duplicated veins, and masses responsible for extrinsic venous compression. Only 40–80% of patients with angiographically confirmed pulmonary emboli have leg phlebograms or duplex studies that demonstrate a venous thrombus. Thus, a negative duplex or color-flow scan of the legs does *not* rule out pulmonary embolism. A *positive* leg scan, however, makes it possible to proceed with anticoagulation even when the diagnosis of pulmonary embolism is uncertain.

10. The answer is **D** (Rutherford, 4th ed., pp. 1744–1748).

Only one published study has correlated pathologic findings to venographic interpretation in order to establish sensitivity and specificity. That study performed intraosseous venography on cadavers. The sensitivity of venography for detection of thrombus in this postmortem study was 86%. The sensitivity of venography for detection of clinically significant lower-extremity DVT in living patients is almost certainly much higher. However, pathologic correlation is impossible because DVT is treated with anticoagulation, not surgical excision. Although contrast venography has been accepted as the "gold standard" for diagnosis of DVT, it also carries a low but measurable rate of potentially serious complications. Additionally, performance of venography usually entails significant patient discomfort. Alternatively, both grey scale compression ultrasound and color-flow duplex imaging have been proven in multiple studies to have a sensitivity and specificity that rival contrast venography for diagnoses of *above-knee* DVT in patients with symptoms suggestive of DVT. Because these modalities involve no significant risk or discomfort, one ultrasound technique ought to be the initial imaging modality employed in evaluation of symptomatic patients. Venography should be reserved, then, for cases in which the ultrasound examination is nondiagnostic. Multiple well-designed studies have shown that considerable interobserver variability exists regarding interpretation of conventional venograms. Overall rates of interobserver variability range from 10 to 30%. Presumably due to differences of opinion regarding the significance of small filling defects, the rate of interobserver disagreement is significantly lower for negative (normal) exams (2%) than for positive (DVT present) exams (30%).

11. The answer is **B** (Rutherford, 4th ed., pp. 1753–1754).

Serious contrast reactions occur in approximately 0.1% of contrast injections administered to the general population and in approximately 1% of patients with a history of a prior contrast reaction. Pretreatment of high-risk patients with a short course of steroids as well as use of nonionic contrast material has been shown to decrease the risk of a subsequent contrast reaction and are measures recommended for patients at high risk for reactions. Although several retrospective series and large-scale surveys have suggested that nonionic contrast material is less likely to cause contrast-induced nephropathy, prospective, randomized studies have found no significant difference in the rate of contrast-induced nephropathy between comparable doses of ionic and nonionic contrast material. Extravasation of contrast material potentially can be serious and may result in slough of adjacent skin. This risk of skin slough is increased in patients with arterial disease. The risk of contrast extravasation is minimized by use of a plastic cannula. Postvenography deep venous thrombosis occurs in 2 to 13% of patients (not 20%). Additionally, the incidence is distinctly higher for more concentrated contrast material (13%) than for diluted contrast (3%).

12. The answer is **A** (Rutherford, 4th ed., pp. 1748–1753, 1755–1769).

Closed system venography essentially renders all of the venous channels free of blood so that filling of venous structures (e.g., a venous malformation) is more complete than with ascending venography, which has physiologic blood flow. Descending venography uses gravity or a Valsalva maneuver to test valvular competence of the superficial femoral, deep femoral, and greater saphenous veins (not the perforating veins). Inflation of a proximal blood pressure cuff permits retrograde opacification of the arteriovenous fistula so as to evaluate arteriovenous or arterial graft anastomosis, not the central veins. The Wright's maneuver is used to provide extrinsic compression of the subclavian vein in a patient with suspected thoracic outlet syndrome, not to distinguish thrombotic from artifactual filling defects.

13. The answers are **B, E** (Rutherford, 4th ed., pp. 1771–1772).

The ambulatory venous pressure (AVP) is defined as the venous pressure in the superficial veins of the foot at the completion of 10 tiptoe exercises performed in the standing position. It has been demonstrated that changes in the venous pressure are identical in the deep and superficial venous systems, that venous pressure is reduced to its minimal levels with leg muscle contraction during ambulation, and that it returns to the resting values when walking stops. A high degree of correlation has been established between increasing levels of AVP and incidence of leg ulceration in patients with chronic venous insufficiency (CVI). The AVP is elevated in most patients with CVI arising in either the superficial or the deep venous systems. Patients with isolated varicose veins and competent communicating veins have a slight elevation in the AVP, whereas patients with deep valvular incompetence, including the popliteal vein and perforators, tend to have the highest levels of AVP. The presence of concomitant proximal deep venous obstruction can further elevate AVP levels. The ambulatory venous pressure reflects the net effects of valvular incompetence, venous outflow obstruction, and calf muscle failure. However, measurement of the AVP cannot separate the individual effect of each component contributing to the presence of CVI. Despite being the hemodynamic standard for comparison with noninvasive venous studies, AVP measurement has some limitations. It does not separate the different components contributing to the presence of CVI, and it remains within normal limits in a significant number of patients who develop venous stasis skin ulceration.

14. The answersare **C, E** (Rutherford, 4th ed., pp. 1772–1775).

Air plethysmography allows the detection of lower-extremity volume changes in relation to gravity and exercise. Volume changes are detected by a calibrated system connected to an inflatable plastic sleeve placed around the calf. Although it has been demonstrated that the residual volume fraction measured with APG correlates directly with ambulatory venous pressure levels, air plethysmography does not *measure* venous pressure changes (see Fig. 133–4). The venous filling index measures the rate of venous refill of the limb, expressed in milliliters per second, and it evaluates *overall* valvular competence. Measurement of the venous filling index, using a tourniquet to occlude the superficial venous system, separates the effect of the latter on the degree of reflux. The one second outflow fraction measured with APG evaluates the presence of venous outflow obstruction. The combination of hemodynamic parameters obtained by APG offers quantitative information about the presence of venous reflux, the integrity of the calf muscle pump mechanism, and the overall venous function.

15. The answer is **D** (Rutherford, 4th ed., pp. 1775–1776, 1778–1779).

The maneuvers used to elicit valve closure during the evaluation of venous reflux are as important as the method employed to document reversed flow. The classic methods using manual compression proximal or distal to the insonation site in either the supine or erect position have been shown to have an extremely high variability and to be very unreliable in eliciting valve closure. The best methods to elicit valve closure in the evaluation of venous reflux are those that consistently elicit valve closure. Venous reflux is in great part determined by gravity. Therefore, the best method to evaluate venous reflux is with the patient in the standing position, using rapid deflation cuffs applied distal to the insonation site and inflated to pressures that upon deflation produce reverse flow velocity above the threshold for valvular closure (i.e., 30 cm/second).

16. The answer is **C** (Rutherford, 4th ed., pp. 1780–1781).

The presence of incompetent calf perforating veins (ICPVs) has great clinical significance. However, the currently available methods for their evaluation remain unreliable. The diagnosis of ICPVs is based on the finding of flow from the deep to the superficial system following release of compression distal to the site under study. Ascending phlebography, considered by many the diagnostic method of reference in the evaluation of ICPVs, has a low incidence of false positive findings but a high rate of false negative findings. In a prospective study comparing ascending phlebography, Doppler evaluation, and physical examination, using the operative findings as the method of reference ("gold standard"), it was shown that neither phlebography nor Doppler evaluation is superior to clinical examination in the diagnosis of the presence or localization of the site of ICPVs. Color-flow duplex ultrasonography has been shown to identify reliably ICPVs. Unfortunately, its sensitivity is not yet established.

17. The answers are **C, D** (Rutherford, 4th ed., pp. 1785–1788).

Pulmonary embolism (PE) continues to be an important clinical problem in the United States. Unfortunately, the mortality rate from pulmonary embolism has not declined during the past decade; therefore, physicians must understand the importance of accurate diagnosis and therapy. Although diminished pulmonary vascular markings in the distribution of a pulmonary embolus may be evident, the classic Westermark's sign is seldom recognized prospectively. Electrocardiographic findings likewise are usually nonspecific. The classic findings of right heart strain (S1Q3T3) are observed in less than 10% of patients. However, the ECG is useful for detecting myocardial ischemia or excluding myocardial infarction and identifying arrhythmias. Arterial blood gases should be routinely obtained to evaluate the degree of hypoxia. Usually patients with pulmonary embolism have some degree of hypoxia associated with hypocarbia. There is usually a widened A-a gradient with a respiratory alkalosis; however, these are not invariable findings. Anywhere from 8–10% of patients can have a normal PaO_2, and in 15% the PaO_2 exceeds 80 mm Hg. The ventilation perfusion (V/Q) scan is the most widely used specific diagnostic test for suspected pulmonary embolism. The Canadian study and the recent PIOPED study (published in 1985 and 1990, respectively) evaluated the appropriate place of ventilation perfusion scans in the diagnostic evaluation of patients with suspected pulmonary embolism. Ninety-six percent of patients with high clinical suspicion who had a high-probability V/Q scan were found to have angiographically demonstrable pulmonary emboli. On the other end of the scale, patients with normal V/Q scans were unlikely to have pulmonary emboli demonstrated by subsequent pulmonary angiograms. However, other V/Q results, such as intermediate or low probability, require additional evaluation, because 16–50% of those patients were found to have angiographically proven pulmonary embolism. Unfortunately, the V/Q scan can be used as the definitive test in less than 30% of patients with suspected pulmonary embolism.

18. The answer is **A** (Rutherford, 4th ed., pp. 1802–1806).

Venous thrombectomy for patients with iliofemoral venous thrombosis is being revisited with renewed interest and when properly performed has shown significantly better short- and long-term results compared to anticoagulation alone. Although a venous thrombectomy can be performed under local anesthesia, regional and general anesthesia is preferred. Autotransfusion devices should be available to salvage blood lost during the procedure to minimize transfusion requirements, because venous engorgement can lead to substantial blood loss. Although pulmonary embolism during the procedure is a theoretical concern, it has been demonstrated in very few patients; therefore, adjunctive measures to protect from intraoperative pulmonary emboli are not required.

19. The answer is **E** (Rutherford, 4th ed., pp. 1799–1802).

Although not widely employed, thrombolytic therapy for acute DVT, when successful, is likely to reduce post-thrombotic sequelae. If successful, thrombolytic therapy clears the thrombus from the deep venous system, restoring patency and potentially maintaining valvular function. Pooled data indicate that thrombolytic therapy restores patency significantly more frequently than anticoagulation alone. Several prospective randomized studies indicate that medium-term function of the deep venous system is better following a successful lysis compared to treatment by anticoagulation alone. However, higher complication rates have been observed with lytic therapy, and high failure rates have also been reported. In most institutions, lytic therapy is reserved for patients with the most extensive deep venous thrombosis; therefore, any method of therapy in these patients is likely to be associated with higher failure rates and more severe post-thrombotic symptoms. In many centers only patients with iliofemoral venous thrombosis are treated with systemic lytic therapy. Because there is no blood flowing through the involved veins, activation of fibrin-bound plasminogen does not occur. Failure of thrombolysis in these patients can be expected because the plasminogen activator cannot reach the thrombus. Other causes for failure include (1) antistreptococcal antibodies (if streptokinase [SK] is the plasminogen activator used), which bind and inactivate SK, (2) failure of the physician to monitor the thrombus resolution, and (3) premature termination of the lytic infusion.

20. The answer is **D** (Rutherford, 4th ed., pp. 1815–1816).

A Greenfield filter can be inserted safely in patients with sepsis and bacteremia, because it has been demonstrated both experimentally and clinically that the entrapped infected thrombus can be sterilized with intravenous antibiotics. The filter can also be inserted safely into a pregnant patient, but it should be placed *above* the level of the renal veins in order to avoid contact between the gravid uterus and the filter in the lower portion of the vena cava. This location also assures protection for emboli that might originate in the ovarian or pelvic veins. Similarly, for the patient with a thrombus extending to the level of the renal veins, the filter can be placed in the suprarenal position with anticipated high level of long-term patency and little or no risk to renal function.

21. The answer is **B** (Rutherford, 4th ed., pp. 1816–1817).

Although there is limited reported follow-up experience for many current filter devices inserted percutaneously, they appear to be relatively equivalent in their ability to protect against recurrent embolism at a rate of 3–5% (see Table 135–2). Similarly, occasional migration and caval penetration have been seen with all of the devices, usually without significant clinical sequelae. The major difference has been in the incidence of caval thrombosis, which has averaged about 20% for the Nitinol, Bird's Nest, and Venatech filters, whereas the titanium and stainless steel Greenfield filters average only 2–5% long-term vena caval thrombosis. The consequences of vena caval thrombosis are significant not only in terms of venous stasis sequelae but also because vena caval thrombosis represents a nidus for new thrombus and potential embolism.

22. The answer is **D** (Rutherford, 4th ed., pp. 1816–1817, 1821–1824).

The titanium Greenfield filter is designed to be inserted percutaneously through a sheath/dilator system that essentially eliminates the possibility of misplacement because any premature discharge of the filter would be into the sheath rather than into the patient. The cost is also considerably reduced because the procedure is done in the radiology suite rather than in the operating room. The time required for insertion is similarly reduced because no operative cut down is required.

23. The answer is **B** (Rutherford, 4th ed., pp. 1825–1826).

Arteriovenous fistulas in association with varicose veins have been described independently by Haimovici in 1987 and Baron in 1986; weakness of the vein wall has been studied extensively by European phlebologists; and valvular incompetence has long been associated with dilated veins. Whereas it might seem that local trauma to veins could be an etiologic agent, it has not been described.

24. The answer is **false** (Rutherford, 4th ed., p. 1826).

Isolated insufficiency of the greater saphenous system is the cause of chronic venous insufficiency more frequently than was previously thought. Darke and Penfold have recently recommended saphenous ligation for this disorder. In a 1992 publication, these authors described brawny edema, subcutaneous fibrosis, cutaneous atrophy, pigmentation, and ulceration due entirely to longstanding *superficial* venous insufficiency.

25. The answer is **false** (Rutherford, 4th ed., pp. 1825–1827).

Isolated incompetence of the greater saphenous vein below the knee, *without* incompetence of the valve at the saphenofemoral junction, has been recognized with increasing frequency. Likewise, incompetence of the valve of the saphenofemoral junction does not *always* cause varicosity of the greater saphenous below the knee. Selective stripping based on Doppler ultrasonic findings was recommended by Koyano and Sakaguchi in a 1988 article.

26. The answer is **D** (Rutherford, 4th ed., pp. 1827–1828).

The best way to prevent stripping the femoral artery is to pass the stripper from bottom to top. This method affords absolute identification of the saphenous vein in the groin. Identifying the saphenofemoral junction is also appropriate, but is not the best answer. There have been cases in which the profunda artery was mistaken for the saphenous vein. Passing the stripper from top to bottom necessitates incision of the vessel before absolute identification has been made. Small arteries in spasm are not uncommonly mistaken for veins, so color and even lack of pulsations are not absolute identifying features.

27. The answer is **D** (Rutherford, 4th ed., pp. 1828–1831, 1833–1835).

There is no doubt that sclerotherapy may be useful in treatment of all the lesions mentioned above (see Table 137–1). However, its *greatest* utility is in the treatment of telangiectasias, also known as venectasias. These are located just below the epidermis and well within the dermis.

28. The answer is **D** (Rutherford, 4th ed., pp. 1829–1830).

Although gravitational reflux is the most publicized of the sources of venous hypertension that leads to varicosities, all of the sources mentioned, including compartmental pressure and reflux through the reticular network, contribute to total venous hypertension in telangiectasias and varicosities.

29. The answer is **B** (Rutherford, 4th ed., pp. 1830–1833).

Ideal sclerotherapy produces endothelial damage and necrosis of significant portions of the vascular wall. Healing of these lesions results in obliteration of the vascular lumen *without* thrombosis. The thrombotic reaction, in fact, may thwart success of sclerotherapy and may contribute to cutaneous pigmentation and leakage of red cells by diapedesis. It is not a desirable result of sclerotherapy.

30. The answer is **C** (Rutherford, 4th ed., pp. 1839–1840).

The data regarding the natural history of CVI involve several prospective and retrospective studies describing the onset of valvular insufficiency and/or symptoms following documented DVT. In addition, multiple studies have examined the anatomic location of valvular incompetence and association to disease severity in patients with known CVI. Most of this information is based on duplex scanning to determine valvular incompetence and venous recanalization. The following conclusions can be made from these studies. Venous recanalization occurs early, within weeks to months after a DVT, but valvular insufficiency appears later. The occurrence and localization of valvular insufficiency after DVT in an individual patient cannot be predicted by the extent and location of the initial thrombus. A small fraction of patients with venous ulceration (up to 17%) have isolated superficial venous valvular incompetence. Popliteal and infrapopliteal valvular incompetence produce a greater incidence of skin changes and/or ulceration.

31. The answer is **A** (Rutherford, 4th ed., pp. 1840–1843).

The evidence that venous ulcers are ischemic in origin is controversial. Elevated magnetic resonance spectroscopy-determined levels of radio-labeled high-energy phosphates from gastrocnemius muscle in patients with CVI supports this etiology. In addition, positron emission tomography (PET scanning) of radioactively labeled oxygen has demonstrated a marked increase in regional blood flow but *reduced* oxygen extraction in areas of venous ulceration. $TcPO_2$ measurements in CVI have been inconsistent. With the probe heated to 43° to induce local hyperemia, perimalleolar $TcPO_2$ levels in CVI limbs have been lower than in controls. Laser Doppler studies have demonstrated a resting cutaneous hyperemia in limbs with CVI compared to controls.

32. The answer is **C** (Rutherford, 4th ed., pp. 1846–1847).

All of the agents listed have been used to treat CVI. Hydroxyrutosides are a class of flavanoid drugs derived from plant glycosides. Their mechanism of potential benefit in CVI is to decrease capillary permeability. Although they have proved marginally beneficial in controlling lower-extremity edema, they have never been shown to improve venous ulcer healing rates. Stanozolol is an androgenic steroid with fibrinolytic activity. Treatment of CVI with this agent has been largely unimpressive. A moderate reduction in lipodermatosclerosis has been reported by some investigators, but others have demonstrated no benefit. Dimethyl sulfoxide, a free radical scavenger, has been used as a topical treatment of venous ulceration in one randomized trial with marked success. Calcium dobesilate acts to increase lymphatic flow and macrophage-mediated proteolysis with a net reduction in edema. Subjective symptomatic improvement in pain and swelling has been demonstrated in a single trial, but its effect on venous ulceration is unknown.

33. The answer is **D** (Rutherford, 4th ed., pp. 1840–1843).

The "white cell trapping" theory of venous ulceration began with the observation that femoral venous blood from normal dependent limbs had proportionally lower white blood cell counts than the same limbs in the supine position. Subsequent studies in CVI limbs confirmed decreased numbers of white cells in femoral venous samples after 30 minutes of dependency compared to control limbs. Capillary microscopy has demonstrated capillary microthrombosis in perimalleolar skin of patients with CVI. These thrombi have been postulated to be due to intracapillary sludging of white cells. Lipodermatosclerotic skin biopsies have demonstrated increased numbers of white cells per mm^3 than in control skin.

34. The answer is **B** (Rutherford, 4th ed., pp. 1851–1853, 1857–1859).

Kistner's internal valvuloplasty technique utilizes direct exposure of the redundant and refluxive valve cusps for placement of reefing sutures that tighten the free edges of the valve and render it competent. "Primary" valve reflux is the most appropriate valvular pathology to perform the procedure. The precise etiology of primary valve reflux is unknown, but the valve cusps are redundant, leading to poor coaptation and reflux. The post-thrombotic syndrome comprises a multitude of pathological elements and may result in obstruction, reflux, or a combination. Reflux may occur through the previously thrombosed axial vein itself that has become recanalized with destruction of the valve apparatus. A valvuloplasty procedure will not be possible under these circumstances. Considerable collateral reflux that is frequently present in this condition will also need to be corrected. Again, a valvuloplasty procedure is an impractical choice to accomplish this goal because the collaterals are frequently small in size and may not contain repairable valves. When a combined obstruction/reflux is present, accompanying stasis ulceration is thought to result from the reflux component, which requires correction for healing of the ulcer. Perforator incompetence can be primary or secondary, the latter associated with deep venous reflux. A perforator interruption may be combined with a valve reconstruction procedure in the latter situation.

35. The answer is **C** (Rutherford, 4th ed., pp. 1853–1857).

Deep venous thrombosis initially results in acute venous obstruction. With recanalization and collateral development, acute venous obstruction resolves to varying degree. A residual obstructive component may be present along with post-thrombotic reflux. Anatomical methods of investigation, including ascending venography and color duplex examination, provide details of collateral development and post-thrombotic changes as well as the location and extent of residual obstruction. However, no *hemodynamic* information is provided. This information can be obtained by measuring arm/foot venous pressure differential in the supine patient. A value of over 4 mm Hg signifies hemodynamic obstruction at rest. When the process of recanalization/collateral development has occurred, a pressure differential may not be present. The adequacy of collateral development can be further assessed by monitoring the foot venous pressure increase that occurs after induced reactive hyperemia. In some patients the recanalization process is incomplete, and the collateral development is inadequate, yielding an abnormal foot venous pressure increase under conditions of increased arterial inflow. Descending venography is utilized for delineating valve *reflux*, not obstruction.

36. The answer is **B** (Rutherford, 4th ed., p. 1861).

The internal valvuloplasty procedure originally described in 1979 by Robert Kistner has superior durability, notably when compared to the axillary vein transfer. As much as a 20% difference in stasis ulcer healing beyond two years has been noted (see Table 139–5). Whereas part of the difference may be accounted for by differences in case selection (i.e., postphlebitic versus cryptogenic valve reflux), a high percentage of axillary vein valves are noted to be incompetent in situ in the axilla. When transferred to the lower limb they are prone to dilatation and recurrent reflux, presumably because of compliance mismatch. A prosthetic sleeve may be applied around the transferred axillary vein valve in an effort to reduce this complication. Experience with the segment transfer procedure has been limited. In one reported series (Bergan and Yao, 1991), a high incidence of recurrent reflux was noted. Sufficient experience with external valvuloplasty technique has not been accumulated to determine its durability.

37. The answer is **E** (Rutherford, 4th ed., pp. 1857–1860).

Initial fears about possible high incidence of serious thromboembolic complications following direct valve reconstructive surgery have proved to be unfounded. Among several reported series, the incidence of pulmonary embolism and thrombosis of the venous repair have been insignificant (see Table 139–4). Following axillary vein harvest it is not necessary to repair the host vein. Cut ends of the vein may be ligated, and no adverse sequelae have been reported. Wound problems are unusual because the skin of the thigh is generally spared from cutaneous manifestation of venous insufficiency.

38. The answers are **B, D, E** (Rutherford, 4th ed., pp. 1862–1867).

The pain pattern of chronic obstructive venous disease is described as a "bursting, stretching ache" in the thigh or calf occurring with vigorous exercise. This venous claudication is usually less severe than arterial claudication and does not commonly limit normal daily activities. The pain is caused by increased intramuscular pressure, both at rest and with exercise, resulting from increased transudation of fluid into muscle as a result of venous hypertension. The increased volume within a fascia-enclosed compartment raises interstitial pressure and reduces capillary flow. The pain is thought to be mediated by Bassini pain receptors associated with the fasciae. The four diagnostic criteria for venous claudication are (1) leg pain with exertion, (2) iliac vein obstruction, (3) venous hypertension at rest, and (4) elevation of venous pressure with exercise.

39. The answers are **A, C, D** (Rutherford, 4th ed., pp. 1864–1868).

If history, physical examination, and noninvasive venous tests indicate significant obstructive venous disease, ascending and descending phlebography and foot and femoral venous pressure measurements are all mandatory before venous reconstructive surgery. Patients with phlebographic obstruction may have normal hemodynamic function because of extensive collateral formation, whereas patients with phlebograms showing patent but recanalized main venous channels may demonstrate significant hemodynamic abnormality. Large, profuse collaterals around an obstructed venous segment on phlebograms can be *hemodynamically inadequate* because of the presence of stenosis or other high-resistance areas not readily seen with phlebography. A hemodynamically significant iliofemoral venous stenosis/obstruction exists if a vertical gradient of >2 mm Hg exists at rest, if the horizontal gradient (compared to the contralateral femoral pressure) is >2 mm Hg at supine rest, and if an exercise venous pressure (with pedal ergometer) increases >3 mm Hg from the resting level. An arm/foot venous pressure differential at rest of >4 mm Hg and a foot venous pressure elevation with reactive hyperemia >6 mm Hg are also indicators of hemodynamically significant venous obstruction.

40. The answers are **A, C** (Rutherford, 4th ed., pp. 1868–1880).

Venous anastomoses have a marked tendency for stricturing because of the thin, nonrigid, highly elastic vein walls that are under greater tension than in the arterial system. To prevent excessive tension, it is advisable to interpose a graft longer than the excised vein segment. There is unanimous agreement that the most nonthrombogenic conduit in the venous system is autogenous vein. However, when autogenous vein is not available or of poor quality, or when large-diameter veins need to be replaced (e.g., thoracic caval or iliocaval), a prosthetic externally supported ringed conduit (polytetrafluoroethylene) can have a patency rate comparable to autologous vein. Adjunctive temporary arteriovenous fistulas improve long-term patency of both autogenous and prosthetic venous bypass conduits. The timing of closure of an adjunctive arteriovenous fistula remains unsettled. Most data support closure of adjunctive fistulas before six months. These can be closed nonoperatively by percutaneous deployment of a detachable balloon in the fistula under direct radiographic control.

18

Lymphatic Disorders

1. The discovery of the lymphatic system is attributed to:
   A. William Harvey.
   B. Gasparo Asellius.
   C. Jean Pecquet.
   D. William Hunter.
   E. E. H. Starling.

2. The most frequent local or regional cause of chronic swelling of the extremity in North America is:
   A. Primary lymphedema.
   B. Secondary lymphedema.
   C. Chronic venous insufficiency.
   D. Congenital vascular malformation.
   E. Acquired arteriovenous fistula.

3. The most important independent risk factor(s) predicting the development of lymphedema following treatment for breast cancer include:
   A. Extensive axillary lymphadenectomy.
   B. Positive pathological nodal status.
   C. Postoperative chemotherapy.
   D. Axillary radiotherapy.
   E. Axillary venous thrombosis.

4. The primary mechanism by which lymph is propelled is:
   A. External muscular squeezing.
   B. Respiration.
   C. Intrinsic lymphatic ("lymphangion") contraction.
   D. Fascial constriction.
   E. Arterial pulsation.

5. Which of the following statements is/are most accurate?
   A. Veins and lymphatics are both thin-walled conduits that propel liquid back to the heart under *high* intraluminal pressure and *high* vascular resistance.
   B. Veins and lymphatics are both thin-walled conduits that propel liquid back to the heart under *low* intraluminal pressure and *low* vascular resistance.
   C. Veins and lymphatics are thin walled conduits that propel liquid back to the heart; but whereas venous blood flows at *low* intraluminal pressure and high vascular resistance, lymph flows at *low* intraluminal pressure and *low* vascular resistance.
   D. Veins and lymphatics are thin-walled conduits that propel liquid back to the heart; but whereas venous blood flows at *low* intraluminal pressure and *low* vascular resistance, lymph flows at *low* intraluminal pressure and *high* vascular resistance.
   E. Veins and lymphatics are thin-walled conduits that propel liquid back to the heart; but whereas venous blood flows at *high* intraluminal pressure and *low* vascular resistance, lymph flows at *low* intraluminal pressure and *low* vascular resistance.

6. With an increase in interstitial volume:
   A. Both lymph and blood capillaries collapse, thereby restricting further accumulation of tissue fluid and protein.
   B. Lymph capillaries dilate and blood capillaries collapse, thereby facilitating fluid and protein resorption into the bloodstream via lymphatics while minimizing further plasma filtration.
   C. Lymph capillaries collapse while blood capillaries open, favoring rapid resorption of protein and liquid into the bloodstream.
   D. Both lymph and blood capillaries dilate, favoring rapid absorption of tissue fluid and protein into the bloodstream.
   E. None of the above.

7. The pathophysiology of secondary lymphedema (chronic lymph stasis) is characterized by:
   A. Progressive loss of lymphatic truncal contractility, intraluminal valve incompetence, and lymphangiectasis; often several months or years pass with no symptoms before edema becomes apparent with progressive deposition of fat, fluid, and collagen in the skin and subcutaneous tissue.
   B. Rapid onset of limb swelling, accumulation of protein-poor edema fluid, and progressive insufficiency of the greater and lesser saphenous venous systems with dermal hyperpigmentation and paramalleolar skin ulceration.
   C. Acute, unremitting extremity swelling, prompt response to diuretic drugs, and gradual remission of edema over many years.
   D. Low-protein edema fluid, progressive improvement with diuretic drugs, and dietary salt restriction, often in conjunction with limb-threatening ischemic foot ulcers.
   E. Progressive limb swelling, hyperpigmentation, subcutaneous fibrosis, and development of painful ulceration.

8. The term "Milroy's disease" should be reserved for patients with:
   - **A.** Primary lymphedema.
   - **B.** Primary congenital hereditary lymphedema.
   - **C.** All patients with lymphedema praecox.
   - **D.** Lymphangiectasia.
   - **E.** Lymphangiosarcoma in a limb with chronic lymphedema.

9. The test of choice to diagnose lymphedema is:
   - **A.** Direct contrast lymphangiography.
   - **B.** Indirect contrast lymphangiography.
   - **C.** Computed tomography.
   - **D.** Magnetic resonance imaging.
   - **E.** Lymphoscintigraphy.

10. The most important signs and symptoms of patients with primary lymphedema include the following:
    - **A.** Nonpitting edema of the ankle and foot.
    - **B.** Squaring of the toes (Stemmer's sign).
    - **C.** Hyperkeratosis.
    - **D.** Multiple punched-out ulcers.
    - **E.** Yellow fingernails.
    - **F.** Constant, severe pain.

11. Which of the following statements about lymphedema is/are true?
    - **A.** Lymphangiosarcoma develops in approximately 10% of all patients with lymphedema of more than 15 years' duration.
    - **B.** Emotional problems are common in patients with lymphedema and should be addressed by the physician when identified.
    - **C.** Severe lymphedema, while unsightly, rarely causes significant physical or emotional disability/limitation.
    - **D.** Nonoperative measures to control lymphedema are generally inferior to surgical treatment.
    - **E.** Ulceration is a common sequela.

12. Which of the following is the *least* common cause of lymphedema in North America?
    - **A.** Metastatic malignancy.
    - **B.** Idiopathic (i.e., primary) lymphedema.
    - **C.** Infection.
    - **D.** Filarial disease.
    - **E.** Treatment of nonmetastatic malignancies (using surgery with or without radiation therapy).

13. Which of the following statements about infection in limbs with lymphedema is/are *false?*
    - **A.** The most common causative agent is group A streptococcus.
    - **B.** Topical fungicides should be used to control cutaneous trichophytoses in limbs with lymphedema.
    - **C.** When treating cutaneous infections, it is essential to use an antibiotic that covers gram negative organisms.
    - **D.** Penicillin is a good first choice for treating cellulitis associated with lymphedema.
    - **E.** Recurrent infections contribute to increasing swelling.

14. Which of the following are not acceptable methods for *reducing* a lymphedematous limb?
    - **A.** Bed rest with limb elevation.
    - **B.** Intensive use of diuretics.
    - **C.** Massage/manual lymph drainage.
    - **D.** Elastic compression stockings or wraps.
    - **E.** Pneumatic compression.

15. Which of the following statements about elastic compression stockings/sleeves is/are *false?*
    - **A.** Stockings are an effective means for reducing limbs with lymphedema.
    - **B.** Pressures of 40–50 mm Hg at the ankle are usually needed to control lower-extremity lymphedema.
    - **C.** Many patients can be fit with over-the-counter, premade garments.
    - **D.** Stockings or sleeves are an effective means of maintaining a reduction in limb size once it has been achieved by other limb-reduction methods.
    - **E.** As a rule, stockings or sleeves should be long enough to cover the edematous portion of the limb.

16. Which of the following statements is/are true regarding the surgical treatment of lymphedema?
    - **A.** Approximately 30% of lymphedema patients require surgery.
    - **B.** The patient with restricted movement from gross extremity enlargement is most likely to benefit from surgical intervention, and functional impairment is the best indication for surgery.
    - **C.** The excisional procedures recognize that lymphedema is limited to the skin and subcutaneous tissue and remove varying amounts of this compartment.
    - **D.** Both the Thompson and modified Homans procedures are intended to be both excisional and physiologic in approach.
    - **E.** All of the above.

17. The Charles procedure:
    - **A.** Is the excisional procedure of choice for the majority of patients.
    - **B.** Produces the best cosmetic results and can be considered as a cure.
    - **C.** Usually limited to the leg, and the graft sites will often become hyperpigmented, hyperkeratotic, and scarred with time.
    - **D.** Is usually performed on both thigh and lower leg.
    - **E.** Is the least extensive of the excisional procedures.

18. Regarding the Thompson procedure, which of the following statements is/are *false?*
    - **A.** It is both excisional and physiologic in approach.
    - **B.** It should never be used in the upper extremities.
    - **C.** Theoretically, the buried dermis permits the formation of lymphatic connections between the subdermal lymphatic plexus of the flap and the deep lymphatics of the muscle compartment.
    - **D.** Postoperative communication between the buried flap and the muscle compartment has been documented using lymphangiography.
    - **E.** Flap necrosis and partial tissue loss are the most common complications.

19. Which of the following statements is/are true concerning the modified Homans procedure?
    - **A.** It is similar to the excisional component of the Thompson procedure.
    - **B.** It provides predictable improvement while minimizing the likelihood of postoperative complications.
    - **C.** It can be offered to most patients as a cure.
    - **D.** Approximately 60–70% of patients experience significant postoperative improvement.
    - **E.** The use of compression stockings is not required after surgery.

20. Surgical lymphovenous anastomosis for the treatment of chronic lymphedema:
    - **A.** Is an established surgical procedure.
    - **B.** Is excellent for patients with primary lymphedema praecox.
    - **C.** Can be attempted in patients with secondary lymphedema if conservative treatment fails.
    - **D.** Has documented long-term patency in humans.
    - **E.** Is best reserved for the late stage of lymphedema.

21. Surgical procedures aimed at improving lymphatic drainage of the lower extremity include:
    - **A.** The Charles operation.
    - **B.** The Homans operation.
    - **C.** The mesenteric bridge operation.
    - **D.** The omental flap operation.
    - **E.** Autotransplantation of lymphatic tissue as a free flap.

22. Symptomatic patients with lymphagiectasia and reflux of chyle:
    - **A.** Should be evaluated by lymphoscintigraphy and possibly with direct contrast lymphangiography.
    - **B.** Are at risk to develop chylous effusions, such as chylous ascites or chylothorax.
    - **C.** Most frequently have *bilateral* lower-extremity lymphedema.
    - **D.** May have associated protein-losing enteropathy.
    - **E.** Can be treated with retroperitoneal ligation of the dilated incompetent lymph vessels.

18

Answers

1. The answer is **B** (Rutherford, 4th ed., pp. 1883–1885).

The discovery of the lymphatic system is attributed to Gasparo Asellius, a professor of anatomy and surgery at Pavia, Italy. On July 23, 1622, he observed the mesenteric lymphatics during vivisection of a well-fed dog. Asellius named the lymphatics *vasa lactea* and recognized their function of absorbing chyle from the intestines. Jean Pecquet, whose name is attached to the receptaculum chyli, described first the exact route of the mesenteric lymphatic drainage to the thoracic duct. William Harvey described the arterial and venous circulation but did not recognize the importance of the lymphatic system. William Hunter was one of the first to emphasize that the lymphatic vessels are the absorbing vessels that are similar to the lacteals, and that with the thoracic duct they constitute one system for absorption dispersed through the entire body. The modern investigation of lymph formation began with E. H. Starling, who at the turn of the 20th century confirmed the relationship between the hydrostatic pressure in the blood capillaries and the oncotic pressure of the plasma proteins. He suggested that lymph was formed by filtration of the blood through the wall of the capillaries.

2. The answer is **C** (Rutherford, 4th ed., pp. 1885–1886).

The most frequent local or regional cause of chronic leg swelling in North America is chronic venous insufficiency, caused either by primary venous valvular incompetence or by a previous deep venous thrombosis. In third world countries, however, secondary lymphedema caused by filariasis is the most frequent. Filariasis, which was eradicated from Europe and North America with public health measures and wide control of mosquito breeding, affects almost 100 million people in the world. In developed countries, however, the most important secondary lymphedema is postmastectomy lymphedema. Primary lymphedema is less common than secondary lymphedema; it occurs in young patients more frequently than secondary lymphedema. Of the conditions listed, congenital vascular malformation and acquired arteriovenous fistula are the least frequent causes of leg swelling.

3. The answers are **A, B, D, E** (Rutherford, 4th ed., pp. 1885–1886).

The most important cause of secondary lymphedema in developed countries is postmastectomy lymphedema. The well-documented study by Kissin et al. in 1986 confirmed that extensive axillary lymphadenectomy, axillary radiotherapy, and positive pathologic nodal status are the most important independent risk factors that predict the development of lymphedema. The use of postoperative chemotherapy does *not* appear to influence the development of swelling. The prevention of infectious complications is also important in patients who have undergone axillary lymph node dissection, because cellulitis further aggravates existing swelling and destroys additional lymphatic channels. The presence of axillary venous thrombosis also aggravates postmastectomy lymphedema in a significant number of patients. Although the treatment of a malignant tumor should not be compromised, surgeons should remember that excision of any lymphatic tissue, either for diagnosis or for therapy, should be restricted to a minimum.

4. The answer is **C** (Rutherford, 4th ed., pp. 1890–1892).

Extensive research in both man and experimental animals has firmly established that intrinsic (lymphangion) contraction is the main mechanism by which the lymphatic system propels lymph back to the bloodstream. The other items listed do not play a major role in lymphatic flow.

5. The answer is **D** (Rutherford, 4th ed., pp. 1892–1895).

Whereas both veins and lymphatics transport liquid back to the bloodstream, the flow-pressure dynamics of the two systems are distinctly different. In contrast to venous flow, which receives its circulatory boost from the thrust of the heart and external compression (e.g., muscular contraction), lymph flow is regulated by lymphatic truncal contraction and responds to an interstitial fluid challenge with an increase in both contractile frequency and amplitude. The pumping capacity of these lymphatics overcomes high vascular resistance by generating pressures in excess of 30 mm Hg. Temperature, alpha-adrenergic agonists, neurogenic stimuli, hormones, and cytokines, in turn, modify vascular resistance and thereby affect lymphatic flow.

6. The answer is **B** (Rutherford, 4th ed., pp. 1889–1895).

Unlike blood capillaries, which collapse and thereby decrease the microvascular surface area for escape of liquid and plasma proteins with an elevation in interstitial fluid pressure, lymph capillaries are structurally designed to *open* with increased tissue fluid volume. Anchoring filaments or elastic fibrils connect the lymphatic endothelium to surrounding collagen bundles. With an increased volume load they contract and open lymphatic capillaries wide, thereby facilitating imbibition of water and macromolecules from the interstitium.

7. The answer is **A** (Rutherford, 4th ed., pp. 1895–1898).

The pathophysiology of secondary lymphedema is described

in (**A**). Edema usually develops gradually, not rapidly. Venous thrombosis or insufficiency may contribute to swelling but does not necessarily coexist. Diuretics and salt restriction are generally ineffective means of treatment, and mechanical compression is required.

8. The answer is **B** (Rutherford, 4th ed., pp. 1899–1905).

The report by Milroy in 1892 described lower limb lymphedema in 22 members of the same family over six generations. In all but two of these patients the edema was present at birth. The term "Milroy's disease," therefore, should be reserved for patients who have primary hereditary lymphedema that was present at birth or was noticed soon thereafter. In a collected series of 291 patients with primary lymphedema, 14% had a family history of lymphedema, but only 5% had true Milroy's disease with congenital hereditary lymphedema. Lymphedema praecox includes patients who develop lymphedema between the ages of 1 and 35 years, and the cause of the swelling is either congenital hypoplasia or obstruction of the lymphatic system or is caused by acquired obstruction of the lymph-conducting elements of the lymph vessels and lymph nodes. Patients with lymphangiectasia usually have congenital valvular incompetence and dilated mesenteric and retroperitoneal lymphatics; they frequently develop chylous effusion and chylorrhea from vesicles of the skin. The term "Stewart-Traves syndrome" is used for patients who develop lymphangiosarcoma in a limb with chronic lymphedema.

9. The answer is **E** (Rutherford, 4th ed., pp. 1905–1918).

Radionuclide lymphoscintigraphy using ^{99m}Technetium-labeled antimony trisulfide colloid or ^{99m}Technetium-labeled human serum alburnin is the test of choice to confirm that edema is lymphatic in origin. Semiquantitative evaluation of lymphoscintigraphic images has an excellent sensitivity (92%) and specificity (100%) for the diagnosis of lymphedema. Direct contrast lymphangiography is now used selectively in patients to diagnose the type and the exact site of the lymphatic obstruction. This test, which is invasive and uncomfortable to the patient, has a small but definite rate of complications that include worsening of lymphedema in some patients. It is restricted now to the perioperative evaluation of patients with lymphangiectasia or is used selectively for some patients who undergo lymphatic reconstructions. Indirect contrast lymphangiography includes the subepidermal infusion of a water-soluble contrast material. At present, only dermal lymphatics and some distal lymph collectors can be visualized with this technique. Computed tomography and magnetic resonance imaging are used mainly to exclude any underlying mass, tumor, or retroperitoneal fibrosis. Magnetic resonance imaging is excellent to evaluate congenital vascular malformation but not very useful to demonstrate lymphatics.

10. The answers are **A, B, C, E** (Rutherford, 4th ed., pp. 1903–1905).

Patients with chronic lymphedema usually present with painless swelling of the limb. The edema is nonpitting or only partially pitting and involves the ankle and, in most patients, the foot. The edema of the dorsum of the forefoot resembles the "buffalo hump," and it is characteristic of patients with lymphedema. Squaring of the toes (Stemmer's sign) is also a characteristic feature and is caused by the high protein content of the excess tissue fluid. Although chronic eczematous dermatitis and excoriation of the skin occur in longstanding lymphedema, as does hyperkeratosis and lichenification (*peau d'orange*), frank ulcerations are rare. Punched-out ulcers are typical of ischemic ulcerations, or they are seen in patients with hypertensive ulcers. Yellow nails may occur in patients with primary lymphedema and together with pleural effusion, clubbing, transverse ridging, friability of the nails, and decreased rate of nail growth are the characteristic features of yellow nail syndrome.

11. The answer is **B** (Rutherford, 4th ed., pp. 1905, 1926).

Cancers such as lymphangiosarcoma occur only rarely in patients with longstanding lymphedema, but when they occur they are often catastrophic. Careful and periodic surveillance of the edematous limb should therefore be performed. More commonly, the complications of lymphedema are related to the disfigurement and limitations caused by the disease. Psychological problems are common in those with lymphedema, especially younger patients, and these should be addressed by the physician caring for these patients. In patients with severe lymphedema the physical limitations caused by limb enlargement may interfere with activities of daily living, job performance, etc. In general, conservative medical measures are more effective and more universally applicable than surgical ones. Whereas ulceration frequently occurs in chronic venous insufficiency, it is unusual in patients with lymphedema.

12. The answer is **D** (Rutherford, 4th ed., pp. 1920–1921).

Filarial disease is not common in North America, although isolated cases do occur. Metastatic disease and, perhaps more important, treatment for malignancies using modalities such as surgery and/or radiation therapy are responsible for most of the secondary cases of lymphedema. Idiopathic, or primary, lymphedema is also a relatively common cause of lymphedema in North America. The swelling may appear (or worsen) in association with episodes of cellulitis or other infections, but the etiology is not infectious.

13. The answer is **C** (Rutherford, 4th ed., pp. 1920–1921).

Recurrent infections contribute substantially to increasing swelling in patients with lymphedema, as noted in question 12. Most episodes of cellulitis or lymphangitis associated with lymphedema are due to group A streptococcus and are responsive to penicillin. More broad-spectrum antibiotics are usually unnecessary, although in clinical practice agents that cover staphylococcus are frequently used. Close adherence to preventive measures, including good skin hygiene, protection of the lymphedematous limb from trauma, and prompt treatment of early infections with antibiotics, are essential adjuncts to combating cellulitis and other types of infections. Topical fungicides are useful for controlling trichophytosis; chronic fungal infections can serve as portals for bacteria to enter the skin. Gram negative coverage is rarely, if ever, required for treating cellulitis in lymphedematous limbs.

14. The answers are **B, E** (Rutherford, 4th ed., pp. 1921–1926).

Bed rest with limb elevation, massage, and pneumatic compression pumping (especially when sequential pumps are used) are all acceptable methods for reducing the size of a lymphedematous limb. The *relative* effectiveness of each of these methods is largely untested; each has its proponents and critics. In contrast, the intensive administration of diuretics does little by itself to reduce the swelling in a limb with lymphedema and may actually cause long-term problems by increasing the protein concentration within the interstitial space. Elastic compression stockings are useful for *maintaining* limb size; they do not effectively *reduce* limb size. Other adjunctive measures, such as limb heating or binding the limb with elastic (or nonelastic) wraps, are useful.

15. The answer is **A** (Rutherford, 4th ed., pp. 1924–1926).

A graduated elastic compression garment must usually provide 40–50 mm Hg (at the ankles in the case of stockings) to control lymphedema, but in patients with limited finger/arm strength stockings of such high compression may be impossible to put on. In these cases, lower compression (30–40 mm Hg) stockings may be prescribed and will sometimes help. Unless the limb is unusually large or distorted in shape, over-the-counter, premade stockings can generally be used. As noted in question 14, although stockings are an effective means of *maintaining* a previously achieved reduction in limb size, they are of little value as agents for *achieving* a reduction in limb size. In general, stockings should be long enough to cover the edematous portion of the limb. However, patient preference and physical limitations must be taken into account; if a stocking or sleeve that is less than optimal from the physician's standpoint provides more patient satisfaction and compliance than the alternatives, that stocking or sleeve is the better long-term choice.

16. The answers are **B, C** (Rutherford, 4th ed., p. 1928).

Nonsurgical therapy is the initial form of treatment for lymphedema, and most patients can be adequately managed without surgical intervention. For the 10% of lymphedema patients who ultimately require surgical treatment, the likelihood of benefit and satisfaction depends in large part on the indication for surgery. The patient with restricted movement from massive extremity enlargement is most likely to benefit from surgical intervention. *Functional impairment* is the best indication for surgery. Less important are cosmetic results. The aim of surgery is to improve limb function and appearance either by improving lymphatic drainage or by excising the lymphadematous skin and subcutaneous tissue. Operations for lymphedema can be divided into two major groups: physiologic procedures and excisional procedures. Excisional procedures recognize that lymphedema is limited to the skin and subcutaneous tissue. These operations involve removal of varying amounts of this compartment. Whereas the Thompson procedure is intended to be both excisional and physiologic, the Homans procedure is purely excisional.

17. The answer is **C** (Rutherford, 4th ed., pp. 1928–1929).

The Charles procedure was described in 1912. This operation is the *most* extensive of the excisional procedures. In the lower extremity, all of the skin and subcutaneous tissue are excised from the tibial tuberosity to the malleoli. Tissues overlying the tibial tuberosity, malleoli, and tendons of the calcaneus are not removed. This operation is usually limited to the leg, and with time the graft sites often become hyperpigmented, hyperkeratotic, and scarred. Because of the hyperpigmentation, cosmetic results are not optimal, and the procedure is not considered curative. Few studies have assessed the long-term efficacy of the Charles procedure. In 1965, Taylor reported that 36% of patients had a "good" result, 36% a "satisfactory" result, and 28% an "unsatisfactory" result. Thus, the procedure is not necessarily the one of choice for most patients. Nonetheless, despite its obvious limitations, this operation is sometimes the only surgical option for patients with extensive swelling and extreme skin changes.

18. The answers are **B, D** (Rutherford, 4th ed., pp. 1929–1931).

In the Thompson operation, a portion of the lymphedematous subcutaneous tissue is resected beneath flaps, a flap edge is de-epithelialized, and the resulting "dermis" flap is buried into the underlying muscle compartment. Thus, theoretically, the Thompson operation permits the formation of lymphatic connections between the subdermal lymphatic plexus of the flap and the deep lymphatics of the muscle compartment, allows muscle contraction, which might increase lymphatic flow rate, and provides a physical barrier against deep fascia regeneration. This operation is therefore intended to be both excisional and physiologic in approach. Thompson's report in 1980 described the use of this procedure in 49 patients for secondary lymphedema of the arm. Operative success is attributed to the formation of lymphatic connections between the flap and the muscle compartments, and radioactive iodine-tagged human serum albumin (RISHA) clearance studies have demonstrated postoperative improvement in the rate of lymphatic isotope clearance. However, postoperative lymphangiography has failed to demonstrate any lymphatic anastomoses. Fat necrosis and partial tissue loss are the most common postoperative complications.

19. The answers are **A, B, D** (Rutherford, 4th ed., pp. 1931–1933).

The modified Homans procedure was actually first described by Sistrunk in 1918 and later modified and popularized by Homans. This may be the most reasonable surgical compromise of the excisional procedures. It offers reliable improvement while minimizing the likelihood of unfavorable postoperative complications. The operation is similar to the excisional component of Thompson's procedure and produces results comparable to the latter but with a lower complication rate. It provides predictable improvement. It can be offered as a palliative procedure to most patients but will not provide cure of lymphedema. Roughly 60–70% of patients experience significant postoperative improvement; however, the use of compression stockings is indicated indefinitely in these patients.

20. The answer is **C** (Rutherford, 4th ed., pp. 1936–1938).

Microsurgical lymphovenous anastomoses have been performed for almost three decades. The procedure, however, is still not an established treatment for lymphedema. Although in animal experiments performed with normal lymph vessels 50–80% patency of the anastomoses were documented several months after the operation, no documentation of long-term patency exists in humans. Although a 1990 report from Australia by O'Brien et al. documents long-term improvement in patients who underwent lymphovenous anastomoses for secondary lymphedema, late patency and function of the anastomosis are not proven. The results of these operations when performed for patients with primary lymphedema are poor. In addition, in the late stages of lymphedema, fibrosis and valvular incompetence of the main lymph vessels develop, the intrinsic contractility of the vessel wall is lost, and interstitial pressure decreases. The likelihood of success with lymphovenous anastomoses in such limbs is diminished. However, cure of lymphedema at present is not available, and this operation can be attempted in patients with secondary lymphedema if conservative treatment fails. Clinical trials to confirm the effectiveness of lymphovenous anastomoses are needed.

21. The answers are **C, D, E** (Rutherford, 4th ed., pp. 1938–1940).

Indirect lymphatic reconstructions have been designed to improve lymphatic drainage by the use of an omental flap, by the mesenteric bridge operation, and by autotransplantation of lymphatic tissue as a free flap. These procedures are based on the ability of the lymphatic system to form spontaneous lympholymphatic anastomoses and to improve collateral lymphatic drainage to the mesentery or to regions of the body where lymphatic drainage is normal. The omental flap operation introduced by Goldsmith has largely been abandoned because of perioperative complications and the paucity of lymphatics in the omentum. The mesenteric bridge operation was developed by Kinmonth and was efficacious in several patients who had primary lymphedema due to proximal (aortoiliac) lymphatic obstruction. Postoperative contrast lymphangiography demonstrated lymphatic drainage of the lower extremity through spontaneous lympholymphatic anastomosis through the mesenteric bridge to the para-aortic lymphatics and the thoracic duct. However, experience with this operation is limited, and the number of candidates is small. Autotransplantation of lymphatic tissue as a free flap is a new operation, and too few procedures have been performed to confirm its effectiveness.

22. The answers are **A, B, D, E** and (Rutherford, 4th ed., pp. 1940–1945).

Congenital lymphangiectasia may result in reflux of the chyle, causing lymphedema and chylorrhea (draining chyle through small vessicles of the skin of the lower extremity or of the perineum). Patients with this disorder may have rupture of mesenteric lymphatics and may present with chylous ascites or (if the thoracic duct or thoracic lymphatics rupture) with chylothorax. The lymphatics in the wall of the mesentery may also rupture, and patients may present with protein-losing enteropathy and diarrhea. The so-called antireflux operation that involves ligation of all dilated retroperitoneal lymphatics effectively decreases reflux of lymph. In most cases, even though the lower-extremity lymphatics are ligated, lymphedema of the lower extremity improves because reflux is prevented. The operation is also effective in reducing chylorrhea from skin vessicles. Frequently bilateral retroperitoneal ligation is required for optimal clinical results. The lower-extremity lymphedema associated with this syndrome is most frequently *unilateral*, not *bilateral*.

19

Extremity Amputation for Vascular Disease

1. The most common cause of death in the perioperative period following amputation is:
   A. Stroke.
   B. Acute renal failure.
   C. Myocardial infarction.
   D. Pulmonary embolism.
   E. Hemorrhage.

2. The best initial therapy in the management of an unsalvageable gangrenous necrotic foot infection in the diabetic patient with hyperglycemia, ketoacidosis, and sepsis is:
   A. Intravenous antibiotics and insulin.
   B. Intravenous antibiotics, insulin, and guillotine amputation.
   C. Intravenous antibiotics and below-knee amputation.
   D. Intravenous insulin drip and foot elevation.
   E. Intravenous antibiotics alone.

3. The most practical method of screening patients for myocardial ischemia prior to performing amputation is:
   A. Arm ergometry with or without dipyridamole-thallium scintigraphy.
   B. Exercise treadmill and dipyridamole-thallium.
   C. Resting EKG and coronary arteriography.
   D. 2-D echocardiography and resting EKG.
   E. Exercise treadmill.

4. Which of the following situations define relative contraindications to above-knee amputation unless there is *objective* evidence of adequate local perfusion to ensure a viable stump?
   A. Acute thrombosis of a combined inflow and outflow revascularization operation.
   B. Superficial femoral artery occlusion in association with an occluded or highly stenotic profunda femoris artery.
   C. A 30° fixed flexion contraction of the ipsilateral knee joint.
   D. Absence of a femoral pulse coupled with no detectable pulse volume recordings at the high thigh level.
   E. All of the above.

5. Which of the following clinical findings is/are contraindications to below-knee amputation?
   A. Age greater than 70 years.
   B. A contralateral above-knee amputation.
   C. Nonviable skin and muscle at the mid-portion of the leg.
   D. A bedridden stroke victim with resultant muscular spasticity and rigidity of the ipsilateral lower extremity.
   E. Nonambulatory patients.

6. Which of the following statements is/are true regarding rehabilitation potential after lower-extremity amputation?
   A. Rehabilitation with successful independent ambulation is nearly 100% after a single toe or ray amputation.
   B. Below-knee amputation results in a successful return to independent prosthetic ambulation in about 50% of all patients.
   C. Bilateral below-knee amputation effectively precludes any reasonable chance of successful independent prosthetic ambulation.
   D. Crutch walking demands *less* energy expenditure than prosthetic ambulation for all levels of lower-extremity amputation and is a good alternative to rehabilitation with prostheses.
   E. From 30 to 70% of bilateral below-knee amputees return to independent ambulation.

7. Which of the following statements is/are true regarding optimal selection of lower-extremity amputation level?
   A. The presence of palpable pulses immediately above the proposed site of amputation is a reliable index for successful wound healing.
   B. A transcutaneous oxygen tension level ($TcPO_2$) of 42 mm Hg is a value suggesting that amputation wound healing will be successful at that level.
   C. An ankle-brachial index of 0.18 in a diabetic patient is not a reliable indicator of poor distal perfusion because the tibial arteries are often calcified in the diabetic patient.
   D. In deciding optimal amputation level, the clinical judgment of an experienced physician should be allowed to contradict and supersede the objective findings of usually reliable noninvasive laboratory assays of distal tissue perfusion.
   E. All of the above.

8. Of the following, the *best* laboratory test(s) for predicting wound healing potential in the amputee is/are:
   A. Serum albumin.

B. Twenty-four-hour urine protein analysis.
C. Hematocrit.
D. Urinary hydroxy protein analysis.
E. Transcutaneous oxygen tension ($TcPO_2$).

9. Verrucous hyperplasia is thought to be caused by:
A. Inadequate blood supply to stump.
B. Venous congestion.
C. Poor lymphatic drainage.
D. Loose prosthetic fitting.
E. Postoperative infection.

10. Salvage of a below-knee amputation stump is possible by:
A. Use of a "skew" flap.
B. Wedge resection.
C. Guillotine amputation.
D. Wound debridement and secondary closure.
E. None of the above.

11. The muscles of the hip are important for both knee and pelvic stability when utilizing a prosthesis. The muscles that provide for most of the knee stability are:
A. Gluteus medius.
B. Gluteus maximus.
C. Hamstrings.
D. Adductor magnus.
E. Iliopsoas.

12. The issues essential to successful prosthetic use for the lower limb amputee include:
A. Adequate cardiopulmonary reserve.
B. Correct gait training.
C. Properly reconstructed stump.
D. Maximum soft tissue shaping and shrinking.
E. Provision of the most modern prosthetic components.

13. The use of an immediate postoperative rigid dressing is felt to be superior to the use of soft dressings because:
A. It is easier to apply and monitor.
B. It better controls wound edema.
C. With it there appears to be less postoperative incisional pain.
D. It provides the best environment for wound healing.
E. It can be utilized for early ambulation.

14. Which of the following statements most correctly characterize(s) current thinking about specific amputation surgery as it relates to prosthetic rehabilitation?
A. Myoplastic closure is preferable to transection of the muscles and permitting the muscles to shorten into the proximal stump.
B. Amputation at the transfemoral level should include bringing the adductors around the distal end of the femur and attaching them laterally to the femur.
C. The best residual tibial length in the transtibial amputation is that which corresponds to the taper of the gastrocsoleus muscles.
D. All residual limb length should always be saved.
E. Split thickness skin graft is as good as full thickness skin coverage if there is adequate underlying soft tissue over the residual bone(s).

15. At the time of primary amputation, techniques that have been recommended for prevention of neuroma include all *except:*
A. Placement of nerve in healthy muscle bed.
B. Cauterization of the nerve end.
C. Chemical ablation of the nerve end.
D. Intraosseus transposition of the nerve end.
E. Long vein grafting with placement of the nerve within the conduit.

16. Of the following, the best indication for single-digit replantation is:
A. Circular saw amputation of nondominant index finger in a 34-year-old male carpenter.
B. Crush amputation of dominant thumb in a 52-year-old male mechanic.
C. Clean-cut amputation of nondominant ring finger in an 18-year-old female college student at mid-middle phalanx.
D. Clean-cut amputation of nondominant long finger in a 68-year-old male retiree at distal-middle phalanx.
E. Clean-cut amputation of dominant small finger in a 28-year-old male electrician at proximal-proximal phalanx.

17. The following procedure would most likely allow the *earliest* return to work for a 52-year-old warehouse worker with amputation of the tip of the nondominant index finger (defect size of 1 cm^2 after debridement):
A. Secondary healing.
B. Cross-finger flap.
C. Skin graft.
D. Thenar flap.
E. Atasoy flap.

18. Options for nondominant distal forearm amputation in a 36-year-old male office worker include all *except:*
A. Closure of amputation and subsequent fitting with hand prosthesis.
B. Closure of amputation, secondary shortening of amputation, and final fitting with myoelectric prosthesis.
C. Closure of amputation and secondary Krukenberg procedure.
D. Closure of amputation and no further reconstruction (prosthetic or surgical).
E. Closure of amputation and subsequent fitting with cosmetic hand reconstruction.

19. Contraindications to attempted limb salvage by femorodistal revascularization include:
    - **A.** Ejection fraction <35% on static radionuclide cardiac scan.
    - **B.** No visualization of infrapopliteal vessels on standard aortography.
    - **C.** Failure of prior ipsilateral in situ femorodistal bypass graft.
    - **D.** Previous harvest of ipsilateral saphenous vein.
    - **E.** Nonambulatory non–self-care status.

20. A 78-year-old resident of a nursing home presents with wet gangrene of the right forefoot, cellulitis to the calf, a fever of 39.5°, and shaking chills. He has not ambulated since a stroke that resulted in right hemiplegia one year before. White blood cell count is 28,500, BUN is 48 mg/dL, and hematocrit is 42%. The best management of this patient would be:
    - **A.** Emergency definitive amputation after intravenous hydration and antibiotics.
    - **B.** Guillotine amputation after intravenous hydration.
    - **C.** Physiologic amputation, administration of broad-spectrum antibiotics, and hemodynamically monitored rehydration and cardiac optimization.
    - **D.** Chopart amputation and femorodistal revascularization after intravenous rehydration and administration of antibiotics.
    - **E.** Intravenous hydration and broad-spectrum antibiotics.

21. A 64-year-old otherwise healthy diabetic man presented with severe rest pain and an ischemic toe; angiography demonstrates occlusion of the below-knee popliteal artery but visualization of a patent posterior tibial artery filling the pedal arch. In offering this patient the alternatives of revascularization or primary amputation, the economic costs of an attempt at revascularization can be characterized as:
    - **A.** An amputation costs more than revascularization.
    - **B.** A revascularization costs more than amputation.
    - **C.** The total costs of either procedure are equivalent.
    - **D.** The overall cost of a failed revascularization is the same as the cost of a successful one.
    - **E.** The costs of either procedure increase with complications.

19

Answers

1. The answer is **C** (Rutherford, 4th ed., pp. 1956–1957).

The perioperative mortality from below-knee amputation is 6–10% and for above-knee amputation 20–25%. The major cause of death is myocardial infarction. This occurs as a consequence of significant coronary atherosclerosis, which has a high prevalence among patients who require amputations. Although stroke and pulmonary embolism may occur following amputation and contribute to mortality, myocardial infarction remains the greatest risk for amputees in the perioperative period. Hemorrhage is a relatively uncommon postoperative complication, particularly in the dysvascular patient.

2. The answer is **B** (Rutherford, 4th ed., p. 1958).

The best initial therapy for a diabetic patient with an unsalvageable gangrenous necrotic foot infection and hyperglycemia, ketoacidosis, and sepsis is (1) intravenous antibiotics sufficiently broad spectrum to cover polymicrobial organisms, (2) intravenous insulin drip to lower blood sugar, and (3) emergent supramalleolar guillotine amputation. Guillotine amputation should be performed as an initial step once it is clear that the foot is not salvageable. This allows debridement of the infected nonviable tissue and facilitates drainage of more proximal infected lymphatic channels. Several authors have demonstrated that performing a *definitive* below-knee amputation in the presence of a major foot infection is associated with a much higher infection rate in the below-knee amputation stump when compared to performing the amputation in two stages.

3. The answer is **A** (Rutherford, 4th ed., pp. 1957–1959).

The most practical method of screening patients for myocardial ischemia prior to performing amputation is either arm ergometry testing or dipyridamole-thallium perfusion scanning. Conventional treadmill exercise testing is not feasible because most preoperative amputation patients are unable to walk or are severely limited to an extent that the required heart rate cannot be achieved. Resting ECG does not provide enough sensitivity in identifying patients with silent myocardial ischemia. Ambulatory ECG (Holter monitoring) is an alternative screening method that may be particularly useful in diabetic patients who are at particularly high risk for silent myocardial ischemia. Several groups have shown that a large amount of ischemia on Holter monitor correlates with perioperative cardiac morbidity.

4. The answers are **A, B, D** (Rutherford, 4th ed., pp. 1980–1983).

Three specific situations constitute relative contraindications to above-knee amputation unless there is *objective* documentation of the adequacy of local blood flow to result in a viable stump: (1) acute thrombosis of a combined inflow and outflow revascularization procedure; (2) superficial femoral artery occlusion associated with an occluded or highly stenotic profunda femoris artery; and (3) the absence of a femoral pulse coupled with no detectable pulse volume recordings at the level of the high thigh. Revascularization to correct any of these situations prior to amputation will result in more successful wound healing at the above-knee level and will minimize the need for hip disarticulation, which is a highly morbid procedure in this setting. A fixed knee-flexion contracture is actually an indication for amputation at the *above-knee* level, rather than below-knee level, because below-knee prostheses require near full range of knee motion to function. Moreover, knee-flexion contractures in the bedridden patient often lead to decubitus ulceration of a below-knee amputation stump with complications that culminate in above-knee amputation. Initial above-knee amputation is thus preferred in the patient with a substantial fixed knee-flexion deformity.

5. The answer is **D** (Rutherford, 4th ed., pp. 1973–1978).

Every reasonable effort should be made to preserve the knee joint in the previously active patient. Age alone is not a contraindication to amputation at the below-knee level. If arterial perfusion is adequate, good healing and rehabilitation results may be anticipated, even in the previously ambulatory septuagenarian. Above-knee amputation in the elderly patient is more likely to result in confinement to a wheelchair, because ambulation using an above-knee prosthesis requires much more energy expenditure compared to below-knee prostheses. For the patient with a contralateral above-knee amputation, preservation of the remaining knee joint is immensely helpful in maintaining some degree of independence. Even for nonambulatory patients, a below-knee level allows turning and moving about in bed more readily, as well as permitting easier transfers from bed to wheelchair. Ambulation using prostheses is more achievable in the bilateral amputee if one knee joint is preserved. Nonviable tissue at the mid-leg level actually is an indication for below-knee amputation, provided more proximal perfusion is assured. The various musculocutaneous flaps available to close a below-knee amputation allow considerable latitude in preserving the knee joint. Atypical and ingenious skin flap design is preferable to amputation at a higher level. Rarely, an open below-knee amputation can be successful in the setting of tissue loss up to the level of the tibial tuberosity. Muscular rigidity and spasticity in the bedridden patient are contraindications to below-knee amputation, particularly if a knee-flexion contracture already exists. Unless rigorous physical therapy is employed such a patient will invariably develop a flexion deformity of the knee with decubitus ulceration of the stump.

6. The answers are **A, E** (Rutherford, 4th ed., pp. 1965–1967, 1973–1978).

Contemporary lower-extremity rehabilitation results are impressive in the formerly active and ambulatory patient. Toe or ray amputation results in virtually 100% successful rehabilitation. Of importance, preventive measures must be undertaken to minimize the significant risk of subsequent amputation in this population. Amputation at below-knee level should result in successful ambulatory rehabilitation in 70–100% of such patients, provided the patient was ambulatory prior to amputation. In fact, for the previously active patient, the bilateral below-knee amputee can successfully return to independent ambulation with bilateral prostheses in 33–71% of cases. Interestingly, except in the instance of above-knee amputation, all other amputee groups are able to walk with *less* energy expenditure using a prosthesis compared to crutch walking.

7. The answers are **A, B, D** (Rutherford, 4th ed., pp. 1961–1966).

Examination of pulses can be helpful in determining amputation wound healing potential if interpreted properly. Although the presence of palpable pulses immediately proximal to the proposed site of amputation is a good prognostic indicator, the absence of such pulses does not necessarily lead to failure of healing. Properly obtained transcutaneous oxygen tension ($TcPO_2$) values, can be helpful for amputation level selection, particularly if the values are >40 mm Hg. If the $TcPO_2$ value is >40 mm Hg at a given site, good wound healing can be expected if no other adverse factors are present. $TcPO_2$ levels <20 mm Hg suggest probable wound healing problems, but this is not immutable. The most difficulty in interpreting $TcPO_2$ results occurs in the range of 20–40 mm Hg. Values in this range should prompt alternative determinations of perfusion and evaluation by a very experienced clinician. Certain provocative maneuvers can enhance the reliability of $TcPO_2$ assays (e.g., inhalation of concentrated oxygen). While calcified leg arteries can yield artificially elevated ankle pressure readings (>300 mm Hg), a *low* ankle pressure is still a reliable finding in this setting. Consequently, an ankle-brachial index of 0.18 is believable in any patient and suggests markedly impaired distal perfusion and predictably poor wound healing after amputation. Finally, if experienced clinical judgment contradicts the noninvasive laboratory findings, the given patient should not necessarily undergo a more proximal amputation based solely on vascular laboratory results. Amputation at a lower level may be attempted in an active, motivated person, even if the objective parameters are marginal; yet such an amputation might be contraindicated in a frailer, sicker patient with limited rehabilitation potential. The role of the experienced, involved surgeon should not be underestimated.

8. The answers are **A, E** (Rutherford, 4th ed., pp. 1987–1990, 1994–1995).

Wound healing is dependent on several factors. These include the surgical technique and the level selected for amputation. Nutrition is important and influences overall healing. A serum albumin <3.5g/dl and/or a lymphocyte count <1,500 per mm^3 predict poor wound healing. The hematocrit does not provide reliable information, and urinary analysis is of no value in assessing nutritional status. $TcPO_2$ greater than 40 mm Hg predicts good wound healing in most cases (see question 7).

9. The answers are **B, C** (Rutherford, 4th ed., p. 1996).

Stump edema that occurs after prosthetic fitting has taken place may result in verrucous hyperplasia, which is the wartlike appearance of the entire distal stump (Fig. 150–10). It results from mechanical factors impeding the venous or lymphatic outflow. A *loose* prosthesis will not cause the problem, nor does infection play a role.

10. The answer is **B** (Rutherford, 4th ed., pp. 1989–1998).

A "skew" flap is a good alternative to the long posterior flap and is used when previous bypass incision precludes the use of a long posterior flap. The guillotine amputation is used in the acute stage in a limb- and life-threatening situation rather than as a salvage operation. Wound debridement and secondary closure delay mobilization and rehabilitation of the amputee and may lead to further problems. Wedge resection offers the best alternative for stump salvage.

11. The answers are **B, C** (Rutherford, 4th ed., pp. 2002–2006).

When using a transfemoral or a transtibial prosthesis, knee stability is enhanced by the action of the posterior hip musculature, which produces extension at the hip. This extension provides for stability of the prosthetic knee. Muscles that pass posterior to the axis of rotation in the frontal plane include the gluteus maximus and the hamstrings. The gluteus medius, another important hip muscle for a prosthetic user, provides pelvic stability while the patient is standing on the prosthesis but only minimally assists with hip extension. The iliopsoas passes anterior to the hip and acts as a hip flexor, whereas the adductor magnus serves predominately as a femoral adductor and does not assist significantly in knee stability. Because the hip extensor muscle group provides for the best functional use of a prosthesis, it is important that it be the focus of any preprosthetic therapy program.

12. The answers are **A, C** (Rutherford, 4th ed., pp. 2001–2012).

Whereas all of the listed items may be desirable, they are not all *essential* for successful use of a prosthesis. The sine qua non for prosthetic success is, first and foremost, adequate cardiopulmonary reserve, because energy expenditure increases from 65 to 100% when walking with a transfemoral prosthesis and from 25 to 40% when using a transtibial prosthesis. Second, a properly shaped stump with stabilized muscles and maximum bone length provided at the time of reconstructive amputation surgery are also essentials for prosthetic success. Although correct gait training, maximum soft tissue shaping, and modern prosthetic components are useful, they are not indispensable to prosthetic usage.

13. The answers are **B, C, D** (Rutherford, 4th ed., pp. 2001–2002).

The use of the immediate postoperative rigid dressing is preferred in many centers. It has been shown that the application of the rigid dressing controls edema better than a soft dressing. With edema control, it is believed that there is better chance of primary wound healing in wounds with compromised blood supply. Also, with edema control, there is less postoperative incisional pain. However, rigid dressings require proper training and significant experience in their application and use. Therefore, the rigid dressing requires a tightly controlled system of postoperative care so that it can be changed for wound inspection or reapplied if it becomes loose. It is not the immediate postoperative rigid dressing itself but a pylon that is applied for early ambulation a few days to a few weeks from the time of amputation.

14. The answers are **A, B, C** (Rutherford, 4th ed., pp. 1990–1993, 1995, 2000–2007, 2016).

Myoplastic closure is the preferred method of handling muscle for amputations because it prevents the muscles from retracting proximally into the stump. Myoplastic closure is more likely to provide a cylindrically shaped residual limb which permits better distribution of pressures when wearing a prosthesis. For the transfemoral amputation, Gottshalk (see Chap. 150) has recommended bringing the adductors over the end of the femur and attaching them laterally in order to keep the femur from drifting into abduction. If the femur drifts into abduction, it is less able to generate the abductor muscle forces necessary for good pelvis stability in stance on the prosthesis. The lowest level of amputation of the leg below the knee should be just above the taper of the gastrocsoleus muscle group. This permits myoplastic closure over the end of the tibial and fibula with adequate muscle mass and results in a more cylindrically shaped residual limb. Whereas some authors suggest that all levels of amputation can be fitted satisfactorily with a prosthesis, certain levels of prosthetic restoration should be individualized. Both the Syme's and the knee disarticulation levels may be biomechanically satisfactory for some persons, but for others prosthetic appearance may be cosmetically unacceptable. Therefore, the amputation level chosen must take into account issues in addition to salvage of maximal limb length. Adequate soft tissue coverage is important for the best prosthetic results, but full thickness skin coverage is always preferable to a split thickness skin graft. The split thickness graft does not hold up as well to the shear and direct pressure forces that are present at the stump-prosthetic socket interface.

15. The answer is **D** (Rutherford, 4th ed., p. 2019).

The primary method of neuroma prevention is placement of the nerve in a relatively protected area (away from stimuli) and in a healthy bed. Thus, the technique of traction (mild) and division is most commonly employed. Other techniques that have been attempted with varying degrees of success are cauterization of the free end of the nerve, chemical ablation, and placement of the nerve in a vein conduit. Intraosseus transposition is used for established neuromata, but should *not* be used for prevention. Placement of a free cut nerve end in a fixed space (bone) can lead to continuous, severe pain if the neuroma tries to outgrow its confines.

16. The answer is **C** (Rutherford, 4th ed., pp. 2019–2021).

Single digit replantation is generally not indicated except in the case of thumb amputations. The impairment from a single finger amputation is relatively minor, and when weighed against the length of time to recovery, the ultimate functional impairment, the possible long-term pain, and the cost, it is usually best not to replant. Nevertheless, there are exceptions, and the cosmetic deformity of the loss of the ring finger in a young woman may certainly be one such exception. A crush amputation (finger or thumb) is rarely replantable strictly on the basis of the injury. Technically replantable border fingers (index or small) are not usually done because of the exposure of these digits to daily trauma. The replanted digit is less mobile and sometimes painful, and constant trauma makes these border fingers more of a nuisance than an amputation. Relatively speaking, an amputation through the middle phalanx (distal to the insertion of the superficialis tendon) is more "replantable" than the same injury through the proximal phalanx (the same issues that distinguish tendon repair in zone I and zone II). Replantation can be done in the elderly, but clearly the indications must be pressing because the rehabilitation time can be lengthy, and secondary stiffness in other digits can be significant.

17. The answer is **E** (Rutherford, 4th ed., pp. 2018–2021).

The controversy as to which distal digital amputation closure technique is best rages on. However, with precise attention to goals, it is possible to narrow the options. If one is directed purely toward most rapid return to work, then the issue of sensibility becomes secondary. Obviously, secondary healing is not the technique of choice; neither is any pedicled flap that will require a second procedure to divide such as a cross-finger flap or a thenar flap. A skin graft must also be immobilized long enough for healing and also for a period of time before direct trauma can be tolerated by the area. An Atasoy flap achieves primary closure at the time of injury and does not require secondary surgery. Also, after a week to 10 days, it can be expected that enough healing has occurred to subject the tip to mild trauma.

18. The answer is **C** (Rutherford, 4th ed., pp. 2021–2023).

Which reconstructive option (if any) should be used for a given patient with a distal forearm amputation depends heavily on the patient's activities and desires. In many cases the simple fitting of a hook prosthesis serves very well and is usually considered the most functional. At the other end of the spectrum, a purely aesthetic passive prosthesis without practical functional capabilities can be "functional" in the social setting. A myoelectric prosthesis requires significant motivation on the patient's part to learn how to use it, but it offers a compromise between the hook and the esthetic prostheses. It is also not unreasonable for the patient to use the stump of the amputation as a sensate assist post to be used with the remaining good hand. The Krukenberg procedure, which produces a sensate pincer, is not indicated in the general population. The cosmetic deformity of the procedure is significant. The best indication for this procedure is a blind, double upper-extremity amputee. This patient cannot rely on vision to direct the use of a mechanical (hook) prosthesis and desperately needs the ability to pinch.

19. The answer is **D** (Rutherford, 4th ed., pp. 2025–2032).

With increasing success rates of distal bypasses as well as improved perioperative care there are no real medical or anatomic contraindications to revascularization. Although previous harvest of an ipsilateral greater saphenous vein precludes an in situ femorodistal bypass, many alternative conduits may be available, including contralateral greater saphenous vein, lesser saphenous veins, and arm veins. The main contraindication to femorodistal bypass is a nonambulatory patient who cannot be expected to benefit directly from the limb salvage effort and is better served by primary amputation.

20. The answer is **C** (Rutherford, 4th ed., pp. 2025–2032).

Acute foot infection requiring amputation and with complicating systemic sepsis should be dealt with expeditiously. Emergency amputation carries a high mortality rate in the elderly, who are better served by controlling the septic focus with physiologic amputation (i.e., applying a tourniquet and packing the extremity in ice). Guillotine amputation, although it also controls the septic focus, is more appropriate for a younger, healthier patient because it requires an emergency operation that the older, sicker patient may not tolerate well. Revascularization would be contraindicated because of nonambulatory status and ipsilateral hemiplegia.

21. The answers are **C, E** (Rutherford, 4th ed., pp. 2025–2032).

The economic costs of primary amputation, including prosthesis and rehabilitation, are not significantly different from the costs of a primary successful revascularization, either as immediate or as follow-up over several years. The costs of either procedure increase proportionately with problems and complications.